Improving the Lives of People With Dementia Through Technology

This book explores the practical application of recent improvements in technology for people living with dementia and highlights the positive outcomes on care, quality of life and services on patients through exploration of 15 research projects to redefine the future of dementia care.

Using research compiled in collaboration with leading universities and organisations across Europe, this book demonstrates how INDUCT's (Interdisciplinary Network for Dementia Utilising Current Technology's) findings resulted in implications for practical cognitive and social factors to improve the usability of technology, evaluating the effectiveness of specific contemporary technology, and tracing facilitators and barriers for implementation of technology in dementia care.

Featuring a unique training programme along with a wide range of patient-public involvement, this state-of-the-art volume will be essential reading for researchers, academics and scholars in the fields of dementia and mental health research, gerontology, psychology and nursing.

Martin Orrell is Director of the Institute of Mental Health, University of Nottingham, United Kingdom.

Déborah Oliveira is Lecturer and Researcher on long-term care, dementia, and stigma, Federal University of Sao Paulo (UNIFESP), Sao Paulo, Brazil, and Universidad Andrés Bello, Chile.

Orii McDermott is Senior Research Fellow at the Institute of Mental Health, University of Nottingham, United Kingdom.

Frans R. J. Verhey is Professor of Geriatric Psychiatry/Neuropsychiatry at Maastricht University, the Netherlands.

Fania C.M. Dassen is Project Manager at the Alzheimer Center Limburg, Maastricht University, the Netherlands.

Rose-Marie Dröes is Emeritus Professor of Psychosocial Care for people with dementia and head of the research group 'Care and support in dementia' at the Department of Psychiatry of Amsterdam University Medical Centers, the Netherlands.

Improving the Lives of People With Dementia Through Technology

Interdisciplinary Network for Dementia Utilising Current Technology

Edited by Martin Orrell,
Déborah Oliveira, Orii McDermott,
Frans R. J. Verhey, Fania C.M. Dassen
and Rose-Marie Dröes

Routledge
Taylor & Francis Group

LONDON AND NEW YORK

First published 2023
by Routledge
4 Park Square, Milton Park, Abingdon, Oxon OX14 4RN

and by Routledge
605 Third Avenue, New York, NY 10158

Routledge is an imprint of the Taylor & Francis Group, an informa business

British Library Cataloguing-in-Publication Data
A catalogue record for this book is available from the British Library

Library of Congress Cataloging-in-Publication Data
Names: Orrell, Martin, editor. | Oliveira, Deborah, editor. | McDermott, Orii, editor. | Verhey, F. R. J. (Franciscus Rochus Jozef), 1955– editor. | Dassen, Fania, editor. | Dröes, R. M. (Rose-Marie), 1956– editor.
Title: Improving the lives of people with dementia through technology : interdisciplinary network for dementia utilising current technology / edited by Martin Orrell, Déborah Oliveira, Orii McDermott, Frans R.J. Verhey, Fania Dassen, and Rose-Marie Dröes.
Description: Abingdon, Oxon ; New York, NY : Routledge, 2023. | Series: Aging and mental health research | Includes bibliographical references and index.
Identifiers: LCCN 2022025970 (print) | LCCN 2022025971 (ebook) | ISBN 9781032226675 (hardback) | ISBN 9781032265933 (paperback) | ISBN 9781003289005 (ebook)
Subjects: LCSH: Dementia. | Dementia—Patients—Care—Technological innovations. | Self-help devices for people with disabilities. | Assistive computer technology.
Classification: LCC RC521 .I493 2023 (print) | LCC RC521 (ebook) | DDC 616.8/31—dc23/eng/20220824
LC record available at https://lccn.loc.gov/2022025970
LC ebook record available at https://lccn.loc.gov/2022025971

ISBN: 978-1-032-22667-5 (hbk)
ISBN: 978-1-032-26593-3 (pbk)
ISBN: 978-1-003-28900-5 (ebk)

DOI: 10.4324/9781003289005

Typeset in Bembo
by Apex CoVantage, LLC

Contents

Figures

Tables

About the Editors and Contributors

Aline Cavalcanti Barroso (MSc) is Researcher in mental health and clinical psychology.

Ana Diaz-Ponce (PhD, MSc) is Project Officer at Alzheimer Europe. She worked for several years as a Senior Social Worker in the field of dementia.

Anders Kottorp (PhD) is Dean at the Faculty of health and society, Malmö University in Malmö, Sweden, and Professor of Occupational Therapy and co-founder of the CACTUS (Cognitive Accessibility and Technology Use when Ageing in home and Society) research group at the Division of Occupational Therapy at Karolinska Institutet in Stockholm, Sweden.

Angie A. Diaz-Baquero is PhD student in Biosciences from the University of Salamanca and Research member of IBSAL, Spain.

Anna Brorsson (PhD) is Assistant Professor and Programme Director in Occupational Therapy at the Division of Occupational Therapy at Karolinska Institutet in Stockholm, Sweden. She is member of the CACTUS (Cognitive Accessibility and Technology Use when ageing in home and Society) and Everyday Matters research groups.

Anne Margriet Pot (PhD) is Strategic Advisor at the Healthcare Inspectorate (IGJ), Ministry of Health, and Professor of Regulation of Person-Centred Long-Term Care at the Erasmus School of Health Policy and Management (ESHPM), Erasmus University Rotterdam, the Netherlands.

Annelien Wendrich-van Dael (PhD, MSc) obtained her PhD in March 2021. Annelien is working at ZonMw, the Dutch funding agency for healthcare research, the Netherlands.

Annemieke van Straten (PhD) is Professor of Clinical Psychology and head of the section Clinical Psychology within the department of Clincial, Neuro and Developmental Psychology at Amsterdam University Medical Centers, location Vrije Universiteit Amsterdam, the Netherlands.

Carlijn Hendriks (MSc) is Human Movement Scientist and is currently working as a Product Owner at SilverFit, a technology company in the Netherlands.

Camilla Walles Malinowsky (PhD) is Associate Professor in Occupational Therapy and co-Principal Investigator in the CACTUS (Cognitive Accessibility and Technology Use when Ageing in home and Society) research group at the Division of Occupational Therapy at Karolinska Institutet in Stockholm, Sweden.

Chris Roberts is current Chair of the European Working Group of People with Dementia, Honorary Lecturer & Fellow Bangor University, United Kingdom.

David Neal (MB, BChir, MA cantab) is Marie Sklodowska-Curie Early Stage Research Fellow in the Department of Psychiatry at Amsterdam University Medical Centers, Vrije Universiteit Amsterdam, the Netherlands.

Déborah Oliveira (PhD, MSc, RN) is Lecturer and Researcher on long-term care, dementia, and stigma, Federal University of Sao Paulo (UNIFESP), Sao Paulo, Brazil, and Universidad Andrés Bello, Chile.

Dianne Gove (PhD, MA) is Director for Projects at Alzheimer Europe. She obtained her PhD on the topic of stigma and dementia from the University of Bradford, the United Kingdom.

Eider Irazoki (PhD, MSc) is doing an internship at Cognitiva, a memory centre specialised in the care of elderly people with cognitive impairment in Donostia-San Sebastián, Spain.

Elisabeth Honinx (PhD, MSc) is post-doctoral researcher in the mental health technology sector.

Ester Parra Vidales works at IBIP Center for Clinical Care in Mental Health and Aging, INTRAS Foundation, Zamora, Spain.

Fania C.M. Dassen (PhD, MSc) works at the Alzheimer Center Limburg (Maastricht University, the Netherlands). She is Coordinator of INTER-DEM Academy and the Training Manager of INDUCT and DISTINCT.

Franka Meiland (PhD, MSc) is Psychologist and she works as researcher and teacher at Amsterdam UMC, VUmc, the Nertherlands, department of Medicine for Older People, the Netherlands.

Frans R.J. Verhey is Professor of Geriatric Psychiatry/Neuropsychiatry at Maastricht University, the Netherlands. He is Neuropsychiatrist by training and Clinical Researcher in the field of Alzheimer's disease and related disorders.

Georgina Charlesworth (PhD) is Associate Professor in the Research Department of Clinical, Educational and Health Psychology, UCL, the United Kingdom and also a Consultant Clinical and Health Psychologist with North East London NHS Foundation Trust, the United Kingdom.

Gianna Kohl (MSc) is Marie Sklodowska-Curie Early Stage Researcher at University College London, United Kingdom.

Harleen Kaur Rai (PhD, MSc) works as a Stretch Digital Research Fellow at the University of Strathclyde in Glasgow.

Hannah Christie (PhD, MSc) is Postdoctoral Researcher at the Alzheimer Center Limburg (Maastricht University, the Netherlands).

Helen Rochford-Brennan is Global Dementia Ambassador and has Honorary Doctor of Laws National University of Ireland Galway.

Henriëtte G. van der Roest (PhD) is Head of the Department on Aging of the Netherlands Institute of Mental Health and Addiction (Trimbos Institute) in the Netherlands.

Huibert J. Tange (MD, PhD) is Associate Professor at the CAPHRI School for Public Health and Primary Care, Maastricht University, the Netherlands.

Iva Holmerová (MD, PhD) is Head of the Centre of Expertise in Longevity and Long-Term Care, Faculty of Humanities, Charles University, Czech Republic. She is also Founding Director and Consultant Geriatrician at the Centre of Gerontology in Prague Czech Republic.

Jean Georges (BA) has been the Executive Director of Alzheimer Europe, the umbrella organisation of national Alzheimer's associations, since 1996.

Joeke van der Molen-van Santen (PhD, MSc) is Psychologist and Dementia Researcher, currently working as Policy Advisor, research & development at an elderly care organisation, and is the link person for the University Network for the Care sector South Holland (UNC-ZH), the Netherlands.

Joni Gilissen (PhD, MSW) is Post-doctoral Researcher at the End-of-Life Care Research Group at the Vrije Universiteit Brussel and Universiteit Gent in Belgium, affiliate postdoc at Harvard Center for Aging & Serious Illness at Massachusetts General Hospital in the United States and Senior Atlantic Fellow for Equity in Brain Health.

José Miguel Toribio-Guzmán (PhD, MSc) works as a Neuropsychologist and Researcher at Fundación INTRAS/IDES and is Professor at the Universidad Internacional de la Rioja (UNIR), Spain.

Justine Schneider (PhD) is Professor of Mental Health and Social Care at the University of Nottingham, the United Kingdom. She is Fellow of the Institute of Mental Health, Nottingham, United Kingdom.

Kate Shiells (PhD, MSc, BA) is currently working as a postdoctoral researcher at the University of Oxford, United Kingdom.

Katrin Seeher (PhD, Dipl-Psych) is Mental Health Specialist at WHO Headquarters in the area brain health, Geneva, Switzerland.

Kieren Egan (PhD) is Senior Research Fellow at the University of Strathclyde in Glasgow, the United Kingdom, and has a number of research interests spanning across: digital health, dementia, informal caregivers and healthy ageing.

Kim Beentjes (MSc) was Marie Sklodowska-Curie Early Stage Research fellow at the Department of Psychiatry of Amsterdam University Medical Centers, location Vrije Universiteit, Amsterdam, the Netherlands from May 2019 until October 2020.

Lara Pivodic (PhD, MSc) is Assistant Professor at the End-of-Life Care Research Group of Vrije Universiteit Brussel & Ghent University, Belgium, and Senior Postdoctoral Fellow of the Research Foundation – Flanders (FWO).

Leslie María Contreras Somoza (MSc) is PhD student in Neuropsychology at the University of Salamanca, Spain.

Lieve Van den Block (PhD, MSc) is Professor of Aging and Palliative Care at the Vrije Universiteit Brussel (VUB) and Chair of the Aging and Palliative Care Research Programme at the VUB-UGhent End-of-Life Care Research Group in Belgium.

Lizzy M. M. Boots (PhD, MSc) is Assistant Professor and Coordinator of psychosocial research at the Alzheimer Center Limburg, Maastricht University, the Netherlands.

Louise Nygård (PhD) is Professor of Occupational Therapy and leader of the CACTUS (Cognitive Accessibility and Technology Use when ageing in home and Society, http://ki.se/en/nvs/the-cactus-research-group) research group at the Division of Occupational Therapy at Karolinska Institutet in Stockholm, Sweden.

Lucas Vroemen is General Manager and Co-owner of EuMediaNet. EuMediaNet is a software development company based in Maastricht, the Netherlands.

Manuel Franco-Martin is Head of Psychiatry and Mental Health Department. Zamora Hospital, Spain. He is Head of Psychosciences Research Group of the Biomedicine Research Institute (IBSAL) and Associate Professor of the Salamanca University (Dpto. PETRA), Spain.

Marian Schoone-Harmsen (MSc) is Industrial Design Engineer and specialised in Technology in Health Care. She is Project Manager and Consultant at TNO, the Netherlands Organisation for Applied Scientific Research.

María Victoria Perea Bartolomé is Doctor in Medicine and Surgery from the University of Salamanca (USAL) (1984), Degree Approved by the University of Porto (Portugal) (2000), Medical Specialist in Neurology (1988) and Professor of Neuropsychology (2012).

Marjolein de Vugt is Professor of Psychosocial innovations in dementia at Maastricht University and chair of the Alzheimer Center Limburg, the Netherlands.

Martin Orrell (PhD, FRCPsych) is Director of the Institute of Mental Health, a partnership between the University of Nottingham and Nottinghamshire Healthcare NHS Foundation Trust, United Kingdom.

Maud JL Graff (PhD, MSc) is Professor of Occupational Therapy at the Radboudumc of Nijmegen in the Netherlands.

Olga Štěpánková is Professor of technical cybernetics at the Czech Technical University in Prague (CVUT), Czech Republic.

Orii McDermott (PhD) is Senior Research Fellow at the Institute of Mental Health, University of Nottingham, the United Kingdom.

Paul Higgs is Professor of the Sociology of Ageing in the UCL Division of Psychiatry, United Kingdom.

Rosalia J.M. van Knippenberg is Postdoctoral Researcher at the Alzheimer Center Limburg and the department of Psychiatry and Neuropsychology of the Faculty of Health, Medicine and Life Sciences, Maastricht University, the Netherlands.

Rose-Marie Dröes (PhD, MSc) is Full Professor of psychosocial care for people with dementia and head of the research group 'Care and support in dementia' at the department of Psychiatry of Amsterdam University Medical Centers, Vrije Universiteit, the Nertherlands.

Rose Miranda (PhD, MSc, BSc) is Post-doctoral researcher at the End-of-Life Care Research Group at the Vrije Universiteit Brussel and Ghent University in Belgium.

Sara Laureen Bartels (PhD, MSc) is Postdoctoral Researcher. She is currently employed by Karolinska Institutet Sweden as well as Maastricht University, the Netherlands.

Sarah Wallcook (PhD, MSc OT, BMus) is Analyst and Postdoctoral Researcher at the Stockholm Gerontology Research Centre in Sweden.

Sébastien Libert (PhD, MSc) is Honorary Researcher in Medical Anthropology at University College London, United Kingdom.

Sophie N. Gaber (PhD, MSc, OT) is Postdoctoral Researcher at the Department of Neurobiology, Care Sciences and Society at Karolinska Institutet and the Department of Health Care Sciences at Marie Cederschiöld University in Stockholm, Sweden.

Steve Course is Development Manager and Co-owner of EuMediaNet. EuMediaNet is a software development company based in Maastricht, the Netherlands.

Tinne Smets is Assistant Professor and Senior Researcher at the End-of-Life Care Research Group at the Vrije Universiteit Brussel (VUB) and Ghent University in Belgium.

Vladimíra Dostálová is Researcher at the Centre of Expertise in Longevity and Long-term Care at the Faculty of Humanities, Charles University, Czech Republic.

Yvonne Kerkhof (PhD, MSc) is Lecturer and Researcher at the Faculty of Health of Saxion University of Applied Sciences, the Netherlands. She is also member of the research group Smart Health of Saxion, the Netherlands.

Chapter 1

An introduction to the INDUCT programme

Martin Orrell, Déborah Oliveira, Orii McDermott, Frans R.J. Verhey, Rose-Marie Dröes

How we started

The development of the INDUCT proposal came from a workshop during a meeting of INTERDEM during the Alzheimer Europe conference in Glasgow in October 2014. Having explored a number of topics, it became clear that research training on dementia care and technology was very much needed in Europe. The Marie Skłodowska-Curie Actions is the European Union's reference programme for doctoral education and postdoctoral training, contributing to excellence in research, boosting jobs, growth and investment by equipping researchers with new knowledge and skills. They foster research cooperation across borders, sectors and disciplines. Following this we worked closely with friends and colleagues in particular Frans Verhey from Maastricht University and Rose-Marie Dröes from VU University medical centre in Amsterdam on designing a start of the art programme and bringing in exactly the right mix of leading academic and other partners to improve our chances of success. We knew all too well that getting a grant of this scale and importance was a very difficult enterprise and would require at least 93% in the rating by reviewers. The three of us went for a special training in Marie-Curie grants run by Yellow Research in Amsterdam, and also we much appreciated the advice provided by Dr. Martin Pickard, one of their consultants from the University of Nottingham EU Office. We heard about the success of the award in May 2015 (our rating was 98%) and since we would expect the Early Stage Researchers (ESRs) to be best placed to start in September registering for a PhD, they were recruited the following year via our special recruitment and interview event in May 2016 in London. The INDUCT programme has been completed now and it has been a wonderful experience. In particular we were able to appoint really excellent ESRs, very many of whom have now gone on to complete their PhDs and get excellent posts in Europe much like the grant intended. So as an introductory chapter we thought going back to the basics of the grant itself would well illustrate how we took the first few steps on the INDUCT journey.

Martin Orrell

DOI: 10.4324/9781003289005-1

The main ingredients

This book hopes to illustrate the diverse and important range of projects making a distinct and lasting contribution to improving dementia care. Initially we have a section on two very innovative aspects of the programme including both a detailed description of our unique training programme and perspectives on the wide range of public involvement activities written in collaboration with Alzheimer Europe. The main research section of the book is divided along the three main themes: (1) technology in everyday life; (2) technology to promote meaningful activities and (3) healthcare technology. To consolidate the best approaches to getting technology into practice, we also had three crosscutting themes which strongly influenced our best practice guidance: (1) determining practical, cognitive and social factors to improve usability of technology; (2) evaluating the effectiveness of specific contemporary technology; (3) tracing facilitators and barriers for implementation of technology in dementia care.

Our programme has also shown the importance of impact and public engagement work including participation in the conferences of INTERDEM and Alzheimer Europe. ESRs have done a range of public engagement events such as presentations to groups of older and younger people to stimulate their interest in knowledge, research and care of people with dementia. Key findings and recommendations and resources from the programme including the Best Practice Guidance are available on our website (www.dementiainduct.eu/guidance/). Better public understanding of the role of technology in dementia care should lead to reduced fear and stigma, and a more proactive approach to seeking help by people worried about their memory and their families. We are delighted to be able to bring so much together in this book and hope you find it interesting and useful to improve research, practice and care.

Background

In Europe there are almost 7 million people with dementia, and this is set to double by 2050 (World Health Organization, 2012). The G7 set an ambitious aim of a cure for dementia by 2025 but with the current state of scientific knowledge, there is no guarantee whatsoever that this will be achieved. If a cure is found it will take at least another 10–15 years to get it widely implemented and many people may not come forward until the dementia is well established. Dementia raises complex challenges for people with dementia, their families and society since it leads to progressive deterioration in cognitive functioning and activities of daily living, resulting in people becoming more dependent on the support of others, social exclusion, carer stress and increasing care costs. Most people with dementia live in their own homes and want to maintain their independence and autonomy for as long as possible with support of informal and sometimes paid carers. It usually costs less to support people at home, but this puts a strain on families. In response to this urgent situation the business and social sectors are struggling to know what technology is needed and what works well. The European Parliament and the Council set the 'European initiative on Alzheimer's disease and other dementias goals' of developing high-quality innovative research and helping people with dementia and their carers to preserve health, quality of life, autonomy and dignity. This means there is an immediate need for research specialists working to improve dementia care and supporting people at home and therefore limiting the economic and societal costs. In this context, the INDUCT programme will develop 15 ESRs, researchers who become experts in the health and social needs of people with dementia and the effective application of technological solutions to support them.

The main aim of INDUCT was to develop a premier quality multi-disciplinary, multi-professional and intersectorial education and training research framework for Europe, aimed at improving technology and care for people with dementia, and to use the coherent themes and interrelated ESRs within INDUCT to provide the evidence to show how technology can improve the lives of people with dementia. The unique collaborative partnership INDUCT – Interdisciplinary Network for Dementia Utilising Current Technology comprised seven world leading research organisations, the World Health Organization, and IDES an SME for technology, research and care, with eight partners who included Alzheimer Europe, the leading non-academic sector organisation representing people with dementia and carers within Europe, Alzheimer's Disease International, the global voice on dementia representing an international federation of Alzheimer's associations, the World OT Federation, two other major universities and three other SMEs. The consortium included interdisciplinary, intersectorial and international perspectives with eight countries, four international organisations, key sectors and the right range of disciplines.

The academic and non-academic partners within INDUCT were closely involved with INTERDEM, a well-established, interdisciplinary European collaborative research network of 130 leading academics and researchers in 20 European countries with an aim to improve early detection and timely psychosocial intervention in dementia (www.interdem.org). INTERDEM was founded in 1999 to foster European interdisciplinary and intersectorial collaborations in psychosocial research in dementia between countries and produce robust evidence of interventions to improve dementia care. Harnessing the strategic excellence of the INTERDEM Academy (Klinkenberg et al., 2019), which was established through the INTERDEM network, the comprehensive research training programme for all ESRs would efficiently equip them with the skills needed for work in the academic world, industry, or the health and social sector. INDUCT aims to drive Europe to lead the world in research and research training in dementia care and technology offering the greatest opportunity to be translated and disseminated into the real world where people with dementia live and are supported in their local communities.

Dementia has been identified by the European Commission as a 'societal challenge', and INDUCT also supported the Horizon 2020 Work Programme PHC18 (ICT solutions for independent living with cognitive impairment), PHC20 (Advancing active and healthy ageing with ICT: early risk detection and intervention) and PHC22 (Promoting mental well-being: in the ageing population). The EU had highlighted the need to 'invest in scientific research and efficient approaches to care systems through the development of more effective, technology-assisted care to anticipate the economic and social impact of Alzheimer's and other forms of dementia' (European parliament resolution 19 January 2011) on a European initiative on Alzheimer's disease and other dementias (2010/2084(INI)). The complex nature of how humans relate to and use technology is reflected in the difficulties of applications which aim to support people with dementia. Three principal challenges meant that so far people with dementia had not been able to properly benefit from technology:

1) There was a poor understanding in research and business of how people with dementia use technology in everyday life, with new applications being designed without an in-depth appreciation of people's needs, preferences and limitations (objective 3).
2) Research has been fragmented, with studies often poorly designed, in-house, and small scale, with technology that does not meet people's needs making it hard to draw any conclusions on the effectiveness of technology (objective 4).
3) There was little knowledge about practical, psychological and social barriers and facilitators to implementation to explain why people with dementia frequently do not use technology and why it has been hard to get useful technology into more widespread practice (objective 5).

By focusing on the improvement of the usability of technology in dementia care and by evaluating its effectiveness and implementation issues, INDUCT would enhance the European Commission's Public Health Strategies (2008) and the European Parliament resolution of 2011 for the 'European Initiative on Alzheimer's disease and other dementias' as an EU health priority and support member countries' national dementia strategies. To meet these challenges, Europe had an urgent need for close interdisciplinary collaborations between academia and non-academia to provide a new generation of ESRs who have a comprehensive research training, a deep understanding of the nature of dementia and are equipped to improve dementia care interventions through creative innovative research and intellectual leadership (ARDE project 2013: European University Association) and have the right skill sets for the future needs of the European workforce. Though the evidence was (and is) limited, policymakers and researchers often mentioned technology applications as promising solutions to promote independence and autonomy in people with dementia showing there was a need for INDUCT and suggesting that stakeholders would take a keen interest in the results.

Research in people with dementia living at home showed that some of the most frequently experienced unmet needs are located in the areas of functioning in everyday life, for example support for memory problems, meaningful activities, social contact and safety (van der Roest et al., 2009). The EU funded the COGKNOW (Meiland et al., 2012) study (Sweden, the United Kingdom, the Netherlands, Spain, France, Malta), which developed, by a user participatory design, personalisable technology to help people with dementia in the areas of memory support, social contact, meaningful activities and safety, to increase their autonomy and quality of life via a touch screen, mobile device, sensors and actuators and was field tested in three countries. The Mylife project (Norway, Germany, the United Kingdom) aimed to support independence for people with dementia by giving them access to simple and intuitive Internet services to support time orientation, communication and entertainment. Mylife is adaptable to the person's needs and wishes through a carers administration website. GRADIOR software can remotely assess neuropsychology problems and allow the professional to tailor interventions to the specific cognitive difficulties (attention, perception, language, reasoning and memory) of the person with dementia. The EU-funded Long Lasting Memories project (www.longlastingmemories.eu/) involved IDES/INTRAS (Spain) and worked with GRADIOR for cognitive and physical training in mild dementia. The system was well accepted by people with dementia, and an opportunity remains for applying these psychosocial approaches in the home.

Everyday technologies (ETs) are increasingly vital in today's activities in homes and communities. Nevertheless, little attention had been given to the consequences of the increasing complexity and reliance on them, for example shops, traffic situations and healthcare services. Technology has a potential to simplify our daily lives and compensate for disability. The rapid growth of the technological landscape and related new services have the potential to improve the cost-effectiveness of health and social services and facilitate social participation and engagement in activities (Orpwood et al., 2007). At the same time, it places people at high risk of exclusion if they fail to upgrade or maintain their competencies to manage technology. This risk pertained to daily life at home as well as at work, in public space, as the complexity of both realms is continuously increasing (Nygård and Starkhammar, 2007). The users' ability to manage products and services had been largely neglected or taken for granted. Our insights into how ET could be best designed and used, and how support and environments, private as well as public, should be designed to facilitate the participation of people with dementia were still limited.

Prior to developing this proposal, we carried out consultations with 40 carers and people with dementia. There was enthusiastic support: 'a splendid proposal the timing of which is absolutely right'. People expressed concerns about lack of access to the right technology and emphasised the importance of being involved in the process to ensure technology was appropriate and acceptable. Via Alzheimer Europe we also consulted the European Working Group of People with Dementia (EWGPWD), who provided feedback with strong support for the proposal.

The aim was to develop a multi-disciplinary, intersectorial educational research framework for Europe to improve technology and care for people with dementia, and to provide the evidence to show how technology could improve the lives of people with dementia with the following objectives:

1   to set up INDUCT, the European multi-disciplinary, intersectorial educational research network;
2   to provide a comprehensive training programme for ESRs to acquire a deep understanding of the nature of dementia and needs in relation to the use of technology and to equip them with the right skills needed for work in academia, industry or the health and social sector;
3   to determine the practical, cognitive and social factors needed to make technology more useable for people with dementia;
4   to evaluate the effectiveness of specific contemporary technology;
5   to trace facilitators and barriers for implementation of technology in dementia care; and
6   to disseminate the knowledge and evidence on how technology can be best applied and implemented in dementia care and can improve the lives of people with dementia.

A key part of the programme was to provide not just a comprehensive training programme for ESRs in dementia care, technology and research skills with five week-long training schools, the INTERDEM Academy, placements and secondments but also additional leadership, management and innovation skills needed for work in industry or the academic, health or social sectors. The research of INDUCT built on existing cross-sectorial work by the beneficiaries involving collaborations between European nations. An emphasis on innovative methodologies such as user involvement and co-design with people living with dementia was required to foster the inclusive rights, independence and self-esteem of people living with dementia while working to transform health and social care practice. The methods were based on the UK Medical Research Council Framework for the development and evaluation of complex interventions, which included phases of theory and development (objective 3); feasibility/piloting and evaluation (e.g. randomised controlled trial (RCT) of effectiveness and cost-effectiveness) (objective 4), and implementation (objective 5). The ESR research programme was organised by three main themes and work packages based on three global need areas of which two focused on needs-based technology to support people with dementia in their daily lives (WP3 Technology to support everyday life; WP4 Technology to promote meaningful activities) and the third on organisational and support systems for

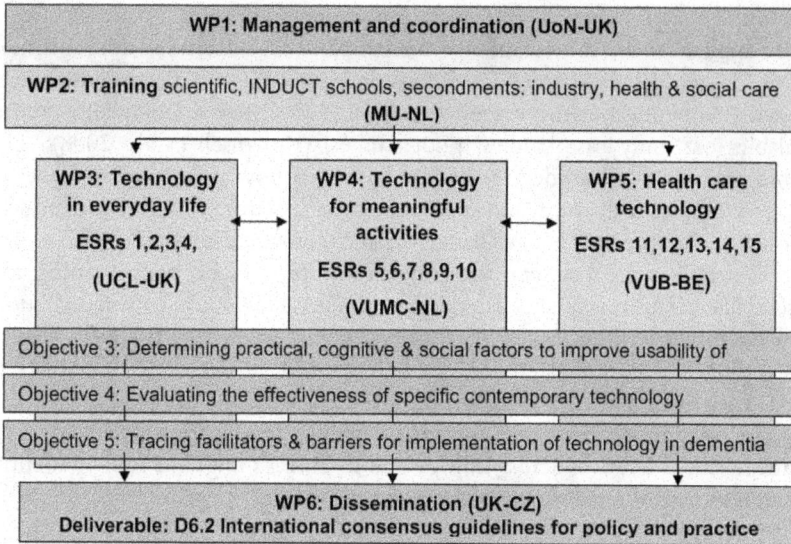

Figure 1.1 Management and Research plan

healthcare (WP5 Healthcare technology). Within each theme different types of technology in different settings and for people with dementia and carers were investigated with different objectives (usability, effectiveness or implementation aspects). The six objectives (including the research objectives 3, 4, 5) cut across all three research themes on the basis that easier use of more adequate technology, which can be attuned to personal abilities, needs, preferences and circumstances, will lead to both personal and societal benefits such as being able to remain at home for longer and reduced overall costs of care. Integration across the 15 individual ESR projects and across the themes produced the synergy required to address the major cross theme research objectives (Figure 1.1: transversal objectives 3, 4 and 5). This generated the main research deliverable: the INDUCT evidence-based international Best Practice Guidance on Human Interaction with Technology in Dementia for policy and practice on improving the usability and effectiveness of technology and understanding how to get technology implemented in practice.

Research theme: technology in everyday life – ESR1, ESR2, ESR3, ESR4

Technology in everyday life comprises ET (e.g. telephones, cell phones, microwaves, cash machines) and assistive technology (AT; e.g. memory aids, safety devices, electronic calendars and reminders). Technology can challenge and hinder older adults with mild dementia in activities at home, at work and in public spaces (Malinowsky et al., 2010). Several studies (Nygård, 2008) have also found that a variety of ETs such as computers, telephones and electronic home appliances are important also for people with dementia, although their use of ET gradually decreases and causes problems. AT is widely used for people with dementia but the evidence is limited with few good-quality studies available (e.g. only case studies, pilot studies) (Brownsell et al., 2008). This theme examined the under-researched topics of how people with dementia relate to ET plus the ethical and social aspects of technology. ESR1 looked specifically at the impact of surveillance on autonomy and dignity. ESR2 examined the relationship between the concept and practice of 'brain training' as a potentially exclusionary and stigmatising process for people concerned about their cognitive abilities. Likewise, for people with dementia, using ET can be demanding and complicated such as being unable to answer cell phones or obtain cash from machines which limits their ability to use public spaces. ESR3 planned to examine how this impacts on public participation and ESR4 will compare the differences across Europe and in Turkish migrants to help identify research strategies for dissemination internationally.

Research theme: technology to promote meaningful activities – ESR5, ESR6, ESR7, ESR8, ESR9, ESR10

Computer-based technology can be used to support and promote meaningful activities for people with relatively mild dementia to improve their quality of life through self-management, meaningful and cognitive activities, social communication and awareness through a range of touch screen-based applications. There is the potential for applications to improve cognition and quality of life. Cognitive Stimulation Therapy (www.cstdementia.com) is the best evidenced psychosocial intervention for dementia and has been used in a manual-based format for groups and carer-delivered modes. ESR5 adapted CST using a touch screen format for iPAD and evaluated the effectiveness of CST touch screen in the United Kingdom, Spain, and the Netherlands. ESR6 examined the use of digital arts and crafts via touch screen tablet computers to enable access to personalised artistic activities. ESR7 scoped the use of exergaming in dementia and conducted a clinical trial compared to usual care. ESR8 used an existing application developed for the iPAD to help people increase their independence and quality of life by online self-management of their needs and leisure activities and evaluated this in a clinical trial to look at effectiveness. ESR9 also looked at how Experience Sampling can be used to enhance people's lives using momentary assessment technology to increase their awareness of the therapeutic process and improve the outcomes of interventions. ESR10 examined how social relationships can be enhanced by assisting people with dementia to use social media technology (e.g. Skype, Facebook). People with dementia often have very limited access to cultural and physical activities.

Research theme: healthcare technology – ESR11, ESR12, ESR13, ESR14, ESR15

Health technology is defined as 'the application of scientific knowledge in health-care and disease prevention' and so dementia care and palliative care are typical examples involving complex processes related to the organisational and supportive systems within which healthcare is provided (Integrate – HTA, EU funded project 2013–2016). This theme builds on the European PACE study extended to evaluate how palliative care can improve quality of dying of people with dementia living in nursing homes (ESR11). ESR12 focused on the specific effectiveness of advance care planning as a complex health technology for people with dementia in nursing homes. Across Europe there is a great variety in the different software applications used to help manage care for persons with dementia in long-term care settings such as nursing homes in terms of quality, content, user-friendliness, data safety, needs assessment and usability for management of care. ESR13 systematically collated and reviewed the most widely used care applications and provided a detailed analysis of their value in practice by studying contrasting applications in nursing home settings in four EU countries, which included an analysis of enabling factors and hurdles in their use. ESR14 developed and trialled an innovative online support system for carers of people with dementia. The GRADIOR, a computer-based cognitive rehabilitation programme, developed by IDES/INTRAS, is used in over 450 centres at national and international levels within the social and health sector but it has not been evaluated in depth. ESR15 developed a clinical trial comparing GRADIOR to usual care in people with dementia.

The involvement of people with dementia throughout the development process has been of great importance in order to develop valuable, user-friendly, support-ive technology for dementia that can be demonstrated to be effective (Span et al., 2013). People with dementia and carers were involved in all phases and across the various different cultural contexts to produce specific international guidelines on how to best involve people with dementia, the specific role of patient/public involvement (PPI), and the impact of involvement on the quality of the tech-nology and on the person with dementia. The outcome is a framework, similar to the guidelines for adapting Cognitive Stimulation Therapy for dementia to other culture (Aguirre et al., 2014). The European Working Group of People with Dementia (Alzheimer Europe, 2021), hosted by Alzheimer Europe, were key partners in this project and reviewed ESR applications and assisted ESRs to design their research with users in mind to maximise impact of their projects.

Transversal objective: determining practical, cognitive and social factors to improve usability of technology

Uptake of technology by people with dementia and their carers is often low with concerns about intrusive devices, aspects of surveillance, devices being hard to use, stigma and the effects on people's dignity (Hanson et al., 2007) so that more evidence is needed about how people with dementia can interact with technology better. People with dementia often do not use the available technology because it does not match their needs and capacities; applications are too difficult to use, contain too many functions, and are not attractive (Lauriks et al., 2007). However, the current cohort of the over 60s are well experienced in the use of computers and other technology so INDUCT was perfectly timed to influence the development of future feasible and effective technologies. The studies used a range of qualitative methods including indepth individual interviews and focus groups as well as questionnaire surveys. This mixed-methods approach provided a detailed picture from the patient, carer and professional perspectives and the international secondments informed cultural issues around the use and acceptability of technology. ESRs closely collaborated with various industrial partners involved in designing technology to better understand the perspectives and needs of technology businesses. ESR3 and ESR4 identified conditions and barriers to use ET along with the first world questionnaire survey of AT (with WFOT). ESR9 assessed the acceptability of momentary assessment technology with PSY-MATE. ESR10 studied the factors that influenced digital engagement of people with dementia and family caregivers to use social media. ESR1 examined the nature of surveillance technologies using a review of the literature and in-depth consultations with experts, staff, family carers and people with dementia and investigated the assumptions behind them since issues such as stigma, ethics and design may make them unpopular.

Transversal objective: evaluating the effectiveness of specific contemporary technology

Lauriks et al. (2007) found that people with dementia could use simple electronic devices for memory support or improving ADL, but most studies were small and uncontrolled. They concluded that more trials were needed for working on integrating and applying existing technologies in real-life situations. Woolham (2005) found in a large controlled study that compared to the control settings, AT was linked with fewer visits, longer residence in the community and decreased carer concerns; however, different settings were used and the study was not randomised. A recent review by Boots et al. (2014) found that Internet interventions for dementia carers may improve well-being, but the evidence lacked methodological quality. More randomised controlled studies assessing interventions performed according to protocol are needed to give stronger statements about the effects of supportive Internet interventions and their most promising elements. This objective used findings of a broad range of clinical trials including qualitative evaluations and process evaluations to identify key themes which are associated with benefit for people with dementia and family carers, and key outcomes (ESR5, ESR9, ESR10, ESR7, ESR8, ESR14). ESR5 developed a touch screen version of CST and evaluated this in a controlled trial. ESR9 used momentary assessment techniques to evaluate benefit in depth in a limited case-control series. ESR12 evaluated advance care planning using quantitative and qualitative outcome and process evaluation. ESR7 conducted an in-depth evaluation and RCT to determine benefits of exergames. ESR8 conducted an RCT of a self-management and leisure iPad-based intervention among people with dementia and carers. ESR14 developed a tailor-made Internet and Mobile Platform for carers of people with dementia and carried out a RCT.

Transversal objective: tracing facilitators and barriers for implementation of technology in dementia care

Living at home means living in a technologically complex society, and research has shown that people with early-stage dementia have decreased ability to man-age ET. Despite the wide variety of AT available, there remains a great debate about what technologies need to be developed and there are concerns about the lack of interactions between industry, health staff and the direct users of AT: people with dementia and their carers. The EU-funded ENABLE study with five countries using prototypes and qualitative methodology concluded that whereas technology could promote independence, it needed to be fully tested and operational prior to use in real life. Moreover, many innovative systems are not commercially available, and there is a need for independent research rather than 'in-house' evaluations. Implementation of technology is not just impeded by lack of evidence of effectiveness but is influenced by stigma, perceptions and people's need for autonomy and dignity. This means many countries and regions provide a disparate range of technology, creating inequality in access, so that implementation is severely limited. Technology studies in care homes cover three main themes: personal living environment (privacy, autonomy and obtrusiveness); the outside world (stigma and human contact); design (indi-vidual approach, affordability and safety), and recommended that ethics should be studied in terms of the underlying concepts of privacy, autonomy, stigmati-sation, human contact, individual approach and affordability.

Network organisation and management structure

The management structure of INDUCT (Figure 1.2) was developed to provide an efficient, transparent framework to fully encourage commitment and commu-nicational exchange between partners across all levels in order to guide, support, coordinate and monitor all activities throughout the network. The Management Board (MB) included the Network Coordinator (NC), Project Manager (PM), Training Coordinator (TC), Secondment Coordinator (SC), Research Coordi-nator (RC), Commercial Exploitation Coordinator (CEC), Recruitment and Equal Opportunities Coordinator (REOC), Ethical Advisor (EA), Financial and Administrative Coordinator (FAC) and the ESR Supervisors (ESR-Ss) and met every three to four months to review all activities (recruitment, training

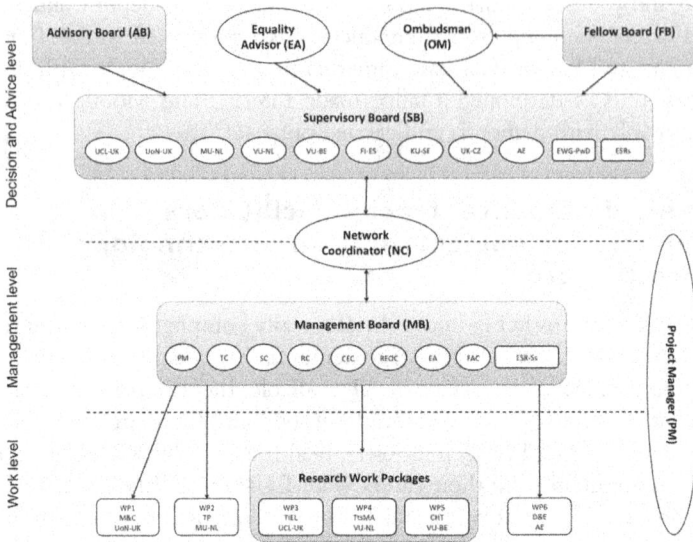

Figure 1.2 Management Structure

programme, research outputs, exploitation and outreach) to ensure that they were progressing towards milestone and deliverable targets. The Supervisory Board (SB) included a representative of each of the beneficiaries and partners, two elected representatives of the ESRs, and two elected representatives of the European Working Group of People with Dementia meeting six times over the project to oversee INDUCT and ensure that ESRs receive the proper combination of academic, transferable skills and on-the-job training through their secondments in the non-academic sector as laid down in the ESRs' PCDP. Moreover, the SB made sure the rights and interests of people with dementia are enshrined by putting them at the heart of the research projects. Also an International Advisory Board (IAB) was convened to provide independent advice and support.

Acknowledgement

The editors would like to thank Christine Bailey for her organizational and administrative support.

References

Aguirre E, Spector A, Orrell M. Guidelines for adapting cognitive stimulation therapy to other cultures. *Clinical Interventions in Aging* 2014; 9: 1003. Retrieved from www.alzheimer-europe.org/Alzheimer-Europe/Who-we-are/European-Working-Group-of-People-with-Dementia

Alzheimer Europe (2021) *European working group of people with dementia*. Retrieved from www.alzheimer-europe.org/Alzheimer-Europe/Who-we-are/European-Working-Group-of-People-with-Dementia

Boots LM, de Vugt ME, Van Knippenberg RJ, Kempen GI, Verhey FR. A systematic review of Internet–based supportive interventions for caregivers of patients with dementia. *International Journal of Geriatric Psychiatry* 2014; 29(4): 331–344.

Brownsell S, Blackburn S, Hawley, MS. An evaluation of second and third generation telecare services in older people's housing. *Journal of Telemedicine and Telecare* 2008; 14: 8–12.

European Commission's Public Health Strategies (2008) EU public health strategy 2008–2013: The EU Council and the Commission urge Member States to focus on health policies: Financing health: OECD reports about health in Denmark and Iceland. *Scandinavian Journal of Public Health* 2008; 36(3): 334–335. doi: 10.1177/1403494808091355

Hanson E, Magnusson L, Arvidsson H, Claesson A, Keady J, Nolan M. Working together with persons with early stage dementia and their family members to design a user-friendly technology-based support service. *Dementia: The International Journal of Social Research and Practice* 2007; 6: 411–414.

Klinkenberg IPM, de Oliveira, D, Verhey, FRJ, Orrell M, de Vugt ME. INTERDEM Academy: A training and career development initiative vital to capacity building of early-stage psychosocial dementia researchers in Europe. *Aging & Mental Health* 2019; 23(8): 929–931.

Lauriks S, Reinersmann A, Van der Roest HG, Meiland FJM, Davies RJ, Moelaert F, Mulvenna MD, Nugent CD, Dröes RM. Review of ICT-based services for identified unmet needs in people with dementia. *Ageing Research Reviews* 2007; 6: 223–246

Malinowsky C, Kottorp A, Almkvist O, Nygård L. Ability to manage everyday technology: A comparison of people with dementia or mild cognitive impairment and older adults without cognitive impairment. *Disability and Rehabilitation; Assistive Technology* 2010; 5: 462–469.

Meiland F, Bouman A, Sävenstedt S, Bentvelzen S, Davies R, Mulvenna M, Nugent M, et al. Usability of a new electronic assistive device for community-dwelling persons with mild dementia. *Aging & Mental Health* 2012; 16(5): 584–591.

Nygård L. The meaning of everyday technology as experienced by people with dementia who live alone. *Dementia* 2008; 7: 481–502.

Nygård L, Starkhammar S. The use of everyday technology by people with dementia living alone. *Aging & Mental Health* 2007; 11: 144–155.

Orpwood R, Orpwood R, Sixsmith A, Torrington J, Chadd J, Gibson G, Chalfont G. Designing technology to support quality of life of people with dementia. *Technology and Disability* 2007: 19; 103–112.

Span M, Hettinga M, Vernooij-Dassen M, Eefsting J, Smits C. Involving people with dementia in the development of supportive IT applications: A systematic review. *Ageing Research Reviews* 2013; 12(2): 535–551.

van der Roest H, Meiland F, Hannie C, Derksen E, Jansen A, van Hout H, Jonker C, Dröes RM. What do community-dwelling people with dementia need? A survey of those who are known to care and welfare services. *International Psychogeriatrics* 2009; 949–965.

Woolham, J. Safe at Home. In: *The effectiveness of assistive technology in supporting the independence of people with dementia: The Safe at Home project*. London: Hawker Publications, 2005.

World Health Organization, Alzheimer's Disease International. *Dementia, a public health priority*, 2012. Retrieved from http://whqlibdoc.who.int/publications/2012/9789241564458 eng.pdf (last accessed 9.11.14).

Part 1

Key components of the INDUCT network

Chapter 2

The unique training programme of INDUCT

Fania C.M. Dassen, Sara Laureen Bartels,
Hannah Christie, Lieve Van den Block,
Marjolein de Vugt, Frans R.J. Verhey

Overview and content of the training programme

High levels of uncertainty with regard to employment and strong competition for funding and resources will eventually force many Early Stage Researchers (ESRs) to leave the research field (Oliveira et al., 2021). Only a minority will end up working in academia, and therefore, preparation for non-academic employment is necessary. The non-academic sector includes all fields of future workplaces of researchers, from industry to business, government, civil society organisations, cultural institutions, hospitals etc. (European Commission, 2019). However, many academics lack experience in the industrial and non-profit sector and may thereby feel ill-prepared to follow those career paths. The need for the development of more effective, technology-assisted care to anticipate the economic and social impact of dementia calls for a hybrid type of researcher – able to combine expertise on dementia care with technological ingenuity, whilst putting the needs and perspectives of people with dementia at the heart of their projects. At the start of the project, to the best of our knowledge, doctoral training programmes available in Europe that offer such specialised education on top of the regular training courses supplied in the academia were non-existent. This makes INDUCT the first to train ESRs using a unique blend of dementia, healthcare, technology and enterprise, thereby bridging the sectors of academy, business, health, non-profit and social care across Europe.

The main goal of the INDUCT consortium was to provide high-quality training and network facilities for ESRs in top-level European Universities and Organisations related to the multidisciplinary area of dementia where technologies would be useful to support people with dementia. INDUCT provided a comprehensive training programme for 15 ESRs to acquire a deep understanding of the nature of dementia and needs in relation to the use of technology, and to prepare them with the right skills needed for work in academia, industry, or the health and social sector.

ESRs were offered a well-rounded training programme. To equip our ESRs with an outstanding education to excel in various occupational settings in dementia care across borders, we envisioned three levels of skills training as

DOI: 10.4324/9781003289005-3

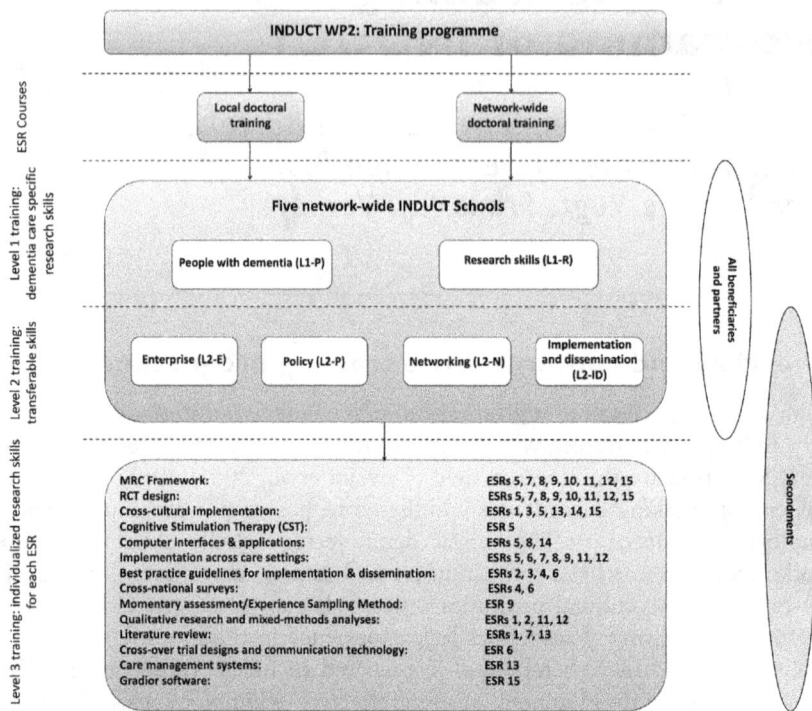

Figure 2.1 Training Programme of INDUCT

detailed later, which were to extend the basic doctoral training to be offered at the local academic partners (see Figure 2.1 for a schematic overview of the training programme). The INDUCT training framework addressed the Marie Skłodowska-Curie policy objective to provide researchers with the right combination of dementia and dementia care research-related skills (Level 1), transferable competencies (Level 2) and the need to extend beyond the traditional academic research training (Level 3), which draws on the intersectoral expertise.

ESRs were recruited in one cohort and were at a similar stage of their scientific career. At the start of their project, a Personal Career Development Plan (PCDP) was identified for each ESR as part of their professional development based on their individual training needs. The ESR's PCDP included an overview and time plan for course, agreed with the supervisor(s). The local and network-wide doctoral training was an integral part of the ESRs PCDP, which was tailored to their PhD research topic and wishes regarding career progression. All ESRs were required to select local and network-wide courses together combining into 240 hours of study. Introductory courses were organised at the start, while more advanced courses were provided later in their trajectories.

Local doctoral training

The local doctoral training was centred on the local PhD courses provided by the doctoral schools of the academic beneficiaries, open to all ESRs and carrying ECTS credits. Participation as an educational tutor in graduate courses offered by the beneficiaries or supervision of undergraduate students was also part of the ESRs local doctoral training. Local trainings varied based on the universities' offers and the ESRs' needs for it; however, ESRs were encouraged to also look at training courses at INDUCT partner universities. The local training programme spanned the following themes: Literature search and management, Analytical and critical thinking, Creativity, Brain training and speed reading, Self-confidence and assertiveness, Time management, Career management and professional development, Good Clinical Practice (GCP), Publishing and Plagiarism, Preparing for your PhD defence, Acquisition of research funding, Academic writing, People management and teamwork, Academic teaching, Equality and diversity, Public media training, Communication and Presenting your research.

Network-wide doctoral training

The network-wide doctoral training was offered through a massive open online course (MOOC) on dementia called Positive about Dementia (POSADEM). POSADEM was funded by the EU Lifelong Learning programme (grant agreement number 2013–3227/001–001; September 2013 to 2016) and led by the University of Salford. POSADEM drew on the strengths of Dublin City University, Carinthia University of Applied Sciences, Maastricht University, Saimaa University of Applied Sciences and Bournemouth University. The main aim of this collaboration was to develop an interdisciplinary masters-level programme with an appreciative view and emphasis on the positive aspects of 'living with' dementia rather than 'being treated for' or 'enduring' dementia, despite its negative effects.

Understanding how dementia is experienced and what promotes quality of life for people with dementia and their families is a fundamental skill for dementia researchers to develop, deliver, evaluate, improve and implement healthcare services and technological innovations for dementia care and support. The first module of POSADEM was therefore offered as a general introduction for the ESRs of INDUCT to get acquainted with the field of dementia care. The module offered a critical appreciation of the key experiences and challenges that individual's living with dementia as well as their carers face on a daily basis, combined with a thorough understanding of (inter)national healthcare policies and psychosocial approaches to improve their quality of life. A variety of learning activities was used to cultivate the ESRs' understanding, discussion and reflection on the themes delivered and to accommodate individual learning styles. ESRs could interact with their peers and teachers on discussion boards, watch online video lectures, read academic literature and case vignettes, complete assignments, fill out online quizzes and/or engage in weekly virtual classrooms. In the final week, an ungraded end assignment was provided to the ESRs requiring them to write a 500-word personal reflection on three important concepts they had learned during the module and three action points for their research projects. ESRs were given a module certificate after completion of the exercises, an end assignment and evaluation survey.

The INDUCT schools

Both level 1 and level 2 training was offered within a core set of five INDUCT schools of five days each, which were physically held in various locations across Europe. Representatives of the European Working Group of People with Dementia (EWGPWD) and speakers and participants from academic and non-academic partners were invited to deliver interactive presentations at the schools. Moreover, ESRs presented their own work to their peers and senior colleagues to receive feedback on their projects and practice their presentation skills. The schools contributed to our public engagement programme entitled 'INDUCT Outreach' and included events open to the general public, which provided updates on the latest research results of the network. As a proof of excellence, all ESR received a certificate confirming attendance of each school organised within INDUCT.

Each school offered an opportunity to learn from the expertise of the INDUCT partners (training sessions), discuss current developments, contributions to transversal recommendations and future plans (INDUCT project meetings), and to network with fellow ESRs, as well as the academic, industrial and health and social care partners in the network (social and networking events). Training sessions offered a comprehensive introduction to INDUCT's expertise when it came to research methodology (academic and industry partners), key projects within or outside the consortium (academic and industry partners), and dementia policies and dissemination of their research (dementia, health and social care organisations). INDUCT project seminars were meant to inform and discuss current developments and future plans with regard to management, roles and communication, research projects, impact, recommendations and dissemination, training, supervision, the PCDPs and secondments. Furthermore, a closed ESR session offered the possibility to vote for an ESR representative and divide tasks, for instance, managing the INDUCT social media accounts. These ESR-only sessions also provided a safe space to receive peer support, discuss workload and work-life balance, and issues related to the project or supervision. An ombudsperson was available for guidance and mediation, if necessary. Finally, social and networking events were meant to get to know one another in a relatively more informal way.

Level 1: Dementia care-specific research skills training

The Level 1 training was offered network-wide within these five INDUCT schools, to enable ESRs to become excellent dementia care researchers able to compete academically at the highest level. To do so, our ESRs needed to be trained how to conduct research with people with dementia. Level 1 network-wide courses were set up around the following two themes and courses:

1   People with dementia: ESRs needed to become aware of challenges regarding people with dementia as advisors to their projects, participant recruitment, informed consent, communication styles and the logistics of working with people with dementia.
2   Research skills: To pursue excellence, INDUCT ESRs needed to understand the methodological aspects of quantitative and qualitative evaluation of care and support interventions, for example trial design, assessment techniques, selecting and developing outcome measures, statistical analysis. Secondly, they needed to be equipped with a cutting-edge overview of the latest developments regarding technological innovations and applications for dementia care and support.

Level 2: Transferable skills training

The Level 2 training was also offered network-wide within the INDUCT schools, preparing the ESRs for future employment in academia, healthcare, industry or the voluntary sector. The Level 2 training was set up around the following four themes and courses:

1   Enterprise – These courses trained a new generation of creative, entrepreneurial and innovative ESRs to be able to face current and future challenges and to convert knowledge and ideas into products and services for economic and social benefit;
2   Policy – These courses provided ESRs with extensive background knowledge regarding national and international policies for dementia care and research as a framework for their own projects;
3   Leadership – These courses enabled our ESRs to become strong leaders in dementia care research equipped with the necessary skills to pursue collaborations and employment across borders;
4   Implementation and dissemination – To ensure sustainability of ESR research projects, it was vital that they became familiar with challenges to successfully implement technological innovations in health and social care, as well as communicating their research findings across employment sectors.

Level 3: Individualised research training specific for each ESR

Additionally, each ESR was required to select courses on specific topics relevant to successfully carry out and finish their individual research project. See Figure 2.1 for an overview of topics per ESR.

Secondments

Intersectoral secondments exposed every ESR to alternate work practices and complementary expertise at other centres or enterprises. Mobility was a key aspect within INDUCT. Secondments organised within INDUCT involved two three-month periods when ESRs worked with another partner, usually in another country than the country of the host institution. In some cases, the duration and form of execution were slightly adjusted to match the ESRs' research project and tasks. By bringing together the expertise of private, public and voluntary sectors, INDUCT considered the participation of the non-academic sector as fundamental to the success of the next generation of creative, entrepreneurial and innovative researchers in dementia care and technology. ESRs developed industry and business experience by conducting secondments as part of their project. Mobility within Europe was key to improve their knowledge about cross-cultural issues in dementia and being mindful of language barriers that may exist. This helped to ensure their increased knowledge about potential employment settings, helped them to identify needs to be addressed and to learn how research translates into non-academic settings, and facilitated a better understanding of where and how expertise and skills would be applicable in non-academic settings. Crossover between industries was also promoted via placements in private, public or the voluntary sector. In such settings, user input could be collected, and unmet needs could be identified to design research studies that would be most beneficial to the end users. For ESRs keen to stay in academia, the knowledge and connections with the secondment experience would ensure the future success of potential collaborations to continue to innovate and change practice to improve life for people living with dementia and their family, as supported by the European Parliament. ESRs were exposed to different industry, health and social care contexts in which to conduct their individualised, personalised research projects with mentorship, support, education and training. The practical settings provided the ESRs with hands-on experience and a variety of potential future employment opportunities.

Contribution of the non-academic sector

The participation of non-academic partners was a vital component of this training network. The non-academic sector was strongly involved in the network-wide training courses as offered within INDUCT, and two intersectoral secondments of three months each as described earlier. Many of the ESRs had non-academic host centres and/or secondments and all partners contributed to specific training workshops over the course of the INDUCT training programme. This presented a clear opportunity for Europe to take a lead in the development of contemporary technology for supporting the lives of people with dementia and their families and to speed their deployment through cooperating closely with healthcare and industrial partners. By sharing expertise and collaborating on cutting-edge research, industrial partners played a pivotal role in the development of next-generation technology systems for enabling cost-effective dementia care and support. The network has enabled the industrial partners to bring in new talent and academic expertise earlier than is typically possible. The ESRs could benefit from becoming familiar with industrial applications of their research, and as a result they better understand how their research relates to care and industry, and future needs for the next generations of technology. Other opportunities included project collaborations between their host institution and a non-academic partner such as writing a joint paper and carrying out a relevant survey or project. In addition to the training and secondments offered within INDUCT, the role of the non-academic sector was also strongly represented in a joint supervision of the ESRs.

Involvement of EWGPWD

Persons with dementia from the European Working Group of People with Dementia (EWGPWD) served as an adviser on the ESR projects regarding the inclusion of people with dementia. The EWGPWD was launched by Alzheimer Europe and its member associations in 2012 (Alzheimer Europe, 2021). The group is formed by people with dementia, and works to make sure that the activities, projects and meetings of Alzheimer Europe reflect the priorities and views of people living with dementia (Alzheimer Europe, 2021).

The EWGPWD as well as the ESRs very much appreciated the opportunity to meet and exchange experiences during the first schools but expressed a need for more time and sessions in smaller groups. Thus, a greater involvement was facilitated and we scheduled more time with the EWGPWD during the second and third schools. For the two final schools, in close alignment with the Alzheimer Europe association, it was decided that representatives of the EWGPWD no longer would attend and present at the schools, as this was considered a too intense setting for the persons with dementia. Instead, to optimally work together with the EWGPWD, in 2019, the group of persons with dementia and their supporters provided input on the ESR projects at a separate one-day EWGPWD event, which focused on the final recommendations resulting from the ESR projects.

The final one-day meeting of ESRs and EWGPWD was a great opportunity for the ESRs to receive feedback from the EWGPWD on the final transversal recommendations, dissemination of results, individual project-related questions, and show their developed technology (demo-market). Both the ESRs and EWGPWD highly valued the event (rated with an 8.8 on average). One member of the EWGPWD commented: '*I was very much surprised how seriously those researchers took their job and also with the empathy. Well done'!* The ESRs were content with the event and provided some positive comments: '*It was a very productive day'.* And '*The small groups worked really well for the type for discussion we wanted to have'*.

Collaboration of INDUCT ITN with INTERDEM and INTERDEM academy

The European INTERDEM (early and timely INTERventions in DEMentia) network emerged in 1999 from the need to collaborate to raise the quantity and quality of the evidence on psychosocial interventions for people with dementia in Europe. INTERDEM is a pan-European network of researchers aimed at improving the quality of life of people with dementia and their supporters. The mission of INTERDEM is (1) to develop pan-European research on early, timely and quality psychosocial interventions in dementia; (2) to actively disseminate this and enhance practice, policy and the quality of life of people with dementia and their supporters, across Europe and (3) to place people with dementia and their supporters at the centre of European research and practice, by actively involving them in developing these activities.

It is the vision of INTERDEM that its future relies on the current generation of early-career researchers, to continue to work on cutting-edge research in psychosocial interventions for dementia (Klinkenberg et al., 2019). Therefore, INTERDEM Academy was established in 2014 as a European training network for early-career researchers to carry out high-quality psychosocial research within Europe, with the goal to stimulate a deeper understanding of the nature of dementia and dementia care and to offer a comprehensive research training (Klinkenberg et al., 2019). INTERDEM Academy aims to develop the careers and to build capacity of young researchers working on psychosocial interventions under supervision of INTERDEM seniors and wants to support the early-career researchers in their pathway to senior posts in the field (Klinkenberg et al., 2019). The INTERDEM Academy is organised by a coordinator and training manager, who is supported by an advisory board, consisting of alternating senior INTERDEM (board) members and both an early-stage and late-stage PhD-student/postdoctoral representative from the Academy network. The capacity building strategy of the network involved a biannual programme of Summer and Winter schools, in close collaboration with the INDUCT network, to stimulate opportunities to discuss ongoing work with fellow researchers, attend workshops and learn from expert masterclasses. Additionally, the Academy offers travelling fellowships for early-career researchers to visit an affiliated INTERDEM institute for three to six months, facilitating knowledge exchange, skills training and network building.

Since the start of the COVID-19 pandemic, the Academy started to offer online network meetings, to stimulate an exchange of experiences and knowledge with fellow Academy members. Also, an annual publication award has been initiated in 2020, with the goal to stimulate early-career researchers and provide a stage to share results with each other and senior INTERDEM members. To date, the INTERDEM Academy has grown to a network of 200+ members (circa. 50% are PhD students), based at INTERDEM centres all over Europe, and even beyond the European borders (e.g. Australia, Brazil, China).

The 15 ESRs of INDUCT joined the INTERDEM Academy, thereby interacting with this large research network focused on psychosocial interventions for people with dementia. Most workshops in the INDUCT training programme were thus also open to the INTERDEM Academy, and (parts of the) schools could be attended by INTERDEM Academy fellows. Established INTERDEM members contributed to the school programmes with invited talks sharing their expertise. After completion of their project within INDUCT, all ESRs remained a member of the INTERDEM Academy, to continue to profit from the network infrastructure and support for future career development. This close collaboration and synergy between INDUCT, INTERDEM and the INTERDEM Academy has enabled a major impact on research capacity development in Europe. To conclude, INTERDEM Academy forms a high-quality, multi-disciplinary, capacity building and dementia care research network in Europe (Klinkenberg et al., 2019). To better understand dementia globally in the future, we need to focus on improving research capacities, and this depends on the investment made on the career development of the ESRs of today (Oliveira et al., 2021). The INTERDEM Academy offers the opportunity to share expertise, create awareness for academy talent and stimulate collaboration.

Evaluation results of ESR training programme

An online evaluation questionnaire was distributed at the end of each training event, allowing quantitative and qualitative data to be collected relating to the attendance outside and inside the network, to ensure openness, transparency and accountability. Open evaluation questions made it possible for ESRs to make suggestions on what the INDUCT training team could provide for the ESRs, and to inform how INDUCT could further support their educational and professional ambitions. All responses sent in by the ESRs were dealt with discreetly and were only used to improve the quality of our training events. Suggestions were carefully considered and implemented at future events whenever possible. For example, a comment provided by an attendee during fourth school showed that the ESRs appreciated the integration of previous suggestions: 'Extremely well organised – concise practical advice e.g., travel/accommodation as well as the content recommendations. This school most clearly showed that our feedback was being listened to'.

Network-wide POSADEM training

Regarding the network-wide POSADEM training, ESRs' satisfaction with the weekly content and learning materials was rated favourably. The general grade of the module (1 = very poor, 10 = excellent) and the likeliness to recommend it to a fellow student working in the field of dementia research (1 = not at all likely, 10 = extremely likely) were both rated a 7.6 (SD = 1.01, range = 6–9; and SD= 1.40, range = 6–10, respectively). Due to various intrinsic (e.g. high student motivation, focus on asynchronous activities) and extrinsic factors (e.g. compulsory participation in the module as part of their doctoral training), the module had a high completion rate, with the majority of the ESRs completing the learning activities after six weeks. ESRs appreciated the international and interdisciplinary setting, the use of different multimedia resources and technical support. Suggested improvements included deadlines on participation, suboptimal timing of delivery, high workload, better fit with target group needs and technical issues during virtual classroom sessions.

Five network-wide INDUCT schools

Overall, the rating (1 = very dissatisfied, 5 = very satisfied) for the organisation of the five schools could be perceived as high, with a mean of 4.5 for the first school, 3.6 for the second school, a 4.9 for the third school, a 5 for the fourth school and a 4.7 for the fifth school. Moreover, the quality of the INDUCT schools was perceived as high. On a scale ranging from 1 (very poor) to 10 (excellent), ESRs rated the first INDUCT school with an 8.1, the second INDUCT school with a 7.9, the third INDUCT school with an 8.1, the fourth INDUCT school with an 9.2 and the fifth INDUCT school with an 8.7.

The combination of sessions focusing on both theoretical underpinnings of dementia (care) and learning specific, transferable skills (e.g. the combination of level 1 and level 2 training elements) was highly valued. ESRs expressed after the first school that they would like to have more time and particularly, more personal and/or ESR-only time during the INDUCT project seminars. ESRs also found the programme of the first INDUCT schools rather intense, and the schedule quite tight. Therefore, additional time was scheduled in between sessions to talk to fellow ESRs and professors to solve issues, ask questions or have in-depth discussions. Each school included a networking day or session organised by the ESRs, to address a topic considered important by the ESRs (e.g. an intercultural theme during the fourth school). We offered more diverse work forms to avoid information overload. Sessions were more focused on discussions and reflections and less offered as passive lectures. Presenters were asked to reflect on preparatory assignments or readings prior to their sessions, and to only include materials essential for understanding the content. This improvement was acknowledged by an ESR in the evaluation of a later school:

'There were clear outlines to prepare and not too much unnecessary preparation which encouraged involvement and interactivity on the day'.

The INDUCT experience: ESR perspectives

As ESRs in the INDUCT project, co-authors HC and SLB describe the environment as fulfilling and stimulating. The vast intersectoral network, together with a very substantial travel and training budget, made for a very rewarding PhD experience. They described a steep learning curve in intercultural communication, both professionally and personally. The sense of community and peer support between the ESRs was very important, as they derived encouragement and advice from other ESRs having similar experiences. HC and SLB explained that the value of this international, intersectoral network became even more apparent when it was time to think about their careers after INDUCT, for instance when it came to collaborations for grant applications, recommendations for non-academic jobs, and postdoc opportunities both inside and outside Europe. They reported that they knew of several INDUCT ESRs who had started postdoc positions in new countries, one ESR who had started an industry job in her host country, one ESR in health policy and one ESR who had started a consulting business in academic writing.

Lessons learned

We see an important role for online learning like the network-wide POSA-DEM training at the start, to foster the sharing of expertise between professionals flexibly and without requiring the need to travel: 'the overwhelming advantage for this group of learners is that the medium has allowed many to study when work, geography or personal commitments would have prevented them from enrolling on a traditional course' (Innes et al., 2006 p. 315). However, we also would like to stress the value of bringing the consortium together *in person* during the network-wide schools. Social and networking events during these weeks were essential to get to know one another in a relatively more informal way, and to provide the ESRs with a strong network for future collaborations. Schools also provided an important opportunity to start collaborations between ESRs; to do so it was important to dedicate time during the schools to initiate this. By allowing ESRs to join training preparations (organisation of schools and sessions), they were able to adopt and practice with senior roles. This way, ESRs also could provide direct input regarding topics of importance (e.g. grant writing, career transition in the final school). It was clear that secondments could be challenging to ESRs as it required them to be very mobile and flexible. Nevertheless, secondments were also highly appreciated by many ESRs as it increased their horizons in the academic and non-academic sectors. Important facilitators of successful secondments included that host and home institutions would be flexible in terms of timing and content, and supported the ESRs in their research, practically and emotionally.

Conclusion

INDUCT had the unique ability to provide exceptional research training including relevant cross-national and cross-sectorial collaboration, which helps to bridge the gaps between science, business, health and social care across Europe where different companies, sectors, cultures and languages have resulted in a patchwork of approaches to technology without a coherent model. The advanced multidisciplinary scientific expertise and the complementary partnerships with industry, the healthcare and social sectors, plus user representative organisations enabled INDUCT to develop and empower future leaders in technology and dementia care research and enterprise. The experience of participating in innovative, excellent and vibrant interdisciplinary research groups, transnational mobility, and in-depth research training and secondments maximised the ESRs' prospects.

Given that the progressive increase in the number of people with dementia, the lack of a cure and the high impact of the disease on the European economy, there will be a high demand for well-trained researchers to bring dementia care technology in Europe to the 21st century, and thereby improving the lives of people with dementia and their carers. Moreover, INDUCT enabled the partners to leverage further academic investment from their universities and attract additional national and international research funding. This European ITN leads the world in providing a model for interdisciplinary knowledge transfer into non-academic sectors and is best placed to disseminate the knowledge across the EU and beyond through its international partners.

Acknowledgements

We are grateful to the ESRs that have taken the time to fill out the quality assurance surveys and to give recommendations for future courses during the INDUCT project.

References

Alzheimer Europe (2021). *European working group of people with dementia.* Alzheimer Europe. www.alzheimer-europe.org/about-us/european-working-group-people-dementia.
European Commission (2019). *Marie Skłodowska-Curie actions, guide for applicants innovative training networks 2020.* https://euraxess.ec.europa.eu/sites/default/files/policy_library/principles_for_innovative_doctoral_training.pdf
Innes, A., Mackay, K., & McCabe L. (2006). Dementia studies online: Reflections on the opportunities and drawbacks of eLearning. *Journal of Vocational Education and Training, 58*(3), 303–317. DOI: 10.1080/13636820600955567

Klinkenberg, I.P.M., de Oliveira, D., Verhey, F.R.J., Orrell, M., & de Vugt, M.E. (2019). INTER-DEM Academy: A training and career development initiative vital to capacity building of early stage psychosocial dementia researchers in Europe. *Aging & Mental Health, 23*(8), 929–931. doi:10.1080/13607863.2018.1442415

Oliveira, D., Deckers, K., Lidan, Z., Macpherson, H., Ishak, W.S., & Silarova, B. (2021) The career development of early- and mid-career researchers in dementia should be a global priority: A call for action, *Aging & Mental Health.* DOI: 10.1080/13607863.2021.1875193

Chapter 3

Perspectives on public involvement activities

Ana Diaz-Ponce, Dianne Gove, Sébastien Libert, Chris Roberts, Helen Rochford-Brennan, Georgina Charlesworth, Paul Higgs, Jean Georges

Introduction

Public Involvement (PI) is often described as a research that 'is done with and by patients and/or the public, rather than to, for or about them' (INVOLVE, 2012), whereby patients and/or the public contribute towards the design, conduct and dissemination of research. PI has gained recognition in the field of dementia with different methods and approaches being used and developed recently (Burton et al., 2019). This chapter describes some of the PI activities organised by Alzheimer Europe (AE) in the context of the INDUCT project. One of the novel aspects of this work is that it involved providing mentoring and support to early stage researchers (ESRs).

The chapter is divided into three main sections. The first section refers to AE's experience of organising this work, the motivation, what was done, the challenges encountered and how these were overcome. In the second section, similar issues are addressed but from the experience and perspectives of two members of the European Working Group of People with Dementia (EWG-PWD) who were involved in the PI activities. In the third section, one of the INDUCT ESRs, who was involved in the PI and who did his secondment at AE, reflects on his experience and lessons learnt. At the end of the chapter there are some final conclusions and recommendations for future similar work.

The perspectives of Alzheimer Europe

Alzheimer Europe and the European working group of people with dementia

AE is the umbrella organisation of 37 national Alzheimer's associations from 33 European countries. The mission of the organisation is to change perceptions, policy and practice in order to improve the lives of people affected by dementia. AE set up the EWGPWD in 2012. The EWGPWD is composed of 10–15 people with dementia from different European countries and with different types of dementia. Since 2012, the EWGPWD has been providing valuable

DOI: 10.4324/9781003289005-4

support to the organisation, having regular meetings to discuss key issues and supporting internal research, policy and communications work. The Chair of the group has a seat on the AE Board, thereby influencing key decisions surrounding the functioning, funding and strategic objectives of the organisation. This includes decisions surrounding participation in European research projects. Such involvement is in keeping with AE's long-standing objective, which is to involve people with dementia and ensure that the voices and perspectives of people with dementia are heard in all aspects of its work. The group is supported by members of AE staff with backgrounds in psychology and sociology and doctorates in qualitative research in the field of dementia, as well as by supporters of their choice (usually partners, adult children or friends).

Working to promote PI in dementia research and motivation to participate in INDUCT

Over the years, the EWGPWD and AE staff have established a good working relationship together and gathered experience in conducting PI in European research projects. This has been a process of mutual learning and adaptation.

This learning process refers to the approach and methods most suitable for involving people with dementia in a meaningful way in PI activities and also to the type and scope of such activities. This is particularly important due to the variety of research projects and the type and level of involvement, which may be more relevant for each, as well as the needs and wishes of the members about their involvement. Typically, in several projects, the PI activities are related to providing feedback on different aspects of the project or to different materials for research participants. However, we also felt that there was a need to reflect on how we could make researchers more aware of the value of PI in dementia research and confident to use and promote it. A possible way to achieve this could be by introducing this into their education or training as, for example during their PhD work. This could be an ideal time, as during this period, researchers can work in a fairly independent and flexible manner and can also make decisions about and spend time on issues of interest to them. This usually occurs at the beginning of their careers and could potentially influence their later work.

INDUCT's aim was to develop a multi-disciplinary, inter-sectorial educational research framework for Europe to improve technology and care for people with dementia. INDUCT involved a network of 15 ESRs who were conducting their PhD in this area. It was essential for people with dementia to be involved not only as research participants, but also in the context of PI and in the development of the framework itself. AE and members of the EWG-PWD were interested in the idea of supporting and mentoring ESRs as this could help ensure that future researchers have a better understanding of the lived experience of dementia and of its relevance in research.

AE's role in INDUCT

An important role of AE in INDUCT was to support and facilitate some of the PI activities of the project. From a theoretical perspective, AE provided some speeches during the INDUCT schools and suggestions for relevant literature on PI in dementia research as, for example the position paper that AE had developed with the EWGPWD and INTERDEM in 2017 (Gove et al., 2017b).

From a practical perspective, AE facilitated the interaction between the EWGPWD and the 15 ESRs. Most of these interactions involved meetings or workshops with several ESRs and members of the EWGPWD. In these workshops, different topics were addressed such as issues related to the recruitment strategy and interview guide, ethical or pragmatic issues related to their research projects, or how to involve people with dementia in their projects. In addition, on a few occasions, some ESRs contacted directly to seek input on specific tasks or activities and this was organised individually (e.g. for feedback on the text for a website).

Approach and challenges

AE's approach in INDUCT was two-pronged. Firstly, we wanted to create a safe environment in which the members of the EWGPWD could support the ESRs in their research through PI work and act as mentors. Secondly, we wanted to create an atmosphere in which ESRs could feel confident to ask questions or share their concerns, and be open to receiving not only the perspectives and experience of the members of the EWGPWD but also constructive feedback. Whilst we had ample experience in conducting PI and had published a position paper on this topic, this did not include specific guidelines or recommendations about conducting PI in this particular context. Many of the overall principles of PI were also relevant in this context, but there were also some specific issues that needed to be considered.

We had to find an approach where we could provide the appropriate environment for productive and meaningful meetings whilst relinquishing control over various factors and measures that needed to be taken into consideration or implemented (e.g. the structure of the ESRs' training, the need for people with dementia to travel and time constraints which limited what was actually possible).

Another important aspect was to provide the right level of support to the ESRs, whilst at the same time not taking over, thereby allowing the ESRs to learn from their own experience of these interactions. For some ESRs, it was the first time they had interacted with people with dementia on a personal level (i.e. not as patients or research participants but as people they could talk to and who could help them improve their research).

To enable members of the EWGPWD to contribute in a meaningful way in meetings, they need to receive information in advance, the topics and questions should be appropriate and clear, and language used should be accessible (e.g. avoiding the use of jargon). Relevant support provided by AE to ESRs was therefore related to the preparation of materials for members of the EWGPWD and to the specific questions that could be addressed in the meetings. It was also important to think about topics that could be sensitive (e.g. palliative care) and to discuss with the ESRs their plans to ensure the well-being of the people involved after the meeting. This helped the ESRs to understand the level of preparation needed for the PI work to run smoothly and for people with dementia to be able to contribute meaningfully.

Another complex aspect of the PI work was the logistics of bringing ESRs and members of the EWGPWD together. The ESRs met regularly on the occasion of their INDUCT schools and that was important for their exchanges with each other and their supervisors. Similarly, members of the EWGPWD also had regular meetings in Brussels. The initial plan was for members of the EWGPWD to join the INDUCT schools. However, after a few schools, it became evident that this was not the best approach as it did not ensure sufficient time and space for ESRs and people with dementia to meet, it only involved a few members of the EWGPWD and there was an imbalance between the time spent travelling and the extent of their involvement and interaction with the ESRs during the schools.

Overcoming challenges

Before and after the INDUCT schools, discussions were held between the INDUCT team and AE to assess how the PI activity had gone and what needed to be changed. In 2018, a meeting was held in Barcelona with representatives of the Project Management team, the ESRs, AE and the then Chair of the EWGPWD (Helen Rochford-Brennan). Together, we discussed the best way forward and agreed that in future the ESR students would attend one of the regular meetings of the EWGPWD. This would facilitate the participation of all members of the EWGPWD in this exchange within a familiar environment. It was also decided that if the schools were being held in a location where there was already a member of the EWGPWD, that person would be invited to attend a session with the ESRs. We were pleased not only with the outcome of this meeting but also with the enthusiasm from all involved and the recognition of the need to decide how to find a solution together with the EWGPWD and not on its behalf.

In addition to the direct interaction with ESRs, the representatives of the EWGPWD were invited to participate in steering committee meetings. This was laudable on the part of the research partners in attempting to involve people with dementia on the same level as the various research partners and in seeking their perspectives on broader issues. However, the format and scheduling of the meetings were not particularly conducive to a meaningful exchange of views or contribution from people with dementia, and this was not pursued.

The INDUCT project was also the first time that AE had accepted a PhD student (Sébastien Libert) on a secondment. We had some concerns about how to organise this as the EWGPWD met quarterly. For some European projects, AE had to seek authorisation for Sébastien's involvement. His flexibility in terms of time and willingness to travel frequently to Brussels, as well as the openness of the external researchers, led to an involvement in AE's PI work that was valuable and greatly appreciated. He was also involved in AE's ethics work on disability. Attending regular meetings over the space of a few years and joining the group in the evenings for meals together gave him the opportunity to interact also more informally with the members of the group, with AE and with external researchers. This created a bond of mutual respect and under-standing which fed back into his PI work with the group.

Lessons learnt

This approach to developing the most effective and mutually beneficial method of PI was in keeping with the principle of reasonable accommodation, atten-tion to the well-being of people with dementia (in terms of beneficence and non-maleficence) and respect for their autonomy. It required a continuous dia-logue between AE, members of the EWGPWD, ESRs and the INDUCT management team. It was rewarding for AE to have been involved in this pro-cess. We learnt about the needs, priorities and challenges of ESRs which we have been able to build upon for other similar research projects. Some of the contacts established between the ESRs and members of the EWGPWD have continued beyond the completion of the ESRs' work and demonstrate the genuine interest and human relationships that were formed in the context of those exchanges.

In the next part of this chapter, we look at the PI work in the INDUCT pro-ject from the perspective of two members of the EWGPWD, namely Helen Rochford-Brennan and Chris Roberts (who are, in addition, the former and current Chairs of the EWGPWD).

The perspective of members of the European working group of people with Dementia

Helen Rochford-Brennan

As the Chair of the EWGPWD at the time of the INDUCT project, I was very proud that the group was invited to play such an active role. As a group, we participated in different events and meetings with the students. In addi-tion, I was also personally involved in decisions about how to best conduct the activities and organise this work between the EWGPWD and the students. It was important that they also involved the Chair in this way, as it ensured that the perspectives of people with dementia were included in the management and planning of the PI work. I felt I was listened to and that my suggestions were properly taken into account.

Meeting ESRs in technology was exciting for both, the EWGPWD and the researchers. It gave everyone an opportunity for learning. Learning and education impart more than just knowledge and skills; they also transmit values, attitudes and behaviours. As these students develop and design technology for people living with dementia, it is vital that they have a good understanding of the lived experience of people with dementia. A person's personality does not change overnight just because they have had a diagnosis of dementia. They are still the same person. Modern technology can provide important tools for someone to live well with dementia. I am grateful to INDUCT for their vision and work in this project.

As this was very new to us, we found that having face-to-face research with students created a positive and friendly atmosphere for all at the early stage of the project. It was important for the group to have a safe environment. This requires careful planning, skills and resources. Thanks to AE for having ensured this.

INDUCT is aimed at developing a multi-disciplinary educational research framework to improve technology and care for people with dementia, and to provide the evidence to show how technology can improve the lives of people with dementia. Needless to say, we were delighted to help INDUCT achieve their goal.

As there is no cure for dementia so far, technology can indeed play a very important role in promoting quality of life. It can help people with dementia and their supporters to cope better with the disease, understand its symptoms or promote independence for as long as possible. All of this is very important to us. However, the technology developed has to be appropriate and meaningful. PI at an early stage gives a clear path to researchers; and in this case, like in some other projects, many of the PhD students had never met anyone with dementia. If the people creating the research do not meet people living with dementia at the very beginning, they only have assumptions to work with, which will inevitably lead to a costly waste of resources.

When you assume, you impart your own perspective, motivations and values upon a situation as that is all you know. When INDUCT met with us, it gave them a good perspective from the beginning. People living with dementia can engage and we are all different in our thoughts, so assumptions should never be made.

We welcomed their vision and presentations; the discussions were thought provoking. Many diverse topics and types of technologies were presented. There were also issues addressed related to palliative care for people with dementia in nursing homes. This is an important topic to all of us. Palliative care is explicitly recognised under the human right to health. It is an extremely sensitive subject for everyone but especially for people with dementia. Throughout this project, we have all learned the importance and potential of technology. Thank you INDUCT for giving the EWGPWD the opportunity to learn together and involving us at different levels and in different ways.

Chris Roberts

As a member of the EWGPWD, I was very curious and interested in the idea of mentoring PhD students. INDUCT was the first project for which the EWG-PWD supported PhD students, or ESRs as they were called in the INDUCT project. This was new for everyone and many members of the EWGPWD thought this could be a great opportunity. Some members had, in their professional lives, mentored or trained students, whilst for others, like myself, this was a relatively new activity. The initial plan was for people with dementia to travel to the INDUCT schools, which we did. We visited two INDUCT schools (in Maastricht, the Netherlands, and in Salamanca, Spain).

It was agreed that two members of the EWGPWD would participate in the school in Maastricht. I was travelling with my wife from Wales and the other member, from Norway. Getting to Maastricht took many hours, driving and flying. We were very warmly welcomed by the organisers and students. However, there was only one quite short session planned with the students. Although there was time for networking during the lunch, this was short as, understandingly, the day was very busy for them and the lunch break was short. We felt that it had involved a lot of travel and effort compared to our more usual opportunities for working together. In the school in Salamanca, we were very pleased to see that the time planned for the formal interaction with students was longer and that the session had been carefully planned; we received a summary of their projects and questions in advance. This helps a lot to prepare and feel confident during the meeting. It was also nice to meet some of the students again; some had contacted us after the first meeting and it was nice to catch up with them. This time, in Spain, it was three of us (from the EWGPWD) attending. Also, some of our supporters (like my wife Jayne) were happy to take part in some discussions. Despite enjoying a very nice time in Spain, it was still not ideal that many of us had to spend several hours travelling to get there for a one- to two-hour workshop. The social time spent with the ESRs was rewarding and we felt it could help, but it was only a few people with dementia and during a time which was very intense and busy for the ESRs. These meetings were in addition to our regular EWGPWD meetings, so for some members and supporters it could be quite a lot of travelling.

It was then decided that if the INDUCT school was in a country where there was a member of the EWGPWD, this member would be invited to attend to avoid long travelling, which worked a lot better. This was the case for our member from Germany who attended the school organised there. I missed the interaction with the students, but I felt this was a better and more practical way of organising this work.

I was very glad when I learnt that the last meeting would be planned in a different way where the ESRs would come to a meeting of the EWGPWD in Brussels. This was a regular meeting for us so no extra travelling was needed. All members of the group were able to take part in this. The main focus of the day was the work between the ESRs and the EWGPWD, so the PI was not just one hour of their very busy schedule in the schools. We had the opportunity to see how the different projects had evolved and also to contribute towards the recommendations they were developing. Some of the sessions were more informal. They had prepared different stands in a big room and we could just walk from one to another and have a chat with the ESR who was working on the project. Other sessions were more formal and in those, some ESRs presented their work and asked us specific questions.

The whole project was based on the collaboration and assistance of people living with, and affected by dementia, because we are experts by experience in our own right. We can bring our own unique contribution, which can only add to the expert knowledge of everyone involved in the project and it was refreshing to see that INDUCT, with the help and assistance of AE and INTERDEM, acknowledged this, and fully involved the members of the EWGPWD.

The project was very exciting and new. It was amazing to be involved and see some of the end results that will show how technology can support people with dementia in their daily lives, how it can be used to support and promote meaningful activities and will improve care and quality of life of people with dementia living at home or in residential care settings. It was a good experience for us and the ESRs to work 'with us', instead of 'for us'. Being involved, assisting by using our own experience of dementia and having honest conversations not only helped them but also allows for our needs and wishes to be heard now, and also in the future. It's even more paramount that our opinions are heard now for the future, as we may not be heard in the same way as we are right now, if at all.

This involvement gave us value and a purpose, which sadly, after a diagnosis you can lose. It was daunting at first, we weren't sure what we could offer or assist with, but we soon realised the value of sharing knowledge. We actually became good colleagues and friends. We continue to share, promote and assist still through our social media connections. It also stimulates the brain and senses, giving our brains extra exercise, which we know is so important for those affected by dementia. I found everything very interesting; even though, I had never considered or knew about a lot of the topics discussed. It was good to take part, learn and share for all of us.

With this collaboration between researchers, people with or affected by dementia, we can and do make a difference. It helps to increase understanding, which then enables ESRs to adapt and revise their projects where new learning has taken place. PI can save money and time, provide valuable insight and advice that you can only receive from someone living with a life-changing condition like dementia. Overall, I felt that the experience was very positive and mutually beneficial for all involved. I would advise people thinking about organising this type of work to go for it, just try to find what works best for the students and for the people with dementia involved. There is no recipe that works for everyone, but asking all involved about their experience and being open to adapt and find new ways will definitely help. In the case of people with dementia who have been asked to mentor students or researchers, do not be shy, the experience can be very interesting and rewarding. My thanks to everyone who made this project possible and successful.

We now look at the perspective of Sébastien Libert, who was an ESR in the INDUCT project and has since obtained his PhD from University College London. Sébastien reflects on his experience of PI in the INDUCT project and shares some of his key impressions and what he learnt from that experience.

The perspectives of an early stage researcher

Sébastien Libert

Between the years 2017 and 2019, I was involved as a social science researcher with AE and the EWGPWD during my PhD research as part of INDUCT. My anthropological research explored aspects of identity, social inclusion and belonging as a person with dementia. My involvement with the group was multiple. I was an ESR learning from my experience in conducting research with people with dementia. I attended, and helped co-moderate, meetings with the group spread over multiple days every four months or so. I made occasional presentations on my findings and related topics and provided feedback on different projects related to the activities of the group. I was also involved as a delegate with members of the group at the fourth European Parliament of Persons with Disabilities (6 December 2017, EU parliament, Brussels). Finally, I co-authored a report on the ethical implications of recognising dementia as a disability (Gove et al., 2017a) together with a group of experts including researchers in the field of dementia, ethics and disability, staff from AE and members of the EWGPWD.

As an anthropologist with experience in participant observation and ethnography, spending time with members of the group prompted me to reflect on group members' perspectives on belonging, ageing and dementia. I gained an understanding of group members' relationships to advising, expertise and advocacy, and the social significance of their actions. My participation allowed me to learn from experience the important *relational* dimension of PI in research.

Benefits of public involvement

Involvement with the EWGPWD was an opportunity for me to be simultane-ously intellectual, experiential and emotional in the kind of appreciation and affection that I developed with group members. I vividly recall many enjoyable moments with the group – cheerful conversations, taking pictures together, sharing meals, singing, saying goodbyes and looking forward to the reunions. Such connections combined with an empathy for the people I encountered, getting some insight into their life circumstances, learning from them and their experience of dementia and life in general. These connections gave an addi-tional depth and contextualisation to the questions I explored for my research. They helped to support my understanding of the complex circumstances in which people live with dementia. I could envision to some extent how the condition impacts people's life, sense of self and identity. In my opinion, this understanding and empathy is probably one of the most important contribu-tions that PI can make to research.

While an anthropological approach can facilitate this type of connection, involving appreciation, understanding and empathy, other modes of PI in research can arguably foster similar insights into people's life circumstances. The relational nature of PI can re-connect researchers with prime research beneficiaries, therefore bridging the fields of science and society.

Challenges of public involvement

Meanwhile, PI can also be a challenging endeavour for researchers. In creating a relationship between stakeholders and researchers, PI implies a commitment to reciprocity. Reciprocity is a logical corollary to the benefits I described ear-lier. Reciprocity is essentially linked to moral accountability, and the notion of *doing the right thing*. PI is not only an act that can support research findings but one that is accompanied by the expectation of a return on investment for members of the public who dedicated time and energy to supporting research, an expectation voiced at multiple occasions by members of the EWGPWD. The people with dementia I encountered spent hours travelling to meetings often by plane, being far away from home, prone to disorientation and fatigue in unfamiliar places, sometimes exposing themselves to judgement and misun-derstanding when being in public spaces. I inevitably felt concerned to meet their engagement with an equally valuable research output. This feeling can be challenging, especially because of the subtle differences in objectives, rules and expectations between the agendas of research and public participation (Poland et al., 2019). I was participating in the activities of the group while also being, to a degree, separate, having to observe the distinct rules of academia (e.g. divergent timelines, ethics committees classifying people as vulnerable as soon as they receive a diagnosis of dementia). The existence of this tension has often been discussed in anthropology, a discipline particularly engaged in the two separate spheres of academia and advocacy (Beck & Maida, 2013). I found myself questioning the most adequate and feasible ways to give back what I had gained from contributions of the group while also satisfying the imperatives of academic research. Simultaneously sustaining this reciprocity and overcoming these obstacles is especially challenging for ESRs given their limited resources and uncertain career prospects.

Meanwhile, reciprocity can also be difficult to implement due to the granularity of expectations among the public involved. 'The public' is not a monolithic entity (Oliver et al., 2015). As I discovered, expectations and objectives can diverge among members of the group themselves – some I met were strongly influenced by advocacy (linked to their activities outside of the EWGPWD PI work) while others perceived their role as merely advisory or informative. Beyond this, life circumstances can vary greatly according to a multiplicity of factors relating to socio-economic situation, age, co-morbidities, stage of dementia and type of diagnosis, availability of support for people with dementia in different national contexts, family configurations etc. Involving members of the public in research requires navigation of this heterogeneity of understandings, motivations and expectations and the need to shape the direction and outcomes of the research accordingly.

In addressing these challenges of reciprocity and heterogeneity in PI, I can offer the following advice. These challenges point to the importance of adopting a relational model of PI rather than utilising a simply transactional one. It is essential for researchers to understand that the tensions generated by heterogeneity and the diverging agendas of research, PI and advocacy can only be resolved through a continuous dialogue between actors composing these spheres and a realisation of the moral commitment that this relation implies. PI is a complex negotiation between researchers and members of the general public. Understanding this relational aspect can help to resolve possible tensions and differences of opinion across academic and public spheres in order to find mutually beneficial solutions. PI should not merely be a desirable add-on to research activity. Done successfully, it is committed to finding compromises and solutions together. While being challenging, PI is crucial to meaningful and ethical research. Emphasising the relationality of PI and stressing the importance of reciprocity when training early career researchers offer a significant entry point into the role of public trust in science and the moral responsibility that research carries towards society.

Conclusions

There is growing evidence of the relevance and value of PI in dementia research. In some countries, some funders require PI in research projects. However, many researchers are still unaware of PI or do not feel confident to plan and organise PI activities in a meaningful way. This chapter has provided an example of how to provide ESRs with opportunities to conduct PI activities in their research projects and presents the perspective of the organisation responsible for the activities (AE), two members of the EWGPWD and one ESRs involved in the PI activities in INDUCT.

This type of involvement in training networks, such as INDUCT, can help to ensure that PI is considered as a key component of future research. We have all learnt a lot from this project, but particularly with regard to the flexibility and constant listening needed to be able to organise PI activities in a way that is meaningful and valuable to the different people involved. This echoes some of the principles of PI with people with dementia such as reasonable accommodation and respect for well-being and autonomy. It has also shown that these activities can be very beneficial and rewarding to both people with dementia and ESRs at personal and professional levels. Nevertheless, it also entails some challenges as creating and maintaining strong relationships and ensuring reciprocity can be demanding and requires sufficient resources. People with dementia and dementia research merit such an investment.

References

Beck, S., & Maida, C.A. (2013). *Toward engaged anthropology*. Edited by Sam Beck, Carl A. Maida. New York, NY: Berghahn Books.

Burton, A., Ogden, M., & Cooper, C. (2019). Planning and enabling meaningful patient and public involvement in dementia research. *Current Opinion in Psychiatry, 32*(6), 557–562. doi: 10.1097/YCO.0000000000000548. PMID: 31306247.

Gove, D., Andrews, J., Capstick, A., Geoghegan, C., Georges, J., Libert, S., . . . Williamson, T. (2017a). *Dementia as a disability: Implications for ethics, policy and practice*. www.alzheimer-europe.org/Ethics/Ethical-issues-in-practice/2017-Dementia-as-a-disability-Implications-for-ethics-policy-and-practice/Preface.

Gove, D., Diaz-Ponce, A., Georges, J., Moniz-Cook, E., Mountain, G., Chattat, R., Øksnebjerg, L., & The European Working Group of People with Dementia (2017b). Alzheimer Europe's position on involving people with dementia in research through PPI patient and public involvement. *Aging & Mental Health*, DOI: 10.1080/13607863.2017.1317334

INVOLVE (2012) *Briefing notes for researchers: Involving the public in NHS, public health and social care research*. Eastleigh: INVOLVE.

Oliver, S., Liabo, K., Stewart, R., & Rees, R. (2015). Public involvement in research: making sense of the diversity. *Journal of Health Services Research & Policy, 20*(1). https://doi.org/10.1177/1355819614551848

Poland, F., Charlesworth, G., Leung, P., & Birt, L. (2019). Embedding patient and public involvement: Managing tacit and explicit expectations. *Health Expectations, 22*(6). https://doi.org/10.1111/hex.12952

Part 2

Improving the usability of technology in everyday life

Chapter 4

Digital diaries to understand and support everyday life in ageing and dementia

Sara Laureen Bartels, Rosalia J.M.
van Knippenberg, Camilla Walles Malinowsky,
Marjolein de Vugt, Frans R.J. Verhey

Why are digital diaries needed in ageing and dementia?

Retrospective questions are commonly part of clinical appointments, may it be with a general practitioner, neurologist, psychologist or occupational therapist. Questions like *'How often during the past weeks did you experience pain?'* will likely sound familiar to any individual who has ever been in contact with healthcare. People with dementia (PwD) or cognitive problems and their spousal carers specifically might be asked how often in the past weeks or months they or their partner had memory problems. These kinds of questions may appear fairly easy to answer and relying on such self-reports presents a solid way to inquire about someone's state of well-being. However, there are several issues that decrease the usefulness, reliability and accuracy of the respondent's answer.

Retrospective self-reports rely on memory functions, and human cognition is prone to biases. Forty-eight forms of bias related to the design or administration of questions and questionnaires are presented in the literature (Choi & Pak, 2005): for instance, general recall bias may occur referring to 'a systematic error of accuracy or completeness of recall to memory of past events or experiences' (p. 153 (Porta, 2014)), and this bias might be even greater in people who experience memory issues in general. The peak bias, also known as peak-and-end-rule, suggests that 'the most intense or final moments of an experience disproportionally influence retrospective judgements, which may bias self-reports' (p. 228 (Schneider et al., 2011)). Thus, influenced by cognitive biases, individuals tend to over- or under-report when retrospectively recalling symptoms (Van den Bergh & Walentynowicz, 2016).

Furthermore, the level of well-being fluctuates throughout the day, days of the week and over weeks. Research shows, for instance, that the 'Thank God It's Friday' feeling is not just an expression, but levels of happiness are actually greater on Fridays compared to other workdays (Stone et al., 2012). Obviously, one retrospective question might be complemented with follow-up inquiries at clinical visit, which improves the accuracy of self-reports to a certain degree and set a symptom into context. *'Is there a specific time of day on which your memory*

DOI: 10.4324/9781003289005-6

problems occur? Did you notice any specific circumstances that trigger these issues?'. However, everyday life is complex and daily well-being is multi-facetted. Any form of ill health, dysfunction or disorder is likely to be the result of an interplay of a number of internal as well as external factors. Cognitive functioning, for example, can fluctuate from hour to hour influenced by an individual's emotions, sleep quality or even food intake (DijK et al., 1992; Gómez-Pinilla, 2008; Mitchell & Phillips, 2007). Thus, retrospective questions are likely to miss out on contextual aspects of a specific situation, resulting in an incomplete picture of reality with low ecological validity (Scollon et al., 2003).

Similarly, neuropsychological assessments, screening tools or test batteries targeting cognition, which is an important aspect of ageing and dementia, are usually performed periodically in clinical settings, and miss out on contextual factors and fluctuations. On one hand, these assessments are an important part of diagnostic processes in neurology and psychiatry and can tell normal cognitive functioning from impaired cognition (Casaletto & Heaton, 2017). On the other hand, the periodical conductance and sterile environments with low-stimuli surroundings inevitably neglect daily and situational fluctuations and fail to capture dynamics of cognition in natural environments (Chaytor & Schmitter-Edgecombe, 2003).

Proxy reports from informal carers such as partners, children or close friends might be gathered when the healthcare professional thinks an external report adds value, or in cases where the individual is generally unable to provide a self-report. At memory clinics, proxy reports are an important element of the diagnostic process and are seen as beneficial (Gruters et al., 2019). Nevertheless, proxy reports face the same dilemma of retrospectivity and memory bias mentioned earlier. For example, a carer might report in a clinical setting that their partner left the stove on as an illustration of their memory issues due to the fact that this situation was perceived as dangerous, representing a peak. Additionally, strong emotions, such as feeling burdened as a carer (Persson et al., 2015), may contort the accuracy of proxy reports.

Finally, observations can be conducted to provide information on an individual's state of well-being, specifically in advanced stages of dementia when verbal communication may be difficult. Here, the issue lies with the interpretation of the observations as those depend on the observer (Ryd et al., 2015). Therefore, the overt can be captured, whereas subjective experiences may be missed. Taken together, traditional methods are important to understand the health-related needs and experiences of PwD and their carers and add value, but the challenge persists to apply an innovative method that monitors and captures the dynamics and complexity of everyday life even better.

Sampling of experiences in everyday life

The experience sampling method (ESM) (Larson & Csikszentmihalyi, 2014), also known as ecological momentary assessment (EMA) (Shiffman et al., 2008) or ambulatory assessment (Trull & Ebner-Priemer, 2013), is a structured diary technique to gather information of an individual's life right there and then,

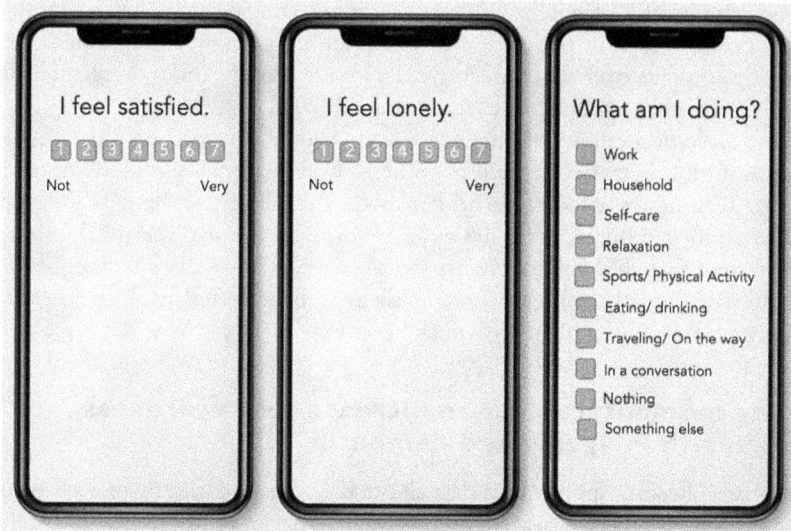

Figure 4.1 Example of a smartphone interface with ESM questions

when the emotion is felt and the behaviour is performed, in specific and unique situations. Using paper-based or digital diaries, a person is prompted to reflect on their current mood, activities, location, stress, pain or fatigue level, and other variables of interest. The diary is typically completed several times a day by rating simple questions in the moment (see Figure 4.1). Morning, lunch or evening questionnaires might ask to recall a couple of hours (*'Today, I experienced memory problems.', 'Last night, I woke up frequently.'*); however, the period of time is usually still rather short, limiting the recall bias.

The ESM allows to depict fluctuations of daily well-being and functioning and provides a fine-graded picture of everyday life (Verhagen et al., 2016). Using the ESM in research studies enables scientists from various disciplines to 'open the black box of daily life' and examine psychological models, biomedical mechanisms, treatment effects or gene-environment interactions in psychopathology (Myin-Germeys et al., 2009). The area of interest in momentary sampling questions commonly lies on physical and emotional aspects (i.e. sleep, medication adherence, mood, stress), whereas social health (i.e. social company, relationship) remains often neglected and requires prospectively more attention, as our narrative synthesis systematic review of 26 ESM-based interventions for middle-aged and older adults reveals (Bartels et al., 2019).

For various target populations including young children, people with severe mental disorders and older adults, including carers of PwD, the ESM appears feasible (Cain et al., 2009; Myin-Germeys et al., 2009; Van Knippenberg et al., 2017; Vilaysack et al., 2016). The author's research adds to the body of knowledge by investigating if the ESM is also feasible and usable in a memory clinic sample of 21 people with mild cognitive impairment (MCI). Results show promise for this population to complete up to eight smartphone-based diary assessments over six consecutive days with a satisfactory compliance rate of 78.7% in study completers (Bartels et al., 2020c).

The ecological validity of the ESM is high, allowing researchers as well as clinicians to test their theories and hypotheses in real-life settings (Scollon et al., 2003). Techniques such as internal consistency reliability assessments and multilevel confirmation factor analysis can be used to confirm the psychometric properties of the ESM items (Gabriel et al., 2019). Thus, diary techniques are an interesting methodology for academia as well as clinical practice to gain a deeper understanding of an individual's context.

Using momentary data to increase self-awareness and health in ageing and dementia

Next to collecting momentary data illustrating the fluctuations of well-being in everyday life, utilising paper-based or digital diaries can have health benefits for the respondent in different ways. According to the social cognition theory, self-monitoring of one's behaviour, its determinants and effects – for instance, by filling in a diary several times a day – stimulates self-regulatory mechanisms (Bandura, 1991). In line with this theory, research shows that experience sampling over six weeks, without a tailored intervention or ESM-based feedback, can increase well-being in carers of PwD (Van Knippenberg et al., 2018). On the basis of self-reports in our aforementioned feasibility study, 71% of the participants reported to become more aware of their mood and memory problems after using the ESM. This increase of awareness was mostly experienced as 'pleasant' or 'neutral', while four participants found it 'unpleasant' (Bartels et al., 2020c). Being conscious about one's cognitive issues might be confronting for some individuals; however, it also represents an opportunity to ask for support and develop self-management techniques. Thus, purely by pausing and reflecting on one's cognitive, emotional, behavioural and social status several times a day, a person can enhance the attention of the elements in life that are meaningful.

To stimulate not only awareness but also a behavioural change towards positive and meaningful activities, ESM-based interventions can provide feedback based on the momentary data. Specifically, feedback focused on positive affect can stimulate well-being, for instance in people with depression (Kramer et al., 2014). In carers of PwD, this form of feedback did not only enhance health on an emotional but also behavioural level, as evaluated by the author and colleagues (Bartels et al., 2020d). In our systematic review of digital self-monitoring interventions for middle-aged and older adults highlighted in the previous section, the momentary data collected through digital diaries are often feedbacked to the individuals, in 23 out of the 26 reviewed ESM-based interventions, either directly by healthcare professionals or by automated technology; however, a combination of both appears recommended (Bartels et al., 2019).

Currently, no guideline is available on how ESM-based feedback should be provided, but researchers from the Belgian-Dutch ESM network are exploring expert opinions and working on comprising an overview of ongoing studies that give feedback based on momentary data.

Stimulating behavioural adaptations is a challenging task for healthcare professionals. Our follow-up study of an ESM intervention involving 50 carers of PwD shows that long-term effects need to be evaluated, as short-term positive treatment effects may fade (Bartels et al., 2020b). The necessity for sustainable treatment effects is emphasised and future studies may apply booster sessions to maintain improvements in well-being and health (Bartels et al., 2020b).

Finally, ESM-based interventions can be seen as add-on interventions to cognitive behavioural or acceptance- and commitment-based therapy (ACT). In emerging adults with psychosis, this paradigm appears feasible even though the effectiveness could not be confirmed yet (van Aubel et al., 2020). ACT itself holds promise as a transdiagnostic approach to increase psychological flexibility and enable self-management of distress in older adults (Petkus & Wetherell, 2013), and available platforms such as www.m-path.io allow clinicians and researchers to prospectively develop and evaluate low-cost, personalised ecological momentary interventions following a blended care approach (Mestdagh et al., 2022).

Measuring cognition in everyday life

Cognition is an important aspect of ageing and it is of interest to assess cognitive functioning in everyday life as neuropsychological tests are thought to have low ecological validity (Chaytor & Schmitter-Edgecombe, 2003). Momentary items such as '*Since the last beep, I experienced memory/language/ concentration problems.*' can be applied (see Figure 4.2). These items are included in the author's ESM study in people with MCI and may be useful to reveal

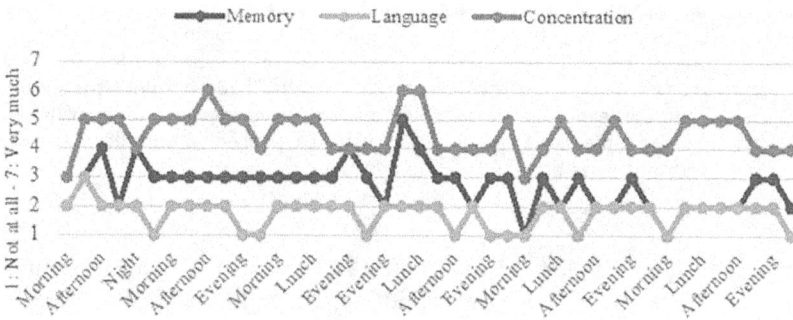

Figure 4.2 Case example of subjectively experienced cognitive problems in a person with MCI.

Source: The specific assessment times were grouped into 'Morning/Lunch/Afternoon/ Evening/Night' for simplicity (Bartels et al., 2020c).

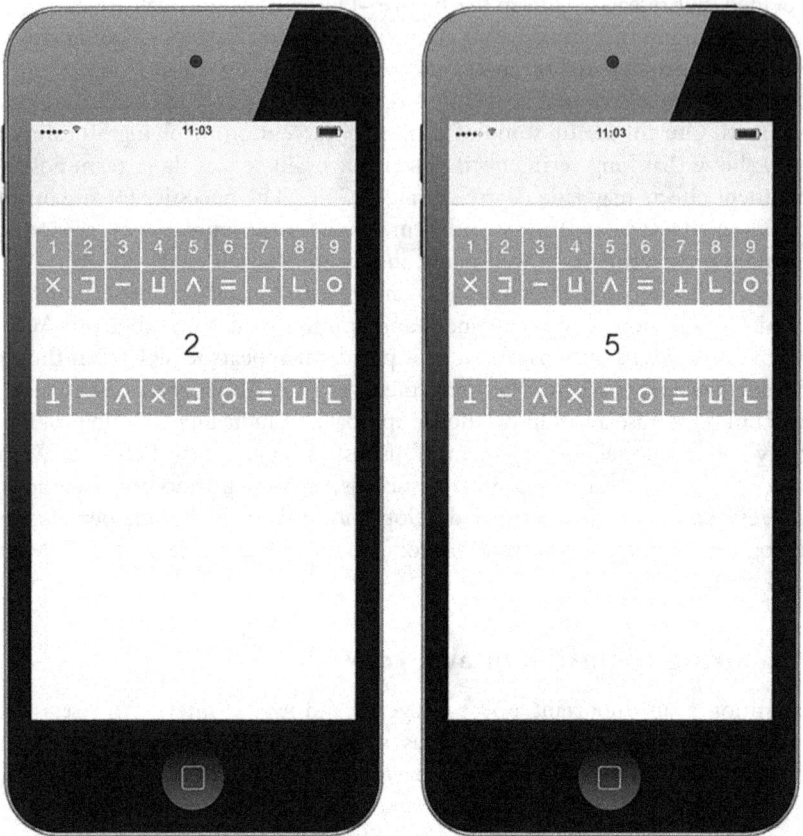

Figure 4.3 Example of a momentary cognition task: the mobile Digit Symbol Substitution Task to assess information processing speed in everyday life. (Explanation: At the top of the screen, numbers from 1 to 9 with corresponding symbols are presented for encoding. In the middle of the screen, different numbers are displayed one-by-one for each trial. At the bottom of the screen, participants had to select the symbol that corresponds to the number presented in the middle. Within a 30-sec timeframe, participants have to correctly complete as many trials as possible.)

Source: (Daniëls et al., 2020).

moment-to-moment fluctuations, contextual patterns and individual differences in subjectively experienced cognitive problems (Bartels et al., 2020c).

Alternatively, short momentary cognition tasks as part of the ESM could be added. Momentary cognition tasks are still in their infancy, and we add to the evidence with two studies, namely a pilot study and a feasibility and validity study (Daniëls et al., 2020; Verhagen et al., 2019). Specifically, the mobile digit symbol substitution task (see Figure 4.3), performed by 49 healthy adults eight times per day on six consecutive days, is perceived as pleasant and easy to use, and shows age sensitivity (Daniëls et al., 2020). Prospectively, momentary cognition tasks could become part of remote assessments at the memory clinic, thus complementing standard neuropsychological assessments and informing neuropsychological and medical doctors on cognitive functioning in everyday life; however, further testing in PwD is still outstanding. Then, tailored support to manage everyday life can be provided in an informed and needs-based way.

Who might – and might not – benefit from the ESM?

Nowadays, the ESM is usually delivered through digital diaries. While this approach has advantages over the paper-based ESM, as the exact moment of diary completion can be determined and the respondent cannot fill in multiple entries retrospectively, a technology-driven assessment also has limitations. First of all, testing the use of technology in older adults is likely to result in a recruitment bias. Eighty-five percent of the individuals with MCI not eligible for our ESM feasibility study were not in possession of a smartphone, or not feeling confident in using it (Bartels et al., 2020c). Furthermore, three of the 21 people that joined the study forgot the study instructions or to carry their smartphone with them. Prospectively, at least the age-related limitation might decrease as smartphone ownership is increasing in seniors aged 65 and above (Pew Research Centre, 2021). Nevertheless, the usability of technology-based ESM needs to be handled with care and other alternatives needs to be present, as not everyone will be able or willing to engage with it.

It is important to emphasise that people with MCI or mild to moderate stages of dementia have adequate insight to express their own ability in handling technology, and that this ability can be depicted through both self-reports and observations as shown in our cross-sectional, non-experimental study involving 38 PwD and 41 people with MCI (Bartels et al., 2020a). Our findings furthermore highlight that it is beneficial to combine self-reports and observations when determining the ability of an individual to use everyday technology, as these methodologies are complimentary. Specifically, observations provide a detailed picture of the stepwise interaction with a specific technology, whereas self-reports reveal the personal relevance of the technology and potential needs for assistance (Bartels et al., 2020a). Older people with and without cognitive impairments are often interested and motivated to learn and engage with new technology, which can even result in feelings of empowerment (Span et al., 2013). To facilitate the use of technology and to avoid frustration or confusion in older people with and without cognitive impairment, adequate training is needed (Mitzner et al., 2008).

Innovative methods such as digital diaries need to be relevant to the user, feasible and usable. 'One way fits them all' is not a realistic view on using technology to understand and support older adults with and without dementia, but instead a person-centred approach including needs assessments and adequate support should be taken. Only then can technology-based ESM have more advantages than drawbacks in healthcare and academic.

The future is inter-sectorial and person-centred

Looking ahead, the ESM still has a long way to make it into clinical practice and be available internationally for PwD, carers and healthcare providers. A number of aspects should be considered along this way. Firstly, next to monitoring physical and emotional well-being through ESM, social health is an important factor for the well-being of older adults with and without cognitive impairments. The relevance of social interactions and support has been highlighted in the field of dementia before (de Vugt & Dröes, 2017) and digital diaries need to ensure to take a holistic approach when studying and supporting the health of PwD and their carers.

Secondly, academics developing and testing technologies and technology-based interventions in university setting take the outer setting and long-term implementation process rarely into account (Christie et al., 2018). Applying a more agile framework combining the rigour of traditional research methods with the iterative flexibility and focus on practicalities applied in industry, such as the mHealth agile research lifecycle, can facilitate the production of effective, evidence-based and sustainable digital products (Wilson et al., 2018). A stronger collaboration between academia, healthcare and industry is thus necessary. Input from not only patients but also healthcare providers ensures that user needs are met, whereas the design of technologies, such as ESM smartphone apps, can be improved through the expertise of industry developers. Gamification elements and reward systems, for instance, can improve data collection and quality of mobile settings (Van Berkel et al., 2017), thus making digital diaries and momentary tasks more enjoyable and positively contributing to adherence.

Finally, randomised controlled trials aiming to evaluate the effects of interventions have been seen as 'the golden standard' for many years. However, real-world evaluations in a heterogeneous manner permit individuals to receive customised treatments (Verhagen et al., 2016). N-of-1 trials and single-case studies utilise repeated measurements, such as the ESM, to provide a more fine-graded, time and context-sensitive view of within-person patterns, thus represent a useful tool for enhancing prevision in a range of conditions (Gabler et al., 2011). For instance, applying a network analysis to N-of-1 ESM data in a person with Parkinson's disease reveals longitudinal associations between symptoms and mood, which can be taken into account to determine individual treatment strategies for this individual (van der Velden et al., 2018). N-of-1 and single-case clinical trials should therefore be considered more often in the context of the ESM and ageing and dementia.

The challenge remains for the ESM and other technology-based innovations to ensure that all older individuals can use new eHealth services and tools, not only in terms of physical and cognitive capacity, but also in terms of personal relevance and sustainable implementation. The author's studies involving healthy adults, people with MCI, PwD and carers contribute to the field of research by testing the feasibility and validity of the ESM and momentary cognition tasks, providing insight into the evidence related to ESM-based interventions and evaluating their beneficial effects, and highlighting ways to promote the usability of digital diaries in the future. If facilitated in an inclusive way, digital diaries may prospectively improve our understanding of real-life experiences and daily challenges of ageing populations, and thus offer a highly personal and unique approach to treat, prevent and rehabilitate.

Note

1   Parts of this chapter were previously published in Bartels, S. L. (2020). Monitoring everyday life in aging & dementia: perspectives from experience sampling and technology use. [Doctoral thesis: Maastricht University]. Maastricht. DOI:10.26481/dis.20200917sb

References

Bandura, A. (1991). Social cognitive theory of self-regulation. *Organizational Behavior and Human Decision Processes*, *50*(2), 248–287.

Bartels, S., Assander, S., Patomella, A.-H., Jamnadas-Khoda, J., & Malinowsky, C. (2020a). Do you observe what I perceive? The relationship between two perspectives on the ability of people with cognitive impairments to use everyday technology. *Aging & Mental Health*, *24*(8), 1295–1305.

Bartels, S.L., Van Knippenberg, R.J., Dassen, F.C., Asaba, E., Patomella, A.-H., Malinowsky, C., Verhey, F.R., & de Vugt, M.E. (2019). A narrative synthesis systematic review of digital self-monitoring interventions for middle-aged and older adults. *Internet Interventions*, *18*, 100283.

Bartels, S.L., van Knippenberg, R.J., Köhler, S., Ponds, R.W., Myin-Germeys, I., Verhey, F.R., & de Vugt, M.E. (2020b). The necessity for sustainable intervention effects: Lessons-learned from an experience sampling intervention for spousal carers of people with dementia. *Aging & Mental Health*, *24*(12), 2082–2093.

Bartels, S.L., van Knippenberg, R.J., Malinowsky, C., Verhey, F.R., & de Vugt, M.E. (2020c). Smartphone-based experience sampling in people with mild cognitive impairment: feasibility and usability study. *JMIR Aging*, *3*(2), e19852.

Bartels, S.L., van Knippenberg, R.J., Viechtbauer, W., Simons, C.J., Ponds, R.W., Myin-Germeys, I., . . . de Vugt, M.E. (2020d). Intervention mechanisms of an experience sampling intervention for spousal carers of people with dementia: A secondary analysis using momentary data. *Aging & Mental Health*, 1–9.

Cain, A.E., Depp, C.A., & Jeste, D.V. (2009). Ecological momentary assessment in aging research: A critical review. *Journal of Psychiatric Research*, *43*(11), 987–996.

Casaletto, K.B., & Heaton, R.K. (2017). Neuropsychological assessment: Past and future. *Journal of the International Neuropsychological Society*, *23*(9–10), 778–790.

Chaytor, N., & Schmitter-Edgecombe, M. (2003). The ecological validity of neuropsychological tests: A review of the literature on everyday cognitive skills. *Neuropsychology Review*, *13*(4), 181–197.

Choi, B.C., & Pak, A.W. (2005). Peer reviewed: A catalog of biases in questionnaires. *Preventing Chronic Disease*, *2*(1).

Christie, H.L., Bartels, S.L., Boots, L.M., Tange, H.J., Verhey, F.R., & de Vugt, M.E. (2018). A systematic review on the implementation of eHealth interventions for informal caregivers of people with dementia. *Internet Interventions, 13*, 51–59.

Daniëls, N., Bartels, S., Verhagen, S., Van Knippenberg, R., De Vugt, M., & Delespaul, P.A. (2020). Digital assessment of working memory and processing speed in everyday life: Feasibility, validation, and lessons-learned. *Internet Interventions, 19*, 100300.

de Vugt, M., & Dröes, R.-M. (2017). Social health in dementia. Towards a positive dementia discourse. *Aging & Mental Health, 21*(1), 1–3.

DijK, D.J., Duffy, J.F., & Czeisler, C.A. (1992). Circadian and sleep/wake dependent aspects of subjective alertness and cognitive performance. *Journal of Sleep Research, 1*(2), 112–117.

Gabler, N.B., Duan, N., Vohra, S., & Kravitz, R.L. (2011). N-of-1 trials in the medical literature: A systematic review. *Medical Care*, 761–768.

Gabriel, A.S., Podsakoff, N.P., Beal, D.J., Scott, B.A., Sonnentag, S., Trougakos, J.P., & Butts, M.M. (2019). Experience sampling methods: A discussion of critical trends and considerations for scholarly advancement. *Organizational Research Methods, 22*(4), 969–1006.

Gómez-Pinilla, F. (2008). Brain foods: The effects of nutrients on brain function. *Nature Reviews neuroscience, 9*(7), 568–578.

Gruters, A.A., Ramakers, I.H., Verhey, F.R., Köhler, S., Kessels, R.P., & de Vugt, M.E. (2019). Association between proxy- or self-reported cognitive decline and cognitive performance in memory clinic visitors. *Journal of Alzheimer's Disease, 70*(4), 1225–1239.

Kramer, I., Simons, C.J., Hartmann, J.A., Menne-Lothmann, C., Viechtbauer, W., Peeters, F., Schruers, K., . . . Delespaul, P. (2014). A therapeutic application of the experience sampling method in the treatment of depression: A randomized controlled trial. *World Psychiatry, 13*(1), 68–77.

Larson, R., & Csikszentmihalyi, M. (2014). The experience sampling method. In *Flow and the foundations of positive psychology* (pp. 21–34). Dordrecht: Springer.

Mestdagh, M., Verdonck, S., Piot, M., Niemeijer, K., tuerlinckx, f., Kuppens, P., & Dejonckheere, E. (2022, January 25). m-Path: An easy-to-use and flexible platform for ecological momentary assessment and intervention in behavioral research and clinical practice. https://doi.org/10.31234/osf.io/uqdfs

Mitchell, R.L., & Phillips, L.H. (2007). The psychological, neurochemical and functional neuroanatomical mediators of the effects of positive and negative mood on executive functions. *Neuropsychologia, 45*(4), 617–629.

Mitzner, T.L., Fausset, C.B., Boron, J.B., Adams, A.E., Dijkstra, K., Lee, C.C., Rogers, W.A., & Fisk, A.D. (2008). Older adults' training preferences for learning to use technology. *Proceedings of the Human Factors and Ergonomics Society Annual Meeting* (Vol. 52, No. 26, pp. 2047–2051). Los Angeles, CA: Sage Publications.

Myin-Germeys, I., Oorschot, M., Collip, D., Lataster, J., Delespaul, P., & Van Os, J. (2009). Experience sampling research in psychopathology: Opening the black box of daily life. *Psychological Medicine, 39*(9), 1533–1547.

Persson, K., Brækhus, A., Selbæk, G., Kirkevold, Ø., & Engedal, K. (2015). Burden of care and patient's neuropsychiatric symptoms influence carer's evaluation of cognitive impairment. *Dementia and Geriatric Cognitive Disorders, 40*(5–6), 256–267.

Petkus, A.J., & Wetherell, J.L. (2013). Acceptance and commitment therapy with older adults: Rationale and considerations. *Cognitive and Behavioral Practice, 20*(1), 47–56.

Pew Research Centre. (2021). *Mobile phone ownership over time*. Retrieved from www.pewresearch.org/internet/fact-sheet/mobile/

Porta, M. (2014). *A dictionary of epidemiology*. Oxford: Oxford university press.

Ryd, C., Nygård, L., Malinowsky, C., Öhman, A., & Kottorp, A. (2015). Associations between performance of activities of daily living and everyday technology use among older adults with mild stage Alzheimer's disease or mild cognitive impairment. *Scandinavian Journal of Occupational Therapy, 22*(1), 33–42.

Schneider, S., Stone, A.A., Schwartz, J.E., & Broderick, J.E. (2011). Peak and end effects in patients' daily recall of pain and fatigue: A within-subjects analysis. *The Journal of Pain, 12*(2), 228–235.

Scollon, C.N., Kim-Prieto, C., & Diener, E. (2003). Experience sampling: Promises and pitfalls, strengths and weaknesses. *Journal of Happiness studies, 4*(1), 5–34.

Shiffman, S., Stone, A.A., & Hufford, M.R. (2008). Ecological momentary assessment. *Annual Review of Clinical Psychology, 4*, 1–32.

Span, M., Hettinga, M., Vernooij-Dassen, M., Eefsting, J., & Smits, C. (2013). Involving people with dementia in the development of supportive IT applications: A systematic review. *Ageing Research Reviews, 12*(2), 535–551.

Stone, A.A., Schneider, S., & Harter, J.K. (2012). Day-of-week mood patterns in the United States: On the existence of 'Blue Monday', 'Thank God it's Friday' and weekend effects. *The Journal of Positive Psychology, 7*(4), 306–314.

Trull, T.J., & Ebner-Priemer, U. (2013). Ambulatory assessment. *Annual Review of Clinical Psychology, 9*, 151–176.

van Aubel, E., Bakker, J.M., Batink, T., Michielse, S., Goossens, L., Lange, I., . . . van Amelsvoort, T. (2020). Blended care in the treatment of subthreshold symptoms of depression and psychosis in emerging adults: A randomised controlled trial of Acceptance and Commitment Therapy in Daily-Life (ACT-DL). *Behaviour Research and Therapy, 128*, 103592.

Van Berkel, N., Goncalves, J., Hosio, S., & Kostakos, V. (2017). Gamification of mobile experience sampling improves data quality and quantity. *Proceedings of the ACM on Interactive, Mobile, Wearable and Ubiquitous Technologies, 1*(3), 1–21.

Van den Bergh, O., & Walentynowicz, M. (2016). Accuracy and bias in retrospective symptom reporting. *Current Opinion in Psychiatry, 29*(5), 302–308.

van der Velden, R.M., Mulders, A.E., Drukker, M., Kuijf, M.L., & Leentjens, A.F. (2018). Network analysis of symptoms in a Parkinson patient using experience sampling data: An n= 1 study. *Movement Disorders, 33*(12), 1938–1944.

Van Knippenberg, R., De Vugt, M., Ponds, R., Myin-Germeys, I., van Twillert, B., & Verhey, F. (2017). Dealing with daily challenges in dementia (deal-id study): An experience sampling study to assess caregiver functioning in the flow of daily life. *International Journal of Geriatric Psychiatry, 32*(9), 949–958.

Van Knippenberg, R., De Vugt, M., Ponds, R., Myin-Germeys, I., & Verhey, F. (2018). An experience sampling method intervention for dementia caregivers: Results of a randomized controlled trial. *The American Journal of Geriatric Psychiatry, 26*(12), 1231–1243.

Verhagen, S.J., Daniëls, N.E., Bartels, S.L., Tans, S., Borkelmans, K.W., de Vugt, M.E., & Delespaul, P.A. (2019). Measuring within-day cognitive performance using the experience sampling method: A pilot study in a healthy population. *PLoS One, 14*(12), e0226409.

Verhagen, S.J., Hasmi, L., Drukker, M., van Os, J., & Delespaul, P.A. (2016). Use of the experience sampling method in the context of clinical trials. *Evidence-based Mental Health, 19*(3), 86–89.

Vilaysack, B., Cordier, R., Doma, K., & Chen, Y.W. (2016). Capturing everyday experiences of typically developing children aged five to seven years: A feasibility study of experience sampling methodology. *Australian Occupational Therapy Journal, 63*(6), 424–433.

Wilson, K., Bell, C., Wilson, L., & Witteman, H. (2018). Agile research to complement agile development: A proposal for an mHealth research lifecycle. *NPJ Digital Medicine, 1*(1), 1–6.

Chapter 5

Social participation and everyday technology use

A mixed-methods study among people living with and without dementia

*Sophie N. Gaber, Louise Nygård, Anna Brorsson,
Anders Kottorp, Georgina Charlesworth,
Sarah Wallcook, Camilla Walles Malinowsky*

Introduction

Social participation is a modifiable determinant for health and well-being among older people (World Health Organization, 2016). The World Health Organization (2016) states that whilst policymakers cannot create participation, more can be done to create 'spaces' that enable and encourage social participation, especially involving marginalised communities, such as older people living with dementia. Social participation refers to the person's involvement in activities that provide interaction with others in society (Levasseur et al., 2010), and it is linked to improved physical functioning and psychosocial well-being (Bai et al., 2020), reduced social isolation (Evans et al., 2019), and prevention of cognitive decline (Fallahpour et al., 2016). By identifying barriers and motivators to social participation, marginalised communities may be empowered to access 'spaces' and places in society where they can harness the benefits of social participation for their health and well-being (World Health Organization, 2016).

Living within an increasingly digitalised society means interacting with technology to engage in social participation (Nygard, 2008). Digital technology can enhance social participation (Barbosa Neves et al., 2019), reinforce existing social relationships (Ten Bruggencate et al., 2019), and mitigate social isolation (Pinto-Bruno et al., 2017) among older people living with dementia. Few studies have explored social participation in relation to technology use, and these have focused on novel technological innovations, such as gaming and self-monitoring, which have been limited by low uptake in the everyday lives of older people with and without dementia (Pinto-Bruno et al., 2017; Thordardottir et al., 2019).

To develop technologies that are assistive for older people with and without dementia, it is important to gain further insights into how existing everyday

DOI: 10.4324/9781003289005-7

Table 5.1 List of abbreviations

Explanation	Abbreviation
ACT-OUT	Participation in ACTivities and places OUTside Home Questionnaire
DSM-IV	Diagnostic and statistical manual of mental disorders, fourth edition
ET	Everyday technology
ETUQ	Everyday technology use questionnaire
IMD	Index of multiple deprivation
MoCA	Montreal cognitive assessment

technologies (ETs) that the older person already uses are assistive or inhibitive to participation in their chosen activities and places in public spaces (Mannheim et al., 2019). This study conceptualises ETs as electronic, digital and mechanical devices that typically exist in an older person's environment and that are embedded in their habits and routines of everyday life (Nygård et al., 2016).

There is no consensus definition of social participation, its component dimensions, or its relationship to technology, places and spaces. This study builds on earlier research to operationalise social participation as 'participation in activities that are embedded within places for social, spiritual and cultural activities as well as those places for recreation and physical activities, in public space' (Gaber et al., 2020).

A review of the literature indicates that barriers within one's living environment should be considered when investigating social participation or technology use (Donkers et al., 2019). Earlier research regarding barriers in one's living environment revealed a negative association between digital engagement, specifically access and use of information and communication technologies, and higher social deprivation of the living environment based on the English Index of Multiple Deprivation (IMD) (Longley & Singleton, 2009). Social deprivation encompasses various aspects, including access to housing and services. Increasingly, research suggests that social deprivation of the living environment is related to less social participation, which requires further exploration.

Our objective was to investigate social participation in relation to total ET use outside home and social deprivation of the living environment among participants with and without dementia in the United Kingdom. This motivated the following research questions:

• In what ways does social participation, as reported by older participants living with and without dementia, relate to total ET use outside home and social deprivation of the living environment?
• What are the motivators, considerations that require extra attention and, strategies for managing social participation of older people with and without dementia, in relation to the role of ET use outside home?

Methods

Study design and ethics

A cross-sectional, convergent, mixed-methods design was utilised. Interview-based tools were used to simultaneously collect quantitative data and free text responses (i.e. participants' replies to open-ended questions). Different types of data were integrated through analyses and interpretation of the findings (Creswell & Creswell, 2018). Participants gave their informed consent for inclusion before they participated in the study. Ethical approval was granted from the Health Research Authority (IRAS project ID: 215654, REC reference: 17/SW/0091).

Participants

Data were collected across urban and rural environments in the United Kingdom, including five National Health Service research sites (London, Cumbria, Greater Manchester regions). Participants living with dementia ($n = 64$) were recruited through the National Health Service and community-based groups. Participants without dementia (i.e. no known cognitive impairment) ($n = 64$) were recruited through local networks (e.g. community-based activity or social groups). Participants living with dementia had a diagnosis of mild-stage dementia from a physician based on the standardised Diagnostic and Statistical Manual of Mental Disorders, fourth edition (DSM-IV) criteria, or as a major neurocognitive disorder (American Psychiatric Association, 2000, 2013).

Procedure

Two occupational therapists (SNG and SW) collected data through one-to-one interviews with participants in their homes or another location chosen by the participants, between May and December 2017. Free text responses were written down on paper by the interviewer and consisted of a couple of sentences. In-depth information about recruitment and data collection is available elsewhere (Gaber et al., 2020). Interviews included the following tools:

(1) The Participation in ACTivities and Places OUTside Home Questionnaire (ACT-OUT) (Margot-Cattin et al., 2019) maps self-reported current participation in four Domains: (A) places for purchasing, administration, and self-care ($n = 6$); (B) places for medical care ($n = 5$); (C) places for social, spiritual and cultural activities ($n = 6$); (D) places for recreation and physical activity ($n = 7$). This study focused on Domains C and D. To capture detailed information about the activity performed in a place and the journey to and from the place, open-ended questions were also used.
(2) The Montreal Cognitive Assessment (MoCA) (Nasreddine et al., 2005) was used to describe current levels of cognitive function, according to the score range of 0–30, with higher scores indicative of higher cognitive status.

(3) A non-standardised demographic questionnaire was developed to gather information about demographic factors that may be relevant according to earlier research (Kottorp et al., 2016). An Index of Multiple Deprivation (IMD) score was determined using information about where the participants lived, as a measure of relative deprivation applied to small geographic areas or neighbourhoods in England (Ministry of Housing, 2015).

(4) The Everyday Technology Use Questionnaire (ETUQ) (Nygård et al., 2016) was used to gather information about the total ET use outside home variable for 49 ETs–16 ETs, which can be used outside home (e.g. ATM, self-service checkout) and 33 portable ETs that can be used both at home and outside home (e.g. smartphone, eBook reader).

Data analysis

The mixed-methods approach involved three sequential steps: (1) statistical analysis of the ACT-OUT and ETUQ data; (2) content analysis of the free text responses from the ACT-OUT using the ATLAS.ti software program and (3) integration of the results from these two types of analyses in a graphical joint display and discussion section (Creswell & Creswell, 2018). The rationale for performing a content analysis was to identify words, categories and concepts within the free text responses and to make inferences about the contexts of their use. To promote trustworthiness, two researchers (SNG and AB) coded a sub-sample of the data separately, and then engaged in critical discussions to review and refine the initial coding system and to reach a consensus draft code. The codes were collated and assigned to overall categories and sub-categories, with ongoing discussions until no new categories were identified.

Differences between the two sub-samples' demographic factors were tested (Table 5.2) and correlations (Spearman's rank correlation coefficients) were calculated. Cohen's guidelines for social sciences were used to interpret the strength of correlations: small = 0.1–0.3, medium = 0.3–0.5 and large effect = 0.5–1.0 (Cohen, 1988). For all analyses, the alpha level was set to 0.05.

Results

Statistical results

Participants

No statistically significant differences were identified in the demographic factors between the two sub-samples, except for age, which was significantly higher among participants living with dementia, as well as years of education and the number of people driving a car which were both significantly lower among participants with dementia (all $p < 0.01$) (Table 5.2). As expected, the MoCA score for participants living with dementia was significantly lower than participants without dementia ($p < 0.01$). There were also statistically significant differences in ethnicity between the groups.

Table 5.2 Demographic characteristics, Montreal Cognitive Assessment (MoCA) and Index of Multiple Deprivation Score (IMD)

Characteristics	Sub-sample with dementia (n = 64)	Sub-sample without dementia (n = 64)	Comparison test	p-value
Age, years			Mann–Whitney	<0.001
Median (Min, Max)	79.0 (62.0, 96.0)	71.0 (55.0, 89.0)	U-test	
IQR [1]	74.0–83.0	64.0–80.8		
Gender, n (%)			Pearson's chi-squared test (χ^2)	0.377
Female	29 (45.3)	34 (53.1)		
Male	35 (54.7)	30 (46.9)		
Living arrangement, n (%)			χ^2	0.856
Cohabiting	39 (60.9)	40 (62.5)		
Lives alone	25 (39.1)	24 (37.5)		
Geography, n (%)			χ^2	0.404
Urban	51 (79.7)	47 (73.4)		
Rural	13 (20.3)	17 (26.6)		
Education, years			Mann–Whitney	0.002
Median (Min, Max)	11.0 (7.0, 21.0)	13.0 (9.0, 19.0)	U-test	
IQR	10.3–13.0	11.0–16.0		
Ethnicity, n (%)			Fisher's Exact test	0.025
White	56 (87.5)	49 (76.5)		
Mixed/multiple ethnic group	0 (0.0)	2 (3.1)		
Asian/Asian British	1 (1.6)	9 (14.1)		
Black/African/Caribbean/Black British	5 (7.8)	3 (4.7)		
Other ethnic group	2 (3.1)	1 (1.6)		
Driving, n (%)			χ^2	<0.001
Driving	26 (40.6)	46 (71.9)		
Not driving	38 (59.4)	18 (28.1)		
Functional impairment, n (%)			χ^2	0.611
Functional impairment	54 (84.4)	56 (87.5)		
No functional impairment	10 (15.6)	8 (12.5)		
MoCA score			Mann–Whitney	<0.001
Median (Min, Max)	21.0 (12.0, 28.0)	26.0 (21.0, 30.0)	U-test	
IQR	18.0–23.0	25.0–28.5		

Characteristics	Sub-sample with dementia (n = 64)	Sub-sample without dementia (n = 64)	Comparison test	p-value
Index of multiple deprivation (IMD)			Mann–Whitney U-test	0.887
Median (Min, Max)	5.0 (1.0, 10.0)	5.5 (1.0, 10.0)		
IQR	3.5–8.0	4.0–7.0		

[1] IQR: Interquartile range. One to ten deciles of the Index of Multiple Deprivation (IMD); one refers to the most deprived 10% of neighbourhoods in England. Rural-urban and ethnicity classifications according to the Office of National Statistics (Office of National Statistics, 2011, 2013).

Social participation in relation to total ET use outside home

Descriptive statistics showed that social participation in Domain C was significantly lower for participants with dementia; however, the median social participation in Domain D was equal for the two sub-samples (Table 5.3). Total ET use outside home was significantly lower among participants with dementia ($Md = 10.0$) than participants without dementia ($Md = 21.0$; $U = 556.50$; $Z = -7.114$; $p < 0.001$). Spearman's rank correlations revealed no statistically significant association between social participation in Domain C and total ET use outside home for participants with or without dementia. Conversely, a small but statistically significant positive association was found between social participation in Domain D and the total ET use outside home for participants with dementia, and a small to medium, statistically significant, positive association was identified for participants without dementia.

Social participation in relation to social deprivation of the living environment

Both sub-samples included a minimum and maximum range across all ten deciles of the IMD. The IMD was lower but not significantly for participants with dementia compared to participants without dementia (Table 5.2). This corresponds to a slightly higher proportion of participants with dementia living in more deprived areas of England, compared to participants without dementia. No statistically significant association was found between social participation in Domain C and IMD for the two sub-samples. A small, statistically significant, positive association was determined between social participation in Domain D and IMD (i.e. lower social deprivation of the living environment) for participants with dementia but not for those without dementia.

Table 5.3 Graphical joint display to visualise the integration of mixed-methods results

Domain	Variables	Participants with dementia (n = 64)	Participants without dementia (n = 64)	Comparison
Domain C (Social, spiritual and cultural places)	Total social participation (places = 6)	Median: 3.0; Min–Max: 1.0–6.0; IQR: 3.0–5.0	Median: 5.0; Min–Max: 1.0–6.0; IQR: 3.0–5.0	$U = 1434.0$; $Z = -2.996$; $p = 0.003$
	Places in Domain C and examples of activities performed in the places	**Places:**	**Activities:**	
		Activities: 1. Drive to daughter's place, a trip 2. Going into the village, sit down, cup of tea, chat 3. Dementia care group and socialise, art group, crossword, singalong 4. Socialise, worship, church duties 5. N/A 6. Go and watch live music	1. Socialise and see grandchildren 2. Breakfast different place each week 3. Gujarati centre. 150 people go. Meet people there, see friends, prayer, pass time, enjoys herself 4. Worship, play guitar, pray, enjoy time with dear friends 5. Walk and look around cemetery 6. See a concert with a friend	
		1. Friend or family member's place 2. Restaurant, café, bar 3. Senior centre, social club 4. Building for worship 5. Cemetery, memorial place 6. Entertainment, cultural place		
	Association between social participation and: i. Total ET use outside home; ii. IMD	i. No significant association ($R_s = 0.176$; $p = 0.164$) ii. No significant association ($R_s = 0.035$, $p = 0.785$)	i. No significant association ($R_s = 0.181$; $p = 0.152$) ii. No significant association ($R_s = 0.157$, $p = 0.214$)	

Domain D (places for recreation and physical activities)	Total social participation (places = 7)	Median: 5.0; Min – Max: 0.0–7.0; IQR: 3.0–6.0	Median: 5.0; Min – Max: 1.0–7.0; IQR: 4.0–6.0	$U = 1900.0$; $Z = -0.719$; $p = 0.472$
	Places in Domain D and examples of activities performed in the places	**Places:** 1. Garden 2. Park, green area 3. Forest, mountain, lake, sea 4. Cottage, summer house 5. Neighbourhood 6. Sports facility 7. Transportation centre **Activities:** 1. Garden, admire the garden and the birds 2. Goes with granddaughter so she can play on the swings 3. Walk the dog along the seafront for a friend 4. Visit son and grandchildren and have a break 5. Neighbourhood, sometimes walk and get fresh air 6. Seated exercises 7. Traveling	**Activities:** 1. Sit there with wife and cat 2. Go to park, people watch, go to café, sit on bench, walk 3. Walk and enjoy the scenery and navigate 4. Has 3 days at the timeshare cottage 5. Walking around, thinking alone. Enjoy exercise, time to think, fresh air 6. Swimming, 70 lengths 7. Get underground or buses	
	Association between Social participation and: i. Total ET use outside home; ii. IMD	i. Small significant, positive association ($R_s = 0.247$; $p = 0.049$) ii. Small significant, positive association ($R_s = 0.267$, $p = 0.033$)	i. Small-medium significant, positive association ($R_s = 0.343$; $p = 0.006$) ii. No significant association ($R_s = 0.014$, $p = 0.911$)	

(Continued)

Table 5.3 (Continued)

Domain	Variables	Participants with dementia (n = 64)	Participants without dementia (n = 64)	Comparison
Domains C and D	Motivators for social participation	Purposeful activity; companionship (doing the journey and/or activity with other people)		
	Considerations that require extra attention for social participation	Contextual factors		
	Strategies for managing social participation	Preparation and wayfinding involving ET use		

Content analysis results

The free text responses from participants with and without dementia correspond to their descriptions about motivators, considerations that require extra attention and strategies for managing social participation in Domains C and D.

Motivators for social participation

Purposeful activity

ACT-OUT data showed that participants with and without dementia viewed purposeful activities as a motivator for social participation. The complexity of the purpose of social participation varied. Some places were associated with the purpose of performing a specific activity, for instance, walking in the park or eating in a restaurant. Other places were associated with repertoires of multiple activities such as going to a community centre to meet friends, pray, pass time and for enjoyment. In Domain C, the places and activities most frequently reported for participants with dementia were friend or family member's place, compared with entertainment or cultural places for participants without dementia. In Domain D, participants with dementia most frequently spoke about participation in their garden whilst participants without dementia commonly spoke about participation in the forest, mountain, lake or seaside.

Companionship

Participants with and without dementia described the journey as a natural continuation of the activity itself, rather than as two distinct parts. Participation in the journey and activity were viewed as opportunities to socialise with other people including their spouse, family, friends or as a group member. The rationale for doing the journey or activity together with other people differed between participants, for instance, due to a shared interest in the activity, to support each other with travel arrangements or for the pleasure of companionship as one participant with dementia explained, 'only go with someone else – not so much fun otherwise'. Participation in the journey or activity with other people was viewed as a way of receiving or giving support to other people.

Managing social participation

Contextual factors were spoken about in relation to considerations that require extra attention for social participation. Familiarity with people in one's neighbourhood was considered an additional layer of support and security for social participation, among participants with and without dementia. The participants with dementia recalled that the support of one's social context was a buffer against problematic situations associated with ETs (e.g. misplacing ETs, forgetting to charge ETs).

Conversely, participants spoke about contextual factors pertaining to perceived risks during social participation. Perceived risks ranged from the inconvenience of being distracted and not being able to escape conversations with people to concerns for one's personal safety (e.g. intoxicated people, criminal behaviours, crowds). Participants reported that there would be no concerns at a place and that they felt able to socialise, if the behaviour of other people was 'considerate and reasonable'.

Preparation and wayfinding involving ET use

Participants reported preparatory strategies for assisting them to find their way to a place and several of these strategies involved ET use (e.g. Global Positioning System (GPS)) for navigation and wayfinding. A participant with dementia explained that he had used his iPhone to find his way when he was lost, 'use compass on my iPhone to navigate did get lost once but found my way'. However, a sense of anxiety was associated with the perceived need to plan and prepare. A participant without dementia explained that anxiety about the journey started with the act of planning and preparing: 'Anxiety begins at the point of booking . . .'.

Attitudes towards the need to plan and prepare for social participation, including the use of ETs, conveyed nuanced meanings. Participants with and without dementia reported that they had encountered problems using ETs for planning purposes or limitations in the ability of ETs to support them to manage social participation.

Discussion

This study identified perceived motivators, considerations that require extra attention, and management strategies underlying social participation, which supports earlier research indicating that older people express interest, motivation and perceived well-being in relation to social participation (Levasseur et al., 2010). One explanation for the significant, positive association found between social participation and ET use outside home, in places for recreation and physical activities (Domain D), but not in places for social, spiritual and cultural activities (Domain C), is that in places for social, spiritual and cultural activities, there is more of a social network to support social participation and thus a lower dependency on ET. Participants with and without dementia tended to report being familiar with places for social, spiritual and cultural activities, having visited a specific place of worship or a community centre for many years. Earlier research substantiates the importance of such places for facilitating social connectedness and a sense of familiarity with one's community (Wiley et al., 2012). Social and cultural norms may discourage technology use in cultural and spiritual places out of a sign of respect (Forgays et al., 2014), although ETs may still be encountered in these places.

Participants described ET use in relation to management strategies to assist them to plan and prepare before participating outside home (e.g. online information search) or for wayfinding purposes. This reinforces earlier research, which found that ET use is integral not only to the performance of the desired activity itself but also to preceding activities (e.g. managing public transport, using a ticket machine, operating an ATM). The preceding activities must be performed before the person can master their desired activity (e.g. socialising with friends, visiting the cinema) (Lindqvist et al., 2016). The results suggest that greater support given to older people with and without dementia in preparatory and wayfinding stages, including support using ETs to help preserve energy reserves and mitigate anxiety, or the design and development of more usable wayfinding and preparatory applications within the mainstream ETs that older people already use, may help to assist their ongoing social participation (Mannheim et al., 2019).

A unique contribution of the study is its mixed-methods approach, which affirmed earlier research that older people with and without dementia perceive social participation in relation to their social and physical context (Donkers et al., 2019), and that ETs may enhance social participation (Barbosa Neves et al., 2019). This approach also elucidated potential inconsistencies in statistical and content analyses from the ACT-OUT Questionnaire. The ACT-OUT Questionnaire asks about the activity and place as well as the journey in two discrete parts; however, according to the free text responses, the journey was described as an extension of the activity and places and as an opportunity to socialise with other people for various reasons (e.g. companionship, to give or to receive support). The results confirm earlier research, which identified social support as a potential strategy for managing problematic situations in public space among people with dementia (Brorsson et al., 2020). Knowledge about social factors, such as social support to travel, is particularly important for participants with dementia, to balance capacities and limitations (Lindqvist et al., 2016) and to enable continued social participation, following changes in their mode of participation (e.g. following driving cessation).

Uniquely, this study highlighted the potential susceptibility of people with dementia to the effects of social deprivation of the living environment on social participation; however, this study does not infer any causal relationship since the convenience sample may raise potential issues of confounding for affluence and geographical location. Future research may benefit from using a larger, randomised sample and exploring potential changes in social participation since the Coronavirus pandemic.

Conclusion

The study identified perceived motivators, considerations that require extra attention and management strategies underlying social participation for the journey as well as at the place and activity itself. If as earlier research suggests, social participation is indeed a modifiable determinant of health and well-being among older people with and without dementia, our research indicates that it is equally important to consider strategies for promoting supportive social contexts for the journey as well as at the intended place and activity. Moreover, this study's mixed-methods synthesis revealed a nuanced view of ETs, as both useful in not only planning and preparatory activities but also challenging for social participation.

Funding

This research was funded by the H2020 Marie Skłodowska-Curie Actions – Innovative Training Networks, H2020-MSCA-ITN-2015 under Grant (676265) and the Swedish Council for Health, Working Life, and Welfare (Forskningsrådet om Hälsa, Arbetsliv och Välfärd, FORTE) under Grant (2013–2104).

Declaration

References

American Psychiatric Association. (2000). *Diagnostic and statistical manual of mental disorders* (4th ed., Vol. Text Revision (DSM-IV-TR)). Washington, DC: American Psychiatric Association Publishing.

American Psychiatric Association. (2013). *Diagnostic and statistical manual of mental disorders.* www.psychiatry.org/psychiatrists/practice/dsm

Bai, Z., Wang, Z., Shao, T., Qin, X., & Hu, Z. (2020). Relationship between individual social capital and functional ability among older people in Anhui Province, China. *International Journal of Environmental Research and Public Health*, *17*(8), 2775. https://doi.org/10.3390/ijerph17082775

Barbosa Neves, B., Franz, R., Judges, R., Beermann, C., & Baecker, R. (2019). Can digital technology enhance social connectedness among older adults? A feasibility study. *Journal of Applied Gerontology*, *38*(1), 49–72. https://doi.org/10.1177/0733464817741369

Brorsson, A., Öhman, A., Lundberg, S., Cutchin, M.P., & Nygård, L. (2020). How accessible are grocery shops for people with dementia? A qualitative study using photo documentation and focus group interviews. *Dementia (London, England)*, *19*(6), 1872–1888. https://doi.org/10.1177/1471301218808591

Cohen, J. (1988). *Statistical power analysis for the behavioral sciences* (2nd ed.). L. Erlbaum Associates.

Creswell, J.W., & Creswell, J.D. (2018). *Research design: Qualitative, quantitative, and mixed methods approaches* (5th ed.). London: SAGE.

Donkers, H.W., Vernooij-Dassen, M.J.F.J., Veen, D.J. v. d., Sanden, M.N. v. d., & Graff, M.J. (2019). Social participation perspectives of people with cognitive problems and their care-givers: a descriptive qualitative study. *Ageing and Society, 39*(7), 1485–1511. https://doi.org/10.1017/S0144686X18000077

Evans, I.E.M., Martyr, A., Collins, R., Brayne, C., & Clare, L. (2019). Social isolation and cognitive function in later life: A systematic review and meta-analysis. *Journal of Alzheimer's Disease, 70*(s1), S119–S144. https://doi.org/10.3233/JAD-180501

Fallahpour, M., Borell, L., Luborsky, M., & Nygard, L. (2016). Leisure-activity participation to prevent later-life cognitive decline: A systematic review. *Scandinavian Journal of Occupational Therapy, 23*(3), 162–197. https://doi.org/10.3109/11038128.2015.1102320

Forgays, D.K., Hyman, I., & Schreiber, J. (2014). Texting everywhere for everything: Gender and age differences in cell phone etiquette and use. *Computers in Human Behavior, 31,* 314–321. https://doi.org/10.1016/j.chb.2013.10.053

Gaber, S.N., Nygård, L., Brorsson, A., Kottorp, A., Charlesworth, G., Wallcook, S., & Malinowsky, C. (2020). Social participation in relation to technology use and social deprivation: A mixed methods study among older people with and without dementia. *International Journal of Environmental Research and Public Health, 17*(11), 4022. https://doi.org/10.3390/ijerph17114022

Kottorp, A., Nygård, L., Hedman, A., Öhman, A., Malinowsky, C., Rosenberg, L., . . . Ryd, C. (2016). Access to and use of everyday technology among older people: An occupational justice issue – But for whom? *Journal of Occupational Science, 23*(3), 382–388. https://doi.org/10.1080/14427591.2016.1151457

Levasseur, M., Richard, L., Gauvin, L., & Raymond, É. (2010). Inventory and analysis of definitions of social participation found in the aging literature: Proposed taxonomy of social activities. *Social Science & Medicine (1982), 71*(12), 2141–2149. https://doi.org/10.1016/j.socscimed.2010.09.041 (Social Science & Medicine)

Lindqvist, E., Persson Vasiliou, A., Gomersall, T., Astelle, A., Mihailidis, A., Sixsmith, A., & Nygård, L. (2016). Activities people with cognitive deficits want to continue mastering – A scoping study. *British Journal of Occupational Therapy, 79*(7), 399–408. https://doi.org/10.1177/0308022616636895

Longley, P.A., & Singleton, A.D. (2009). Linking social deprivation and digital exclusion in England. *Urban Studies (Edinburgh, Scotland), 46*(7), 1275–1298. https://doi.org/10.1177/0042098009104566

Mannheim, I., Schwartz, E., Xi, W., Buttigieg, S.C., McDonnell-Naughton, M., Wouters, E.J.M., & van Zaalen, Y. (2019). Inclusion of older adults in the research and design of digital technology. *International Journal of Environmental Research and Public Health, 16*(19), 3718. https://doi.org/10.3390/ijerph16193718

Margot-Cattin, I., Kuhne, N., Kottorp, A., Cutchin, M., Öhman, A., & Nygård, L. (2019). Development of a Questionnaire to evaluate out-of-home participation for people with dementia. *The American Journal of Occupational Therapy, 73*(1), 7301205030p7301205031–7301205030p7301205010. https://doi.org/10.5014/ajot.2019.027144

Ministry of Housing, C.L.G. (2015). *National statistics. English indices of deprivation.* Retrieved from www.gov.uk/government/statistics/english-indices-of-deprivation-2015

Nasreddine, Z.S., Phillips, N.A., Bédirian, V., Charbonneau, S., Whitehead, V., Collin, I. . . . Chertkow, H. (2005). The Montreal Cognitive Assessment, MoCA: A brief screening tool for mild cognitive impairment. *Journal of the American Geriatrics Society (JAGS), 53*(4), 695–699. https://doi.org/10.1111/j.1532-5415.2005.53221.x

Nygard, L. (2008). The meaning of everyday technology as experienced by people with dementia who live alone. *Dementia (London, England), 7*(4), 481–502. https://doi.org/10.1177/1471301208096631

Nygård, L., Rosenberg, L., & Kottorp, A. (2016). *User's manual: Everyday technology use questionnaire (ETUQ) everyday technology in activities at home and in society.* Solna: Karolinska Institutet.

Office of National Statistics. (2011). *2011 Census analysis: Ethnicity and religion of the non-UK born population in England and Wales: 2011.* Office of National Statistics. www.ons.gov.uk/peoplepopulationandcommunity/culturalidentity/ethnicity/articles/2011censusanalysiset hnicityandreligionofthenonukbornpopulationinenglandandwales/2015-06-18

Office of National Statistics. (2013). *Urban and rural area definitions for policy purposes in England and Wales: Methodology (v1.0).* Office of National Statistics. https://assets.publishing.service.gov.uk/government/uploads/system/uploads/attachment_data/file/239477/RUC11methodologypaperaug_28_Aug.pdf

Pinto-Bruno, Á.C., García-Casal, J.A., Csipke, E., Jenaro-Río, C., & Franco-Martín, M. (2017). ICT-based applications to improve social health and social participation in older adults with dementia. A systematic literature review. *Aging & Mental Health, 21*(1), 58–65. https://doi.org/10.1080/13607863.2016.1262818

Ten Bruggencate, T., Luijkx, K.G., & Sturm, J. (2019). Friends or frenemies?: The role of social technology in the lives of older people. *International Journal of Environmental Research and Public Health, 16*(24), 4969. https://doi.org/10.3390/ijerph16244969

Thordardottir, B., Malmgren Fänge, A., Lethin, C., Rodriguez Gatta, D., & Chiatti, C. (2019). Acceptance and use of innovative assistive technologies among people with cognitive impairment and their caregivers: A systematic review. *BioMed Research International, 2019*, 9196729–9196718. https://doi.org/10.1155/2019/9196729

Wiley, J.L., Leibing, A., Guberman, N., Reeve, J., & Allen, R.E.S. (2012). The meaning of aging in place to older people. *The Gerontologist, 52*(3), 357–366. https://doi.org/10.1093/geront/gnr098

World Health Organization. (2016). *Toolkit of Social Participation.* WHO. www.euro.who.int/__data/assets/pdf_file/0003/307452/Toolkit-social-partecipation.pdf

Part 3

Evaluation of the effectiveness of technology

Chapter 6

Conditions of technology use and its interplay in the everyday lives of older adults with and without dementia

*Sarah Wallcook, Louise Nygård,
Anders Kottorp, Georgina Charlesworth,
Camilla Walles Malinowsky*

Chapter introduction

Dementia- and age-friendly initiatives share an aim to optimise participation in everyday life by addressing inclusivity at various levels (World Health Organization, 2007, 2017). These levels include cities, rural settings, communities, neighbourhoods, institutions, groups, single buildings and objects. However, everyday technologies (ETs) remain poorly considered, despite their high and ever-increasing prevalence in society (Marston & van Hoof, 2019). Furthermore, digitised services demand ET use, which places some older adults at greater risk of social exclusion, particularly in countries such as Sweden, where digitalisation has been more rapid (OECD, 2016). ETs are constantly changing and are defined as commonplace and well-known digital, electronic and mechanical objects and services (Patomella et al., 2013). To bring the focus onto everyday life outside home, this chapter presents research findings that primarily investigated *information and communication technologies and their functions* (*EICTs*, i.e. smartphone, computer for messaging, navigation, information searching, Internet banking) and *self-service technologies* (*SSTs*, i.e. fuel pump, cash machine).

The findings of four studies that used multiple methods have been synthesised in a triangulation approach (Farmer et al., 2006, Wallcook, 2021). Home-based interviews collected responses to the Everyday Technology Use Questionnaire (ETUQ) (Nygård et al., 2016) from 315 respondents aged 55+ in the United States, the United Kingdom and Sweden, 99 of whom had a confirmed diagnosis of dementia. Data from the complete set of responses were analysed using modern test statistics to compare by diagnosis and by country (Wallcook et al., 2020). A subsample of this data from Sweden formed matched groups of people with dementia (*n* = 35) and people with no known cognitive impairment (*n* = 34) for comparative and modern test statistical analysis (Wallcook et al., 2021b). Regression modelling was used with another subsample gathered in the United Kingdom (*n* = 128) (Wallcook et al., 2021a) from which ten

DOI: 10.4324/9781003289005-9

rurally dwelling participants were selected for a multiple case study (Wallcook 2021). In addition to the ETUQ, these UK-based studies gathered responses using the Participation in Activities and Places Outside Home questionnaire (Margot-Cattin et al., 2019) and more open data gathering procedures (i.e. observation, memos) were used with the cases.

People with dementia were involved throughout the research process for these studies via the European Working Group of People with Dementia and the Focus on Dementia Network Group Cumbria (the United Kingdom). Through a series of meetings, the latter group challenged the main author's interpretations of findings to contribute and incorporate alternative views. Group members' engagement with the findings extended to acting upon the new knowledge generated. This action confirms the utility of the suggestions given at the end of this chapter and the relevance of this research to the group's everyday lives.

EICT inclusivity

The challenge of smartphones was perceived by participants both with and without dementia to be generally lower than that of pushbutton mobile phones. Despite this, the more challenging to use mobile was used by a greater proportion of the group with dementia in comparison to the group with no known cognitive impairment. Furthermore, we found EICT challenge to be unfeasibly high in some situations so that sensitivity and compassion were warranted when some people with dementia were dealing with computer/laptop functions (refer to Figure 6.1). In these situations, an appropriate strategy was to share and delegate responsibilities for use, possibly as part of a longer term manualising process. For example, one person manages logging in, passwords, entering transaction details, while the other checks the bank account, or selects shopping items (Wallcook, 2021). However, where the challenge was perceived to be lower, people with dementia may benefit from a more rehabilitative approach (Swaffer, 2021). For example, providing occupational therapy interventions to optimise, tailor and adapt existing EICTs for prolonged use (Wallcook et al., 2021b, Fischl et al., 2020).

Our findings highlight the variation and complexity of EICT use among people with dementia, which suggests the need for a cautious but open-minded approach to acquiring new devices. This is particularly the case for people who anticipate difficulties so that more useable EICT choices may be helped by opportunities to *try before you buy* (Damodaran et al., 2018), for example trialling relevant smartphone functions, alongside those of a pushbutton mobile.

While our studies indicate the smartphone appears relatively easier to use, the pushbutton format may better fit some people's habits and provide a greater sense of familiarity (Jakobsson et al., 2019). Where people are habituated to a particular device, then this habit should be left alone or if necessary, tailored to facilitate continued use (Fischl et al., 2020). However, society may hold false assumptions about EICTs (i.e. longer standing technologies are easier to use, e.g. pushbutton) and who those EICTs are for. Being dementia-friendly means noticing and challenging assumptions and the age-related stigma built into ideals of EICT ownership (Köttl et al., 2021). This stigma may hinder people with dementia from accessing easier to use EICTs and compromise their participation in aspects of everyday life (Wallcook, 2021).

A person's reluctance to acquire a challenging EICT may result from accurate appraisal of other essential prerequisites for EICT use. For example, appropriate infrastructure for Internet connection and service, the ability to manage such services and access to ongoing technological support (Damodaran et al., 2018; Hwang et al., 2020; Wallcook, 2021). Although EICTs are internationally pervasive, the rural cases in our study clearly pointed to infrastructural inadequacies. Rural-urban digital inequalities have resulted in unreliable and slower mobile and Internet connections in remoter areas, which are expected to persist in future (Esteban-Navarro et al., 2020; Salemink et al., 2017). This suggests that EICTs may be systematically less useable in rural contexts internationally. Our research connected malfunctioning and unreliable telecommunications connections and devices (i.e. landline telephone, TV, computer) with barriers to services and the threat of imminent driving cessation. In combination, these aspects completely destabilised and made untenable the everyday life of one case so that he needed to relocate (Wallcook, 2021).

Relative deprivation data, indicated by several dimensions including barriers to services, were gathered for all participants' neighbourhoods. Our modelling highlighted that a more deprived living environment together with hampered use of EICTs and SSTs indicated that a person was going to a restricted range of places outside home (Wallcook et al., 2021a). As a counterpoint, neither having a diagnosis of dementia, driving a car, nor living in a rural setting were found to be significant predictors of the places participants went to. Our studies therefore highlight the overlap between technological and social inequalities as critical indicators of participation that warrant being addressed at a structural level. For example, equitable access to high speed Internet should be considered a key feature of a higher quality living environment that is required by housing standards (Olsson & Viscovi, 2020).

Travel technology challenges

We found international variation in the perceived challenge of four SSTs used for travelling: automated ticket barriers, automated airline check-in and bag drop machines and petrol pumps (refer to Figure 6.1). Their challenge may be impacted by international variation in design features and how the SST is sited in relation to other public space features (Malinowsky et al., 2012; Patomella et al., 2013; Petrie & Darzentas, 2018). For example, public transport ticketing barriers were most often described by the group from the United Kingdom in relation to Transport for London (TFL). At the time of

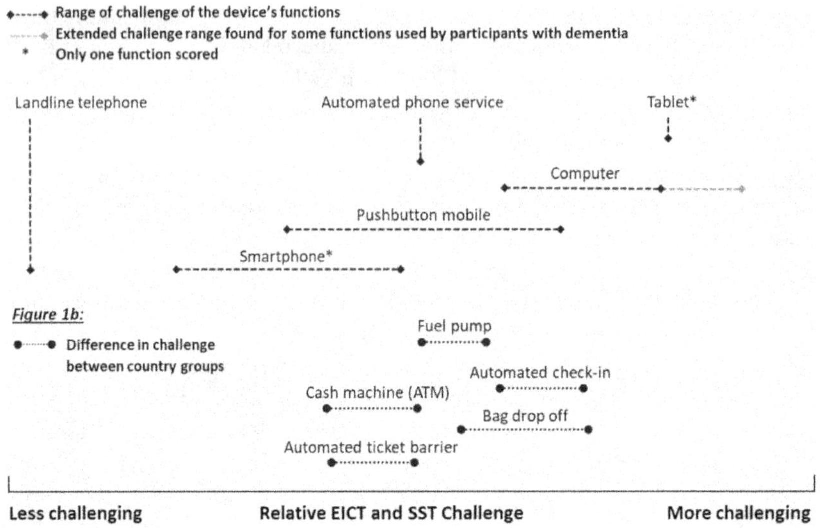

Figure 6.1 Illustration showing the approximate relative challenge of EICTs and SSTs from less to more challenging. Fig. 1a: Gives the range of the challenge relating to all functions on each EICT device. Fig. 1b: Outlines the international variation in SST challenge between Sweden, the United States and the United Kingdom.

data collection, TFL typically placed an onus on passengers to remember to seek out the SST exit touch points. Users must then touch out with access passes or contactless payment cards and failure to comply incurred the maximum daily charge. However, in Stockholm's public transport service (SL), single journeys were fixed price with no requirement to touch out and any exits were funnelled so that all passengers passed the barrier. This variation between automatic ticket barrier design features and siting may explain why this SST was perceived as more challenging for the group from England compared to Sweden. However, differences in the conditions that influence modes of travelling in Sweden, the United States and the United Kingdom may also influence the use of SSTs (Wallcook et al., 2020). For example, we found higher use of ticket barriers, and lower use of fuel pumps among the group from Sweden compared to the United States and the United Kingdom. This finding may be motived by combining accessible, affordable and efficient public transport with climate policy initiatives to reduce private transport use. Additionally, the fuel pump was of high relevance to rurally dwelling cases living with dementia compared to the other country sub-groups both with and without dementia. The cases' reliance on private transport can be linked to limited and often completely unavailable public transport services in rural England (DEFRA, 2019). This highlights how variations in ET use may occur due to *within*-country variation in service provision (Wallcook, 2021).

Design features and siting vary between fuel pumps, particularly the siting of the self-service payment technology and its location adjacent to a non-technologised alternative. Such SSTs may be embedded within a single pump, or standing alone and operable for a number of pumps, and may or may not be sited together with a kiosk, where a responsible attendant provides a face-to-face service (Wallcook, 2021). Experimental studies found, where a choice was presented, using face-to-face services in preference to food ordering SSTs related to older age, even among a sample aged between 18 and 60 years (Wu et al., 2020). While the situation for customer service in our research is fuel rather than food, it may be that co-siting technologised and manualised options together are a key feature of reduced challenge. The rural cases illuminated how such a choice motivated variety in service participation, that is participating with or without others and using or not using the technology. This variety ultimately supported inclusion by providing multiple ways to complete a task (i.e. travel by car) and participate in aspects of everyday life (i.e. attend an appointment, shop) (Wallcook, 2021).

We found that driving-related parking technologies impacted routines regarding where a person went, how often and how long they could remain there. Ultimately, these impacts could thwart the purpose for the trip (e.g. supermarket shopping) leaving the task partially or totally unfulfilled (Wallcook 2021). The importance of being able to park easily in everyday life has been found in wider research into community engagement, leisure and healthcare. However, it is the physical aspects of parking have been in focus, that is sufficient availability of spaces, manoeuvrability within the parking space and proximity to the place (Neville et al., 2018; Parke et al., 2017). From 2019 in the United Kingdom, people with dementia could apply for disability parking permits on grounds that make indirect allowances for cognitive difficulties (i.e. severe psychological distress, being at risk of harm) (Hare, 2019). However, these grounds are insufficiently inclusive of issues such as difficulty with using parking technologies and staying within time limits. This may relate to stigmatised assumptions that a person with dementia experiencing these issues must also be unfit to drive (Byszewski et al., 2013). Although dementia's progression will ultimately lead to cessation, problems with ET use should not be an assumed indicator since the person has a long familiarity with driving but unfamiliarity with new parking technologies. Making such assumptions could lead to pre-emptive and unjust driving cessation with far-reaching consequences to participation in everyday life. These consequences may be exacerbated when public transport is unavailable, as is more often the case in rural areas (Rapoport et al., 2020).

Access to cash

The cash machine (ATM) was relatively easier to use in Sweden, and it is used by greater proportion of participants. This could be indicative of Sweden, the United Kingdom and the United States being located in different phases of a shift towards cashless societies with varying availability of face-to-face, in-bank services (Wallcook et al., 2020). Sweden is at the forefront of this shift where perhaps only two branch locations continue to offer an over-the-counter cash service despite a preference among older people to retain cash (Sveriges Riksbank, 2020). A lack of service plus preference for cash would motivate higher frequency of ATM use, which in turn would facilitate improved performance (Patomella et al., 2011).

The trend of reducing bank branches has also been established in Chicago through a study which highlighted that our research participants came from a suburb of uncommonly high branch density (Hegerty, 2020). Lower ATM use among our US sub-sample may indicate a preference for face-to-face services which are under threat in all three countries (Wallcook et al., 2020). It may also explain the greater difficulty of the ATM to this US group, since having less cause to use a technology may lead to less familiar and higher perceived difficulty in its use (Patomella et al., 2011).

The cashless progression was a prominent issue among the rural cases of our study in England who described using workarounds. These workarounds highlighted the face-to-face role of shop staff combined with chip and PIN devices as an essential route for accessing cash (Wallcook, 2021). The Bank of England envisions that cash will remain essential for supporting financial inclusion (John, 2019). However, disparities are once again noted regarding the disproportional impact of ATM and bank branch closures to older, less well-off and rural-dwelling individuals, potentially undermining the viability of rural communities (Langford et al., 2021).

Reciprocity in personal and customer services relations

As previously exemplified, shared ET use often corresponded with sharing tasks in everyday life. While this in part provides a typical perspective on people with dementia receiving help or support to participate, it also points towards reciprocity as part of stabilising the smooth running of everyday life (Hwang et al., 2020). From the perspective of the person living with dementia, recognition and acknowledgement of delegated or shared ET use and tasks needed to be proportionate and flexible to the situation (Wallcook, 2021). This could mean tacitly downsizing doing to naturally adapt the way that things had long been done (Hedman et al., 2016), that is one pumps the fuel and the other goes in to pay. It could also mean being able to share fears about the impact of failed ET use and being listened to as part of affirming the relationship, giving reassurance and showing appreciation of wanting to put each other first (Wallcook,

2021). This indicates a complex and dynamic state of flux where ET use is co-constituted and entwined in an ongoing process of give-and-take in relationships. As one case highlighted, *doing for others* can be the sole motivation for ET acquisition so that feelings of rejection can follow if this gift of acceptance goes unnoticed. Participants weighed the consequences of failed, or sub-optimal ET use not only financially and practically, but also emotionally to consider ramifications to relationships, for example generating new technology support needs that destabilised participation and created friction regarding closeness and care dynamics (Hedman et al., 2016; Hwang et al., 2020; Wallcook, 2021).

Reciprocity extended to customer services relations in our research, since frequenting local shops and choosing face-to-face services over SSTs were often regarded as contributing to the stability of a fragile rural economy (Wallcook, 2021). Research into SST use among older people frequently acknowledges that non-use can be motivated by not wanting to do people out of jobs or by a preference for human contact (Dean, 2008; Wu et al., 2020). However, it is seldom considered that in some instances taking the manualised choice is about exercising personal responsibility to participate in society in tangible, noticeable ways. For example, making a deliberate choice to use cash in the village and support the local shop. These choices can be reciprocally appreciated and acknowledged as contributing towards stabilising everyday life for others in the community as well as for the choice maker. To continue the example, the custom given by the person supports the shop's viability, secures the service for others and contributes to making cash transactions worthwhile and sustainable (Wallcook, 2021). Taking the manualised choice may therefore produce socially connective interactions that are part of co-constituting and reproducing a stable sense of neighbourhood and familiarity enacted beyond the individual (Clark et al., 2020). These SST interactions implicate the local workforce and their work tasks so that employment opportunities and how businesses deliver services are stabilised in co-constitution with older people.

Stabilising and co-constituting access to banking services could also be seen in how shop and post office staff were drawn into supporting SST use and facilitating access to cash. Staff willingness to be implicated in wider service provision was attested to by several cases which indicates that workers in local amenities and services can and do act in dementia-friendly ways (Wallcook, 2021). However, a spectrum of actions has been found in another study where some workers (i.e. postal workers, public transport drivers, shopkeepers) were reluctant to meet extra-ordinary needs perceiving it was not their responsibility (Zappella, 2019). Equally, we found that it could be other customers who presented a hindrance by creating obstacles with their bodies and trolleys as they stopped to chat in the supermarket. Anticipating a poor response from some staff and customers may partly explain why some cases chose SSTs and EICTs to stabilise their participation behind closed doors and avoid unwanted social encounters. While this indicates a need for better awareness and consideration towards people with dementia throughout the whole community, participants were also sensitive to the intricacies of situations meaning that people cannot always alter how they act. Furthermore, co-constituting an unhindered daily life for others in the community was a focal point for some of the research participants who wanted to cause the minimum of trouble to others (Wallcook, 2021).

Practical suggestions for a human-friendly society

Our research implicates a number of actors in the interplay with ET use whose actions could reduce technological friction for people with dementia in their everyday lives. Practical suggestions for these actors are given in Table 6.1.

Table 6.1 Audience-specific key messages with practical suggestions and examples.

Audience	Key message	
	Suggestions	*Examples*
Households, families and neighbours	*Knowing a person's preferences when choosing and using ET could facilitate uptake of new devices and contribute to a stable, reassuring everyday life*	
	Pay attention to the most comfortable and familiar ETs.	If needing to replace/update, preserve familiar features.
	Think beyond the device to how it is used.	Some people may prefer receiving, while others prefer making phone calls.
	Be open-minded about which devices will be easier to use.	Try specific makes and models of EICTs before you buy.
	Be ready to support, adapt to changes, notice reciprocal efforts and revisit choices/ adaptations.	Facilitate sharing tasks, for example continuing pumping fuel, but not making payment.
	Consider manualised ways to do a task where ET use is problematic.	Make, for example a physical photo album instead of digital.
	Stay aware of ET capabilities as there may also be restrictions and needs in daily life.	Offer support and reassurance through a physical welfare check if a landline is unsuitable/unusable.
Occupational therapy services	*Including participation outside home and ET use within the scope of practice could smooth a person's transition through societal shifts (i.e. cashless societies), support the possibility to remain at home, and aid timely access to support.*	
	Enable continued use of personally relevant ETs connected to participation outside home.	Design and deliver interventions that tailor, adapt and simplify ET use.
	Enable continued participation that avoids ET use if necessary.	Create alternative, non-technologised solutions.

Audience	Key message	
	Suggestions	Examples
	Optimise the fit between the person's ETs and changing circumstances/abilities.	Gain the person's view of their ET and public space environment to identify (non-)modifiable aspects.
	Investigate new difficulties in ET use as part of wider investigations of support needs and housing.	Difficulties with ET can indicate a pattern of instability in wider participation that requires intervention.
Public services – health, social, financial, transport	*Considering and preventing the problems that ETs can cause and involving people with dementia could make services more inclusive and promote participation.*	
	Remain available through simpler, more familiar means; that is direct telephone and face-to-face contact.	Demanding use of EICTs presents high, and sometimes insurmountable, challenge to many older adults.
	Avoid combinations of SSTs and EICTs with complex identification/authentication demands.	Balance efficiency/security with usability, that is parking meter plus SMS code, online service plus e-ID.
	Remove unnecessary ET barriers and reject procurement of ETs that fail to meet cognitive and other accessibility standards.	Identify exclusionary features of ETs that may cause embarrassment, inconvenience, financial penalty, for example surveillance parking technology.
	Involve older people, particularly with cognitive disabilities, in the procurement of new ETs.	User insights can support more accurate appraisal of ETs' inclusivity.
	Consider the siting of the ET in its wider environmental context.	Balance, for example security, distractions, noise, privacy, proximity to help and a non-technologised alternative.
ET designers	*Reducing the challenge of ETs, especially EICTs, can create conditions that support prolonged ET use.*	
	Reduce the challenge of ETs by considering cognitive usability in ET design.	Reduce navigation demands, minimise steps, increase user control beyond personal devices to those encountered publicly.
	Be guided by inclusive design principles to improve the usability of ET.	Adopt forthcoming cognitive accessibility standards and involve people with dementia in testing ETs.

(Continued)

Table 6.1 (Continued)

Audience	Key message	
	Suggestions	Examples
Policy makers – health, social, financial, transport	*Developing policy that addresses social and infrastructural inequalities of ET use would promote participation in everyday life.*	
	Reduce socioeconomic inequalities to improve access to ETs.	Infrastructure between and within rural/urban areas, for example transport, Internet, banking.
	Create resilient/sustainable banking processes that avoid complex cash, payment and banking ETs.	Ensure access to, or develop, inclusive options, for example cards used with signature, rubber stamp.

Conclusion

For multi-level actors implicated in people with dementia's EICT and SST use, our suggestions are intended to positively influence the interplay and reduce technological friction in everyday life. This should be approached as a flexible process of trial and error given the complexity of surrounding infrastructural, societal and individual conditions found in our research. In general, more appropriate suggestions and adaptations to smooth the interplay may come through shifting away from regarding technology as the solution to the problem. Instead, *consider technology as the problem that might need to be fixed*. Doing this may mean ensuring non-technologised options to uphold the participation rights of people who seek a manualised everyday life in society.

References

Byszewski, A., Aminzadeh, F., Robinson, K., Molnar, F., Dalziel, W., Man Son Hing, M. . . . Marshall, S. (2013). When it is time to hang up the keys: the driving and dementia toolkit – for persons with dementia and caregivers – A practical resource. *BMC Geriatrics, 13*(1), 117. https://doi.org/10.1186/1471-2318-13-117

Clark, A., Campbell, S., Keady, J., Kullberg, A., Manji, K., Rummery, K., & Ward, R. (2020). Neighbourhoods as relational places for people living with dementia. *Social Science & Medicine, 252*, 112927. https://doi.org/10.1016/j.socscimed.2020.112927

Damodaran, L., Olphert, W., & Sandhu, J. (2018). Fit for purpose. In A. Walker (Ed.), *The new dynamics of ageing* (Vol. 1, pp. 169–192). London: Policy Press.

Dean, D.H. (2008). Shopper age and the use of self-service technologies. *Managing Service Quality: An International Journal, 18*(3), 225–238. https://doi.org/10.1108/09604520810871856

DEFRA (2019). *Statistical digest of rural England: January 2019 Edition*. Department for Environment, Food & Rural Affairs, Crown Copyright. https://assets.publishing.service.gov.

uk/government/uploads/system/uploads/attachment_data/file/775109/01_Statistical_
Digest_of_Rural_England_2019_January_edition.pdf

Esteban-Navarro, M.-Á., García-Madurga, M.-Á., Morte-Nadal, T., & Nogales-Bocio,
A.-I. (2020). The rural digital divide in the face of the COVID-19 pandemic in Europe –
recommendations from a scoping review. *Informatics*, 7(4), 54. https://doi.org/10.3390/
informatics7040054

Farmer, T., Robinson, K., Elliott, S.J., & Eyles, J. (2006). Developing and implementing
a triangulation protocol for qualitative health research. *Qualitative Health Research*, 16(3),
377–394. https://doi.org/10.1177/1049732305285708.

Fischl, C., Blusi, M., Lindgren, H., & Nilsson, I. (2020). Tailoring to support digital tech-
nology-mediated occupational engagement for older adults – A multiple case study. *Scandinavian Journal of Occupational Therapy*, 27(8), 577–590. https://doi.org/10.1080/11038
128.2020.1760347

Hare, P. (2019). *How can we really make the Blue Badge work for people with dementia?* Innovations
in dementia. www.innovationsindementia.org.uk/2019/06/how-can-we-really-make-
the-blue-badge-work-for-people-with-dementia/

Hedman, A., Lindqvist, E., & Nygård, L. (2016). How older adults with mild cognitive
impairment relate to technology as part of present and future everyday life: A qualitative
study. *BMC Geriatrics*, 16, 73–73. https://doi.org/10.1186/s12877-016-0245-y

Hegerty, S.W. (2020). "Banking Deserts," Bank branch losses, and neighborhood socioeco-
nomic characteristics in the city of Chicago: A spatial and statistical analysis. *The Professional Geographer*, 72(2), 194–205. https://doi.org/10.1080/00330124.2019.1676801

Hwang, A.S., Jackson, P., Sixsmith, A., Nygård, L., Astell, A., Truong, K.N., & Mihailidis,
A. (2020). Exploring how persons with dementia and care partners collaboratively appro-
priate information and communication technologies. *ACM Transactions on Computer-
Human Interaction*, 27(6), Article 46, 1–38. https://doi.org/10.1145/3389377

Jakobsson, E., Nygård, L., Kottorp, A., & Malinowsky, C. (2019). Experiences from using
eHealth in contact with health care among older adults with cognitive impairment. *Scandinavian Journal of Caring Sciences*, 33(2), 380–389. https://doi.org/10.1111/scs.12634

John, S. (2019, 8 April 2019). *Less-cash, but not cashless*. Currency Conference 2019, Dubai.
www.bankofengland.co.uk/speech/2019/sarah-john-currency-conference-2019

Köttl, H., Gallistl, V., Rohner, R., & Ayalon, L. (2021). "But at the age of 85? Forget it!":
Internalized ageism, a barrier to technology use. *Journal of Aging Studies*, 59, 100971.
https://doi.org/10.1016/j.jaging.2021.100971

Langford, M., Higgs, G., & Jones, S. (2021). Understanding spatial variations in accessibility
to banks using variable floating catchment area techniques. *Applied Spatial Analysis and
Policy*, 14, 449–472 https://doi.org/10.1007/s12061-020-09347-2

Malinowsky, C., Almkvist, O., Nygård, L., & Kottorp, A. (2012). Individual variabil-
ity and environmental characteristics influence older adults' abilities to manage everyday technology. *International Psychogeriatrics*, 24(3), 484–495. https://doi.org/10.1017/
s1041610211002092

Margot-Cattin, I., Kuhne, N., Kottorp, A., Cutchin, M., Ohman, A., & Nygard, L. (2019).
Development of a questionnaire to evaluate out-of-home participation for people with
dementia. *American Journal of Occupational Therapy*, 73(1), 7301205030p7301205031–
7301205030p7301205010. https://doi.org/10.5014/ajot.2019.027144

Marston, H.R., & van Hoof, J. (2019). "Who doesn't think about technology when designing urban environments for older people?" A case study approach to a proposed extension

of the WHO's age-friendly cities model. *International Journal of Environmental Research &
Public Health, 16*(19), 3525. https://doi.org/10.3390/ijerph16193525

Neville, S., Adams, J., Napier, S., Shannon, K., & Jackson, D. (2018). "Engaging in my
rural community": Perceptions of people aged 85 years and over. *International Journal of
Qualitative Studies on Health and Well-being, 13*(1), 1503908. https://doi.org/10.1080/17
482631.2018.1503908

Nygård, L., Rosenberg, L., & Kottorp, A. (2016). *Users manual: Everyday technology use
questionnaire, English version.* Stockholm, Sweden: Department of Neurobiology, Care Sciences and Society, Division of Occupational Therapy, Karolinska Institutet.

OECD. (2016). *OECD comparative study: Digital government strategies for transforming public
services in the welfare areas.* OECD. www.oecd.org/gov/digital-government/Digital-
Government-Strategies-Welfare-Service.pdf

Olsson, T., & Viscovi, D. (2020). Who actually becomes a silver surfer? Prerequisites for
digital inclusion. *Javnost – The Public, 27*(3), 230–246. https://doi.org/10.1080/131832
22.2020.1794403

Parke, B., Boltz, M., Hunter, K.F., Chambers, T., Wolf-Ostermann, K., Adi, M.N., Feld-
man, F. & Gutman, G. (2017). A scoping literature review of dementia-friendly hospital
design. *The Gerontologist, 57*(4), e62–e74. https://doi.org/10.1093/geront/gnw128

Patomella, A.-H., Kottorp, A., Malinowsky, C., & Nygård, L. (2011). Factors that impact
the level of difficulty of everyday technology in a sample of older adults with and without
cognitive impairment. *Technology and Disability, 23*, 243–250. https://doi.org/10.3233/
TAD-2011-0331

Patomella, A.-H., Kottorp, A., & Nygård, L. (2013). Design and management features of
everyday technology that challenge older adults. *British Journal of Occupational Therapy,
76*(9), 390–398. https://doi.org/10.4276/030802213X13782044946229

Petrie, H., & Darzentas, J. (2018). Accessibility and usability of self-service terminals, tech-
nologies and systems: Introduction to the special thematic session. In K. Miesenberger &
Kouroupetroglou (Eds.), *Computers helping people with special needs, Part 1* (pp. 291–294).
New York, NY: Springer International.

Rapoport, M., Hyde, A., & Naglie, G. (2020). Transportation issues in dementia. In A.
Innes, D. Morgan, & J. Farmer (Eds.), *Remote and rural dementia care: Policy, research and
practice* (pp. 213). London: Policy Press.

Salemink, K., Strijker, D., & Bosworth, G. (2017). Rural development in the digital age:
A systematic literature review on unequal ICT availability, adoption, and use in rural areas.
Journal of Rural Studies, 54, 360–371. https://doi.org/10.1016/j.jrurstud.2015.09.001

Sveriges Riksbank. (2020, 29 October 2020). *Cash free – not problem-free.* Riksbanken. www.
riksbank.se/en-gb/payments – cash/payments-in-sweden/payments-in-sweden-2020/1.-
the-payment-market-is-being-digitalised/cash-free – not-problem-free/

Swaffer, K. (2021). Chapter 1 – Rehabilitation: A human right for everyone. In L.-F.Low &
K.Laver (Eds.), *Dementia rehabilitation* (pp. 1–13). London: Academic Press. https://doi.
org/10.1016/B978-0-12-818685-5.00001-5

Wallcook, S. (2021). *Conditions of everyday technology use and its interplay in the lives of older
adults with and without dementia.* [Doctoral thesis, Karolinska Institutet]. Stockholm.
https://openarchive.ki.se/xmlui/handle/10616/47651

Wallcook, S., Malinowsky, C., Nygård, L., Charlesworth, G., Lee, J., Walsh, R., Gaber,
S., Kottorp, A. (2020). The perceived challenge of everyday technologies in Sweden, the United States and England: Exploring differential item functioning in the

everyday technology use questionnaire. *Scandinavian Journal of Occupational Therapy, 27*(8), 554–566. https://doi.org/10.1080/11038128.2020.1723685

Wallcook, S., Nygård, L., Kottorp, A., Gaber, S., Charlesworth, G., & Malinowsky, C. (2021a). Kaleidoscopic associations between life outside home and the technological environment that shape occupational injustice as revealed through cross-sectional statistical modelling. *Journal of Occupational Science, 28*(1), 42–58. https://doi.org/10.1080/144 27591.2020.1818610

Wallcook, S., Nygard, L., Kottorp, A., & Malinowsky, C. (2021b). The use of everyday information communication technologies in the lives of older adults living with and without dementia in Sweden. *Assistive Technology, 33*(6), 333–340. https://doi.org/10.10 80/10400435.2019.1644685

World Health Organization. (2007). *Global age-friendly cities: A guide.* World Health Organization. www.who.int/ageing/publications/Global_age_friendly_cities_Guide_English.pdf

World Health Organization. (2017). *Global action plan on the public health response to dementia 2017–2025.* https://apps.who.int/iris/bitstream/handle/10665/259615/978924151 3487-eng.pdf?sequence=1

Wu, R., Liu, M., & Kardes, F. (2020). Aging and the preference for the human touch. *Journal of Services Marketing, 35*(1), 29–40. https://doi.org/10.1108/jsm-09-2019-0366

Zappella, E. (2019). How can we build more inclusive communities regarding individuals with cognitive fragility? An exploratory analysis of the perceptions of members in a Lombardian community. *International Journal of Psychiatric Research, 2*(1), 1–8.

Chapter 7

Thinkability

A new app for cognitive stimulation for people with dementia

Harleen Kaur Rai, Justine Schneider,
Martin Orrell

Background

People with dementia can face difficulties with staying mentally stimulated and often require support with managing their symptoms (National Institute for Health and Care Excellence, 2018). Additionally, dementia care can have a big impact on families and friends with the majority of the care and support provided by unpaid or informal carers which may lead to increased burden and decreased quality of life (QoL) (Alzheimer's Research UK, 2015; Wittenberg et al., 2019). Considering this multi-level impact of dementia and the lack of appropriate resources to reduce disease burden, there is a growing need for more innovative approaches to better support people with dementia in their daily lives (Prince et al., 2015). Cognitive stimulation therapy (CST) is an evidence-based, psychological intervention for people with dementia which offers mentally stimulating activities within a social setting. Findings from previous research have shown that it can lead to improvements in cognition and QoL (Spector et al., 2003). CST is the only non-pharmacological treatment recommended by the National Institute for Health & Clinical Excellence guidelines for treating the cognitive symptoms of dementia in the United Kingdom (National Institute for Health and Care Excellence, 2018). For people who are either unable or unwilling to attend groups, an individual version of CST (iCST) has also been developed and is usually delivered at home by a carer (Yates et al., 2015). Results from a large-scale study have shown that iCST can benefit the QoL of carers and lead to improvements in the quality of the relationship between the person with dementia and carer (Orrell et al., 2017). Other innovations include offering CST groups via Zoom, a video-conferencing software, which has been a result of the social restrictions and suspension of services for older people with dementia caused by the COVID-19 pandemic (Cheung & Peri, 2021). Findings from a systematic review suggest that the effects of cognitive stimulation can indeed be maximised through the added use of computers as their content and platforms can be cognitively stimulating by themselves (Yates et al., 2016). However, in another systematic review, researchers point out that people with dementia have clear unmet needs regarding the availability of computerised resources that offer

DOI: 10.4324/9781003289005-10

independent activities for entertainment and fun, and as a meaningful way to spend time (Joddrell & Astell, 2016). Furthermore, there is a lack of evidence-based technology which can provide remote support such as mental stimulation. There is currently no such resource for people with dementia that is easily accessible from home and can be scaled up to reach a maximum number of users both nationally and internationally. Therefore, researchers at the University of Nottingham developed the Thinkability application (app), which allows people with dementia and carers to engage in a form of CST together using interactive touch-screen technology. The app provides a range of game-like discussion activities and combines elements of CST and iCST with multi-media stimuli to promote mental stimulation, engagement and social interaction for both the person with dementia and the carer.

Road to Thinkability

To successfully implement effective interventions that are fit for purpose, there is a need for a rigorous approach towards development with the help of appropriate frameworks. In line with previous CST and iCST work (Spector et al., 2003; Yates et al., 2015), the Medical Research Council (MRC) Framework for the development of complex interventions was applied in the development of Thinkability (Rai et al., 2020). The MRC Framework offers a rigorous approach for evaluating complex interventions and describes the entire process from development to implementation (Table 7.1) (Craig et al., 2008). For the development of novel technology, van Gemert-Pijnen et al. (2011) have developed the Centre for eHealth Research (CeHRes) roadmap, which includes distinct development phases from contextual inquiry to summative evaluation (Table 7.1). Together with the MRC Framework, this enables a highly systematic approach towards the development of Thinkability to ensure the application is both usable and useful.

The University of Nottingham collaborated with EuMediaNet, a software development company in Maastricht, the Netherlands. The teams decided to adopt an agile approach during which development takes place in an iterative and dynamic manner while collaborating with all relevant stakeholders (Larman & Basili, 2003). This approach was especially suitable as it encourages meaningful involvement of end users throughout the development process. While there are different types agile development approaches, we chose the 'Scrum' method given its focus on efficient project management, iterative development and feedback loops (Dybå & Dingsøyr, 2008). This allowed the research and software development teams, in collaboration with people with dementia and carers, to monitor the development of Thinkability on a regular basis and ensure it met the necessary requirements. The process led to the development of three prototypes over three consecutive stages following the development and feasibility/piloting phases of the MRC Framework, and the contextual inquiry, value specification, design and summative evaluation phases of the CeHRes roadmap (see Figure 7.1).

Table 7.1 Stages and activities of the MRC Framework (Craig et al., 2008) and CeHRes roadmap (van Gemert-Pijnen et al., 2011).

MRC Framework	CeHRes roadmap
Development	Contextual inquiry
• Identifying the evidence base (e.g. systematic review)	• Identifying problems and needs of intended users (e.g. literature review, field observations, interviews, workshops)
• Identifying or developing theory (e.g. scope existing theories and interviewing stakeholders)	
• Modelling the process and outcomes (e.g. pre-trial economic evaluation, focus groups, surveys, case studies)	
Feasibility/piloting	Value specification
• Testing procedures for acceptability, determining appropriate sample size, estimating rates of recruitment	• Determining most favourable solutions based on stakeholders' values
Evaluation	Design
• Assessing clinical and cost effectiveness (e.g. RCT)	• Building prototypes to fit values and user requirements (e.g. focus groups and field-testing)
• Understanding processes (e.g. process evaluation)	
Implementation	Operationalisation
• Getting evidence into practice	• Activities to introduce, adopt and employ the technology in practice (e.g. creating a business model)
• Surveillance, monitoring and long term outcomes	
	Summative evaluation
	• Assessment of the impact of eHealth technologies in clinical, organisational and behavioural terms

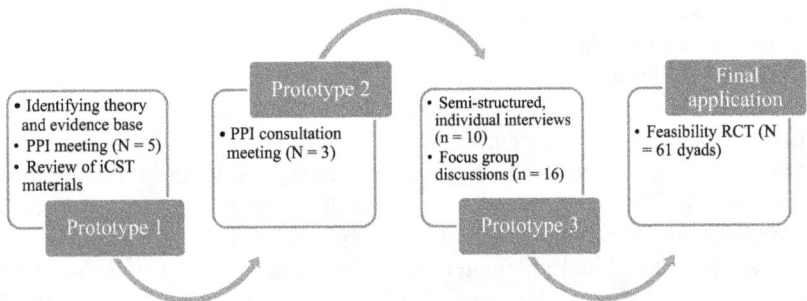

Figure 7.1 Development of Thinkability.

Stage 1: Developing and evaluating the first prototype

To develop the first prototype of Thinkability, the researchers (1) identified the evidence base and theory supporting the use of CST and technology, (2) organised a Patient and Public Involvement (PPI) consultation meeting and (3) reviewed existing iCST materials (Rai et al., 2020). The first prototype was then evaluated in an informal consultation with people with dementia and carers.

Identifying the theory and evidence base

CST is multifaceted and its key principles reinforcing mental stimulation, use of reminiscence, enjoyment and more, contribute to its effectiveness (Spector et al., 2003). Stimulating activities targeting certain neuropsychological domains, like in CST, can improve cognition (Hall et al., 2013). The effects of CST on QoL may be explained through the mediating role of improvements on cognitive functioning (Woods et al., 2012). The large-scale RCT with iCST did not find positive effects on the cognition and QoL for people with dementia (Orrell et al., 2017). Although iCST is as multifaceted as group CST, the trial results may be the result of a lack of adherence to the intervention. Alternatively, the lack of a social setting in iCST may have contributed to the results. Researchers encouraged the exploration of innovative approaches towards delivering iCST such as the use of a computerised platform as it could lead to different results. For instance, there is a potential to increase adherence through monitoring progress on a device and there is more scope for different types of stimulating activities which can include media.

In terms of digital cognitive interventions for people with dementia, Garcia-Casal et al. (2017) concluded that such interventions led to significant improvements in cognition, depression and anxiety among people with dementia. However, considering these interventions vary greatly, there is a need for more research to better understand their effects. Regarding the platform on which an intervention is offered, there is evidence suggesting that touch-screen tablets are highly intuitive for older people with dementia (Lim et al., 2013). Moreover, Tyack and Camic (2017) found that touch-screen interventions, which are simple, intuitive, aesthetically pleasant and error free, can lead to several benefits for people with dementia including mood, mental health and social relationships. The intervention should include slightly challenging content so the user is invited to apply more complex cognitive skills rather than simpler ones (Tyack & Camic, 2017). In addition, these interventions can have a positive impact on the well-being of carers by decreasing their burden and improving the quality of the relationship with the person they are caring for by spending more time together.

The separate findings on the use of CST, iCST and touch-screen technology for people with dementia and carers are promising. By integrating cognitive stimulation within a digital application, Thinkability is therefore well placed to offer better outcomes for people with dementia and carers compared to paper-based CST and iCST. The rationale is that benefits of computer use on cognitive functioning and QoL may add to the overall effectiveness of the intervention as a result of engaging with novel and stimulating activities.

First PPI consultation meeting

A PPI consultation meeting was organised with people with dementia and carers (N = 5) to explore their attitudes towards a potential cognitive stimulation app based on CST, and to identify facilitators and barriers towards using (touchscreen) technology in general. Main discussion topics included willingness to use a cognitive stimulation app, potential benefits and limitations, and practical issues.

Participants were enthusiastic about CST and said they would welcome it in any format whether it was computerised or paper-based. For a computerised version, they suggested that there would be a need for personalisation according to the person's background, and a diverse selection of activities. Some participants mentioned the need for a facilitator to provide support with the activities. This could be an informal or a paid carer. Being able to keep track of which activities were done and when was also considered to be a useful feature.

Attitudes towards technology were diverse with some more willing to use technology than others. A person with dementia mentioned she would not want to be pushed to use technology, which might happen through the involvement of a carer. However, there was consensus among the group that people with dementia need to be empowered and to be made aware of how to handle technology. Lastly, for technology to be useful for people with dementia, it should be free of jargon and difficult terminology as much as possible.

Review of paper-based iCST materials

A second PPI consultation meeting was organised with people with dementia and carers (N = 7) during which participants were given iCST manuals and, in pairs, were asked to review the materials and discuss which qualities they liked or disliked. Participants were also asked to discuss how the iCST manual could best be adapted into a touch-screen version. The group discussion included key topics related to the design, content and feasibility of a potential cognitive stimulation app.

All participants liked the iCST manual in terms of content and usefulness, and the comments for improvements were mostly related to practicalities and some lay-out issues for a potential app. For instance, participants agreed there was too much text on one page and that this would have to be minimised significantly for an app. Keeping with this, although the content was perceived to be useful, participants felt that there were too many activities (75 in total) and that researchers would need to consider which activities could be better for adaptation than others. Flexibility was one of the most important needs for an app. The amount of time needed to complete an activity and the whole app would differ between people with dementia. Therefore, people should be able to use it according to their own pace and decide per day how much time they would like to spend on the app. Participants also emphasised some challenges: it might be difficult for some users to maintain concentration for a certain period of time. In addition, their physical condition might prevent them from using the app (e.g. pains).

After the PPI consultation meeting, the research and software development teams evaluated each iCST activity for its potential to be adapted onto a touch-screen platform. Considerations included the added level of interactivity and novelty, promoting mental stimulation or the sharing of ideas and opinions, and overall enjoyment. On the basis of these considerations, all activities were first categorised per iCST theme and type of activity (e.g. a quiz, picture game, audio) and then ranked according to priority for development by the research and software development teams separately. Following the advice from the PPI group members, the researchers decided to reduce the amount of iCST activities from 75 to 21 for the initial iCST app. This encompassed one activity per theme. After reaching a consensus in terms of priority, a first small selection of activities was developed for the first prototype.

Prototype 1

Content

Following the principles of an agile approach towards development, we developed a working prototype. which allowed end users to operate a device which resembles the final product, and hence to obtain more accurate feedback.

Prototype 1 consisted of several key features: a home screen, welcome/introduction, two activities (Sounds and Past Events) with two levels of difficulty, and a timeline. When opening the app, users were first presented with the home screen (Figure 7.2). From here, users could choose to read the welcome section including some general information and tips about using the app, or choose a new Thinkability activity to start.

A short summary preceded the actual activity to provide some instructions. Within the activity itself, there was a timer, which counted down from 20 minutes to keep track of the amount of time spent, and some buttons to move through the activity or finish it (Figure 7.2). Lastly, each completed activity was added to a timeline on the home screen. This enabled users to keep track of their journey through the app.

Evaluation

A small informal consultation was organised with two people with dementia and one carer. Main discussion topics included the design, navigation and content of the prototype. Each participant was given a touch-screen tablet to use

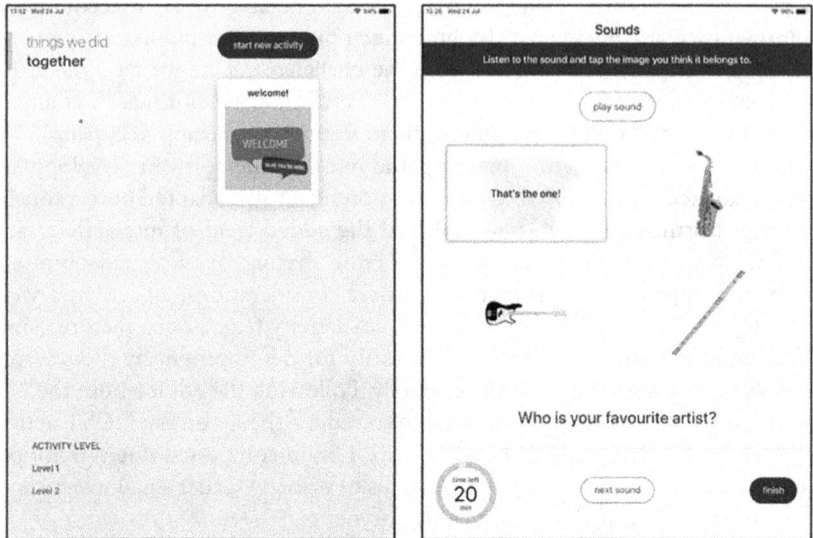

Figure 7.2 Screenshots of Prototype 1: home screen (left) and the Sounds activity (right)

the prototype for 15 to 20 minutes, which was followed by a group discussion of approximately one hour. Researchers made observations and took detailed notes during the meeting which were shared with EuMediaNet.

The design was evaluated positively with a minor suggestion to increase the size of the text. Use of colours was deemed appropriate as well. One example came from a person with dementia who did not seem to have any problems with the colour scheme despite being colour blind. The navigation was intuitive as participants were able to move through different parts of the prototype with little difficulty. However, the purpose of the timeline was not clear and needed additional explanation from the researcher.

In terms of the content, the participants were positive about the type of activities and found them relevant and enjoyable. It was suggested to simplify the discussion questions by directing them to the person with dementia rather than having a general question. Participants also had a look at the introduction section and suggested adding an image of a person with dementia and a carer using the app together to clarify how it is meant to be used. Some changes were suggested to the language to make it more suitable. Suggestions included shortening the sentences and improving on the overall sentence structure. Some words were discussed in more detail for example using 'finish activity' rather than 'stop activity'. Lastly, participants were keen on seeing more levels included in the future.

Stage 2: Developing and evaluating the second prototype

Content

Following the feedback from the PPI consultation meeting, five additional activities were developed leading to seven in total. These new activities (Garland, Hangman, Odd One Out, The Price is Right, Useful Tips) were chosen based on the initial selection of activities during the review of iCST materials. The aim was to have a diverse selection and therefore included several types of activities such as a number game, categorisation activity and a video. The introduction section was simplified and an image displaying two people interacting with a tablet was added. Lastly, some bugs in the system were removed such as incomplete captions within activities.

Evaluation

Prototype 2 was evaluated in four focus groups and ten semi-structured individual interviews with 13 people with dementia and 13 carers. The groups included one with people with dementia ($n = 4$), one with family carers ($n = 4$) and two mixed groups with both ($n = 8$) (Rai, Griffiths, et al., 2020). The interview participants were additionally invited to complete a short usability and acceptability questionnaire (Castilla et al., 2016).

Following thematic analysis of the qualitative data, the following four main themes emerged (Rai et al., 2020): 'approaches to technology', 'quality of Thinkability', 'perceived benefits of Thinkability' and 'involvement of a relative or friend'.

Participants mentioned that it would be helpful for older people to have some prior experience with technology before using something like Thinkability in addition to being familiar with the platform or operating system:

> 'It's like suddenly if you was given a new laptop, how would you feel, because it's now a different system. . . . You've gone over to Apple or something like that . . . you would feel lost I'd tell ya!' – Person with dementia.

The majority of the participants were enthusiastic about the app and found it to be useful. Some participants also appreciated the combination of mentally stimulating and discussion content:

> 'I liked the, sort of, you do one thing with the sounds and there's a second bit and that's a question and that's the conversation, I quite liked that idea'. – Carer.

The variety of the activities was thought to be appropriate, but a clear need for more diverse content was identified for the app to retain its appeal, and to cater towards the interests of as many people as possible.

Observations indicated that the app was intuitive for most participants and although the navigation was generally considered to be appropriate, there was a need for better signposting and clearer button placement. Participants noted that the images and text could both be slightly bigger but they were rated well in terms of clarity:

> 'I understand what each one is showing and that's all that's necessary for it to do. So long as the image is clear I don't see a problem, and generally speaking they are clear'. – Person with dementia.

In terms of possible benefits of Thinkability, participants mentioned mental stimulation, spending quality time together, sharing ideas and opinions, and enjoyment:

> 'I think anything that you do, you do together that stimulates the brain at any time, even if it's a short space of time, I'll have a go at it.' – Carer.

Lastly, some participants with dementia expressed a preference for using Thinkability on their own or at least to have the choice, saying that a family member or friend might not always be available. Others preferred to do the activities with another person and found it more enjoyable.

The usability and acceptability were assessed by five people with dementia and five carers. Thinkability was rated well in multiple areas namely: its ease of use, usefulness and suitability of the letter/button size for both people with dementia and carers, suggesting that the overall design was appropriate (Rai et al., 2020). Carers felt more confident while using the app than people with dementia and were also more willing to use it frequently suggesting that the navigation of the Thinkability may not be as intuitive for people with dementia as it is for carers.

Stage 3: Developing and evaluating the third prototype

Content

On the basis of the findings from the focus groups and interviews, the third prototype was expanded with the full range of 21 activities (Table 7.2). Some suggestions for new activities given by the participants were incorporated in the third prototype such as a word search and a quiz. The majority of the improvements were related to the design of the app and activities. For instance, some participants felt rushed while doing an activity due to the timer counting down

Table 7.2 List of 21 activities included in prototype 3.

Activity name	Activity type
Arts	Discussion
Being Active	Game
Being Creative	Game
Brainstorm	Game
Food	Game and discussion
Globe Trotter	Game and discussion
In Pairs	Game and discussion
iSpy	Game and discussion
My Life	Discussion
Odd One Out	Game and discussion
Old Wives' Tales	Discussion
Past Events	Discussion
Sayings	Game and discussion
Sounds	Game and discussion
Spaceman	Game
Sudoku	Game
The Price is Right	Game and discussion
Toys Are Us	Discussion
Trivia Quiz	Game
Useful Tips	Discussion
Word Search	Game

the amount of minutes. Therefore, the timer was changed to count up to 20 minutes with participants being able to spend more time on it if they wanted to. In addition, the activity level was added in the top right corner so it would be visible while completing the activity. The language was deemed appropriate and free of jargon; however, more changes to the discussion questions were necessary. As a result, the questions were written to be more open and relatable. Furthermore, some participants suggested to add a little prompt above the question saying 'discuss' to clarify the purpose of the questions. Lastly, some more contexts were provided to the Garland activity (renamed as Being Creative) to clarify it is an activity which can be done without the tablet.

Evaluation

A feasibility RCT was conducted with prototype 3 to evaluate the feasibility of conducting a full-scale RCT with Thinkability compared to a treatment-as-usual (TAU) control group. The study set out to assess aspects of usability, feasibility and potential effectiveness for people with dementia and carers including rates of recruitment and retention, acceptability of the outcome measures, and intervention fidelity and usability (Rai et al., 2021b). On the basis of previous iCST research and findings from the development activities, participants in the experimental group were advised to use Thinkability for two or three times a week and to use it for 30 minutes each time (e.g. two or three activities a week). This was monitored through weekly telephone calls from the research team and back-end tracking using analytics. Key outcomes included cognition and QoL for the person with dementia and QoL for the carer which were examined at baseline, and at 5 and 11 weeks post-baseline (Rai et al., 2021b).

A total of 61 people with mild to moderate dementia and their carers were randomised to the Thinkability ($n = 31$) or TAU control group ($n = 30$) for 11 weeks. In the Thinkability group, 77% used the app for 20 minutes or more each week but only 11% used it for 60 minutes per week or more as per the recommendations. Qualitative data suggested that though Thinkability was deemed to be usable and enjoyable, participants found the content too easy and would complete the activities relatively quickly and therefore, spend less time on the app. More tailored and appropriate content may increase fidelity (Rai et al., 2021a). The overall design of the app in terms of the layout, navigation, and colour scheme was considered to be appropriate. In terms of outcomes, carers using Thinkability rated their QoL better at the second follow up (11 weeks post-baseline) compared to the TAU control group. These findings are in line with previous iCST research, which also only found significant improvements for the carer's QoL suggesting that a carer-led cognitive stimulation programme may be helpful to the carer him/herself (Orrell et al., 2017). Such benefits on well-being may be explained through a decrease in burden or an improvement in the quality of the relationship between themselves and the person they are caring for (Tyack & Camic, 2017). For people with dementia, no significant differences were found on any of the outcome measures (Rai et al., 2021a). Astell et al. (2018) investigated the effectiveness of a group-based, computerised reminiscence and conversation tool. Results showed significant improvements in the cognition and QoL of people with dementia following the intervention, which is in line with previous group CST research findings (Spector et al., 2003). This potentially suggests that elements such as a group setting or a structured approach towards delivery may be essential in obtaining benefits on cognition and QoL for the person with dementia.

In terms of qualitative findings and benefits, two dyads in the post-trial interviews mentioned that Thinkability had helped the person with dementia to feel more confident about their cognitive abilities and their abilities to use technology (Rai et al., 2021a). For one dyad, this increase in confidence subsequently led the person with dementia to engage with other cognitive activities which he had previously not done. These findings are in line with previous research: Asghar et al. (2018) found that assistive technology could encourage people with dementia to undertake activities that they were previously unable or reluctant to. Similarly, Tyack and Camic (2017) found that mastery of a touch-screen intervention for people with dementia could lead to increased confidence in own abilities, feelings of empowerment and pride.

Summary and future directions

Given that the prevalence of dementia is set to increase in the coming years, there will be an increased need for sustainable, affordable and scalable solutions to support people with dementia. Thinkability offers such a solution: the app is easy to access from home; it only requires a single download with a one-off payment, and it includes a wide range of activities, which can be updated in real time. Furthermore, the Thinkability app is well placed to reach underserved communities of people with dementia, for example those who live more rurally or those who are uncomfortable with attending groups; this may help to reduce inequalities in terms of care and support received.

The development process, over the course of multiple stages and small-scale studies, has demonstrated that an agile approach towards technology development where all relevant stakeholders are involved can be effective in creating suitable technology for people with dementia and carers. However, within our studies, we found that agile development requires a quick turn-around meaning that when a prototype is developed, it should be evaluated by users as soon as possible. Given the practicalities of conducting research, which require sufficient time for study preparation, this is not always possible. Therefore, to add more value to development, it is recommended to involve one or two people with dementia as co-researchers throughout the development process in order to receive consistent feedback. Furthermore, the development process can be supported by using appropriate frameworks to better understand the process and determine the necessary research activities. These recommendations are useful in creating an intervention which is fit for purpose and has better potential to be successfully implemented into practice.

In terms of the evaluation, feedback from people with dementia and carers indicated that Thinkability could be useful and had good usability. The majority of the participants found Thinkability to be enjoyable; however, for people who had milder dementia, the activities were found to be less challenging and therefore, less mentally stimulating. Adding more relevant content in the form of activities and levels, which are tailored to individual needs and interests, would help make Thinkability more engaging. This is also recommended for future touch-screen interventions for people with dementia to ensure an appropriate level of personalisation. Preliminary results are in accordance with previous iCST research and show improvements in the QoL of carers in a small sample. Furthermore, Thinkability has been deemed to be an enjoyable app appropriate for mental stimulation and engagement. These findings contribute to the existing but limited body of research surrounding computerised cognitive stimulation and will therefore be relevant for multiple stakeholders looking to develop or participate in such interventions. However, large-scale studies investigating the formal effectiveness of such interventions are still lacking. Therefore, it is recommended to conduct a fully powered RCT to determine the cost-effectiveness of Thinkability. If individual benefits on cognition and

QoL can be established, these could lead to reduced excess disability, longer residence at home and perhaps even decrease admissions to care and/or nursing homes, thus affecting overall costs of care.

References

Alzheimer's Research UK. (2015). *Dementia in the family: The impact on carers.* Alzheimer's Research UK. www.alzheimersresearchuk.org/wp-content/uploads/2019/09/Dementia-in-the-Family-The-impact-on-carers1.pdf

Asghar, I., Cang, S., & Yu, H. (2018). Usability evaluation of assistive technologies through qualitative research focusing on people with mild dementia. *Computers in Human Behavior, 79,* 192–201. https://doi.org/10.1016/j.chb.2017.08.034

Astell, A.J., Smith, S.K., Potter, S., & Preston-Jones, E. (2018). Computer interactive reminiscence and conversation aid groups-delivering cognitive stimulation with technology. *Alzheimer's & Dementia, 4,* 481–487. https://doi.org/10.1016/j.trci.2018.08.003

Castilla, D., Garcia-Palacios, A., Miralles, I., Breton-Lopez, J., Parra, E., Rodriguez-Berges, S., & Botella, C. (2016). Effect of Web navigation style in elderly users. *Computers in Human Behavior, 55,* 909–920. https://doi.org/10.1016/j.chb.2015.10.034

Cheung, G., & Peri, K. (2021). Challenges to dementia care during COVID-19: Innovations in remote delivery of group cognitive stimulation therapy. *Aging & Mental Health, 25*(6), 977–979. https://doi.org/10.1080/13607863.2020.1789945

Craig, P., Dieppe, P., Macintyre, S., Michie, S., Nazareth, I., & Petticrew, M. (2008). Developing and evaluating complex interventions: The new medical research council guidance. *BMJ, 337.* https://doi.org/10.1136/bmj.a1655

Dybå, T., & Dingsøyr, T. (2008). Empirical studies of agile software development: A systematic review. *Information and Software Technology, 50*(9–10), 833–859. https://doi.org/10.1016/j.infsof.2008.01.006

Garcia-Casal, J.A., Loizeau, A., Csipke, E., Franco-Martin, M., Perea-Bartolome, M.V., & Orrell, M. (2017). Computer-based cognitive interventions for people living with dementia: A systematic literature review and meta-analysis. *Aging and Mental Health, 21*(5), 454–467. https://doi.org/10.1080/13607863.2015.1132677

Hall, L., Orrell, M., Stott, J., & Spector, A. (2013). Cognitive stimulation therapy (CST): Neuropsychological mechanisms of change. *International Psychogeriatrics, 25*(3), 479–489. https://doi.org/10.1017/S1041610212001822

Joddrell, P., & Astell, A.J. (2016). Studies involving people with dementia and touchscreen technology: A literature review. *JMIR Rehabilitation and Assistive Technologies, 3*(2), 1–9. https://doi.org/10.2196/rehab.5788

Larman, C., & Basili, V.R. (2003). Iterative and incremental development: A brief history. *IEEE Computer, 36*(6), 47–56. https://doi.org/10.1109/MC.2003.1204375

Lim, F.S., Wallace, T., Luszcz, M.A., & Reynolds, K.J. (2013). Usability of tablet computers by people with early-stage dementia. *Gerontology, 59*(2), 174–182. https://doi.org/10.1159/000343986

National Institute for Health and Care Excellence. (2018). *Dementia: Assessment, management and support for people living with dementia and their carers.* www.nice.org.uk/guidance/ng97/resources/dementia-assessment-management-and-support-for-people-living-with-dementia-and-their-carers-pdf-1837760199109

Orrell, M., Yates, L., Leung, P., Kang, S., Hoare, Z., Whitaker, C., . . . Orgeta, V. (2017). The impact of individual Cognitive Stimulation Therapy (iCST) on cognition, quality of life, caregiver health, and family relationships in dementia: A randomised controlled trial. *PLoS Medicine, 14*(3), 1–22. https://doi.org/10.1371/journal.pmed.1002269

Prince, M., Wimo, A., Guerchet, M., Ali, G.C., Wu, Y.T., & Prina, M. (2015). *World Alzheimer report 2015. The global impact of dementia. An analysis of prevalence, incidence, cost and trends.* Alzheimer's Disease International. www.alz.co.uk/research/WorldAlzheimer-Report2015.pdf

Rai, H.K., Griffiths, R., Yates, L., Schneider, J., & Orrell, M. (2020). Field-testing an iCST touch-screen application with people with dementia and carers: A mixed method study. *Aging & Mental Health, 25*(6), 1008–1018. https://doi.org/10.1080/13607863.2020.178 3515

Rai, H.K., Schneider, J., & Orrell, M. (2020). An individual cognitive stimulation therapy app for people with dementia: Development and usability study of thinkability. *JMIR Aging, 3*(2), e17105. https://doi.org/10.2196/17105

Rai, H.K., Schneider, J., & Orrell, M. (2021a). An individual cognitive stimulation therapy app for people with dementia and carers: Results from a feasibility randomized controlled trial (RCT). *Clinical Interventions in Aging, 16*, 2079–2094. https://doi.org/10.2147/cia. S323994

Rai, H.K., Schneider, J., & Orrell, M. (2021b). An individual cognitive stimulation therapy app for people with dementia and their carers: Protocol for a feasibility randomized controlled trial. *JMIR Research Protocols, 10*(4), e24628. https://doi.org/10.2196/24628

Spector, A., Thorgrimsen, L., Woods, B.R.L., Davies, S.B.M., & Orrell, M. (2003). Efficacy of an evidence-based cognitive stimulation therapy programme for people with dementia. *British Journal of Psychiatry, 183*, 248–254. https://doi.org/10.1192/bjp.183.3.248

Tyack, C., & Camic, P.M. (2017). Touchscreen interventions and the well-being of people with dementia and caregivers: A systematic review. *International Psychogeriatrics, 29*(8), 1261–1280. https://doi.org/10.1017/S1041610217000667

van Gemert-Pijnen, J.E., Nijland, N., van Limburg, M., Ossebaard, H.C., Kelders, S.M., Eysenbach, G., & Seydel, E.R. (2011). A holistic framework to improve the uptake and impact of eHealth technologies. *Journal of Medical Internet Research, 13*(4). https://doi. org/10.2196/jmir.1672

Wittenberg, R., Hu, B., Barraza-Araiza, L., & Rehill, A. (2019). *Projections of older people with dementia and costs of dementia care in the United Kingdom 2019–2040.* www.lse.ac.uk/ cpec/assets/documents/Working-paper-5-Wittenberg-et-al-dementia.pdf

Woods, B., Aguirre, E., Spector, A.E., & Orrell, M. (2012). Cognitive stimulation to improve cognitive functioning in people with dementia. *The Cochrane Database of Systematic Reviews, 2*, 1–54. https://doi.org/10.1002/14651858.CD005562.pub2

Yates, L.A., Leung, P., Orgeta, V., Spector, A., & Orrell, M. (2015). The development of individual cognitive stimulation therapy (iCST) for dementia. *Clinical Interventions in Aging, 10*, 95–104. https://doi.org/10.2147/CIA.S73844

Yates, L.A., Ziser, S., Spector, A., & Orrell, M. (2016). Cognitive leisure activities and future risk of cognitive impairment and dementia: Systematic review and meta-analysis. *International Psychogeriatrics, 28*(11), 1791–1806. https://doi.org/10.1017/S1041610216001137

Chapter 8

Participatory visual arts activities for people with dementia

A review

Aline Cavalcanti Barroso, Harleen Kaur Rai,
Lídia Sousa, Martin Orrell, Justine Schneider

Introduction

The 2019 scoping review on arts and health from the World Health Organization (WHO) concluded that the arts have a major role in health promotion across individuals' lifespan while fostering social participation, independence and cognitive stimulation (Fancourt & Finn, 2019). For dementia, it has been argued that the benefits of the arts could include higher sustained attention, slowing of the rate of cognitive decline, as well as increased well-being and self-esteem of people with dementia, and promote social inclusion (Fancourt & Finn, 2019). Art interventions are usually less costly in comparison with other health interventions, so they do show some economic benefits (Fancourt & Finn, 2019).

Being active and engaged in meaningful activities, such as art activities, is an important determinant of quality of life by people living with dementia (Chung, 2004; Phinney et al., 2007). Generally, as dementia progresses, people have fewer opportunities to engage in satisfying activities, and most people eventually require support for daily life activities (MacPherson et al., 2009). This could significantly reduce their quality of life, by means of loss of independence and autonomy, decrease in social participation, and changes in identity and social roles (Chung et al., 2017; Gillies & Johnston, 2004).

Noice et al. (2013) defined participatory arts as making art as opposed to observing art, of any form, for example visual arts, dance, music or theatre (Noice et al., 2013). One problem in finding evidence regarding participatory visual arts interventions benefits in dementia is the lack of standardisation of the interventions reported in the literature. Some reviews (Beard, 2012; Chancellor et al., 2014; Cowl & Gaugler, 2014) include different types of use of art in individual studies, without differentiating the use of visual arts as an isolated intervention, making it difficult to draw conclusions.

Deshmukh et al. (2018) performed a Cochrane review focusing on the effects of art therapy (i.e. type of psychotherapy which uses art as form of expression) in comparison with non-pharmacological interventions for people with dementia. They searched for randomised controlled trials that evaluated

DOI: 10.4324/9781003289005-11

cognition, behaviour, quality of life, emotional and social aspects. They concluded that there was heterogeneity in the studies leading to insufficient evidence on the efficacy of art therapy with people with dementia (Deshmukh et al., 2018). Windle et al. (2017) set out to explain the mechanisms by which art interventions effect change through a realistic review. Their results showed that with visual art interventions, it is possible for people with dementia to have improvements in their well-being, cognitive processes and social connectedness (Windle et al., 2017).

None of the reviews mentioned earlier had a focus on the evaluation of participatory visual art making. However, there are reasons to believe that participatory arts intervention may bring benefits to people with dementia (Beard, 2012; Chancellor et al., 2014; Cowl & Gaugler, 2014). This review aims to weigh up the evidence for the effects of participatory visual arts on individuals with dementia, taking into consideration the quality of the research presented in the articles. This review adopts the narrative synthesis approach by Popay et al. (2006) and builds on recent reviews by Deshmukh et al. (2018) and Windle et al. (2017). This approach permits the interpretation of qualitative and quantitative findings through argument and reasoning, generating inferences that are robust and evidence-based (Popay et al., 2006). It builds on existing knowledge about arts interventions for people with dementia by the process of narrative synthesis systematic review and follow the four elements as described by Popay et al. (2006) by (1) developing a theory, (2) developing a preliminary synthesis of the findings, (3) exploring the relationships in the studies and (4) assessing the robustness of the synthesis (Figure 8.1).

Objective

The aim of this review is to investigate the effects of interventions using participatory visual arts activities on the mental well-being of people with dementia. This review includes evidence from qualitative, quantitative and mixed-methods studies to evaluate what worked, and to investigate why and how the interventions may affect people with dementia.

Methods

Search strategy

A systematic approach to literature search was used to guarantee replicability of the search process. The search was performed in four databases: MEDLINE, EMBASE, PsycINFO and Applied Social Sciences Index & Abstracts (ASSIA). Search terms included dementia, frontotemporal dementia, AIDS dementia complex, vascular dementia, Alzheimer disease, Alzheimer*,[1] cognitive impairment, art therapy, art, painting, drawing, artists, arts, art therap*, draw*, artist*, craft*, pottery, ceramic, sculpt*, paint*, visual art*, digital art,

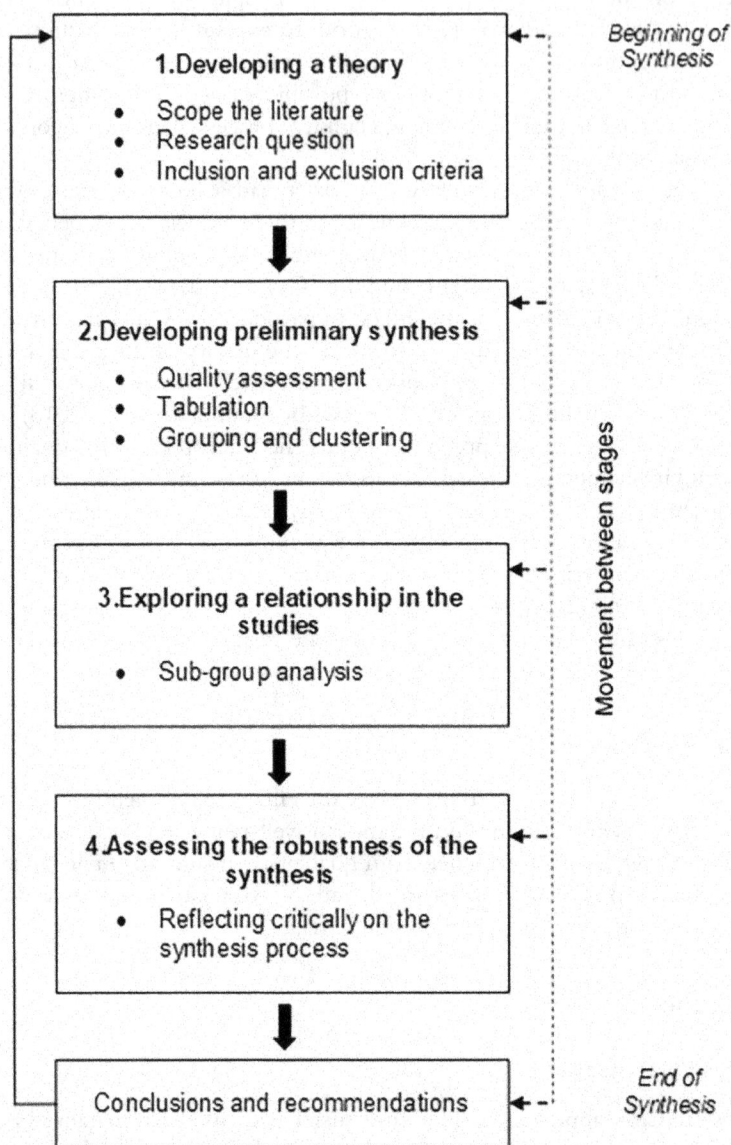

Figure 8.1 Narrative synthesis process
Source: Adapted from McDermott et al. (2013) and Popay et al. (2006)

creative arts therapy and art* creat*. The research search terms were modified to match terms in each database.

Criteria for considering studies

Publications with empirical evidence using qualitative, quantitative and mixed-methods were included.

Types of intervention

The person must be creating something themselves, not just observing and discussing art.

Inclusion criteria

All selected studies involved people living with dementia and participatory artwork interventions, in peer-reviewed English language publications before January 2019.

Quality appraisal

The team used two quality assessment tools to evaluate the studies: the Downs and Black (1998) quality checklist for randomised and non-randomised studies and the Critical Appraisal Skills Programme – CASP (Critical Appraisal Skills Programme, 2017) tool for qualitative and mixed-methods studies. The Downs and Black (1998) checklist contains 27 items in five sub-scales, which includes the reporting of study information, external validity, internal validity (bias), internal validity (confounding) and power. Although this checklist is suitable for the evaluation of randomised and non-randomised studies, four items (8, 13, 14 and 27) were omitted as they were not applicable to the psychosocial interventions evaluated here. The maximum score for the 27 items of the checklist is 31. However, the maximum score that could be obtained for this review was variable according to the study design. For Randomised Controlled Trials the maximum score was 23, while for repeated measures studies (RMS), the maximum was 16.

The CASP checklist consists of ten items. The first nine items have three possible answers: 'yes', 'no' or 'can't tell'. The last item is a general open question about the value of the research. Quality of the studies was rated by number of criteria met. Our quality-related inclusion criteria were as follows:

- For qualitative or mixed-methods studies the threshold for inclusion is met at least 5 of ten items in Critical Appraisal Skills Programme (CASP) criteria (Critical Appraisal Skills Programme, 2017).
- For quantitative studies the threshold for inclusion is met at least 51% of the Downs and Black (1998) checklist criteria.

Exclusion criteria

Exclusions comprised research on participants without dementia or related cognitive disorders, interventions rather than visual arts, case studies, dissertations and conference papers.

Data extraction

The citations found with the search strategy were screened independently by two reviewers (A.C.B. and H.K.R.). The first screening was based on the titles, followed by the exclusion of articles with non-relevant titles, a subsequent screening took place to check the remaining articles' abstracts. After this selection, the same two members of the team evaluated the full text of selected articles and discussed which should be included in the review. The reference lists of included papers were screened to check if other articles needed to be included. The 20 selected studies were classified as Quantitative (*n* = 6), Qualitative (*n* = 8) and Mixed Methods (*n* = 6) (Figure 8.2).

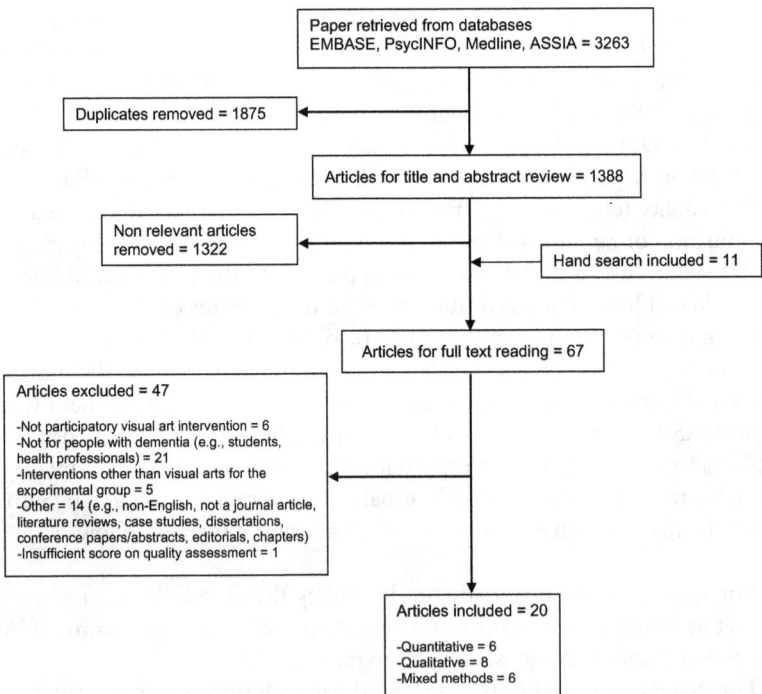

Figure 8.2 Study process selection

Quality assessment

The quality of the studies was independently assessed by three reviewers (A.C.B., H.K.R. and L.S.) to minimise bias. Differences in the scores were discussed and resolved between the three reviewers. Six quantitative studies were appraised using the Downs and Black (1998) checklist and 15 qualitative or mixed-methods studies were appraised using the CASP (Critical Appraisal Skills Programme, 2017) checklist.

Results

For the 15 qualitative and mixed-methods studies, one study (Rentz, 2002) was excluded for not meeting the CASP checklist inclusion criteria and 14 studies were considered valuable and included in the review (Table 8.1). The included studies had appropriate research designs and data collection; considered ethical issues were sufficiently rigorous with data analysis and gave clear statements of findings. None of the studies considered the relationship between researcher and participants and the bias it could have in the research.

Of the six quantitative studies evaluated with Downs and Black (1998) checklist (Table 8.2), none provided information on the confounders. The mean quality score for all qualitative studies was 70.41%.

Characteristics of the studies and interventions

All the 20 studies were classified into five main outcome areas: programme evaluation; cognition; psychological aspects (mood, behaviour, self-esteem); well-being (quality of life, enjoyment, pleasure) and social aspects (Table 8.3). These areas were defined by the researchers conducting this review, rather than being classified by the study authors. Most interventions involved painting or drawing, but clay, collage and printing or photography were also popular. Less common activities were calligraphy, mask making and computer tablet-based art. Table 8.4 provides additional information on the characteristics of each study.

Table 8.5 summarises the characteristics of each intervention and their principal findings. The presence of carers, especially family carers, was also frequent. Eight studies did not have involvement of other people in the activity (Byrne & MacKinlay, 2012; Gross et al., 2015; Kinney & Rentz, 2005; Pérez-Sáez et al., 2018; Rusted et al., 2006; Sauer et al., 2016; Ullan et al., 2013; Windle et al., 2018). Of those, six were art making only.

Among the methods used for data collection were observation of the participants, semi-structured interviews with participants, field journals kept by the facilitators, focus groups with participants and facilitator, satisfaction surveys of the participants, and use of quantitative measures with participants (e.g. scales, inventories and questionnaires). Of these, the most frequent method was the observation of the participants during the activity. Five studies (Gross et al., 2015; Kinney & Rentz, 2005; Pérez-Sáez et al., 2018; Sauer et al., 2016; Windle et al.,

Table 8.1 Methodological quality of the qualitative and mixed-methods studies

CASP Qualitative Checklist (2017)	Belver et al. (2018)	Burnside et al. (2017)	Byrne and MacKinlay (2012)	Camic et al. (2014)	Camic et al. (2016)	Eekelaar et al. (2012)	Flatt et al. (2015)	Hazzan et al. (2016)	Rentz et al. (2002)	Roe et al. (2016)	Schall et al. (2018)	Ullan et al. (2013)	Windle et al. (2018)	Wyatt et al. (2018)	Young et al. (2015)
1. Clear statement of aims?	✓	✓	✓	✓	✓	✓	✓	✓	✓	✓	✓	✓	✓	✓	✓
2. Qualitative methodology appropriate?	✓	✓	✓	✓	✓	✓	✓	✓	–	✓	✓	✓	✓	✓	✓
3. Research design appropriate?	✓	✓	✓	✓	✓	✓	✓	✓	–	✓	✓	✓	✓	✓	✓
4. Recruitment strategy appropriate?	✓	✓	–	✓	✓	✓	✓	✓	–	✓	✓	✓	✓	✓	–
5. Data collected in a way that addressed the research issue?	✓	✓	✓	✓	✓	✓	✓	✓	–	✓	✓	✓	✓	✓	✓
6. Has the relationship between researcher and participants been adequately considered?	–	–	–	–	–	–	–	–	–	–	–	–	–	–	–
7. Ethical issues taken into consideration?	✓	✓	✓	✓	✓	✓	✓	✓	–	✓	✓	✓	✓	–	✓
8. Data analysis sufficiently rigorous?	✓	✓	✓	✓	✓	✓	✓	✓	–	✓	✓	✓	✓	✓	✓
9. Clear statement of findings?	✓	✓	✓	✓	✓	✓	✓	✓	–	✓	✓	✓	✓	✓	✓
10. How valuable is the research?	✓	✓	✓	✓	✓	✓	✓	✓	✓	✓	✓	✓	✓	✓	✓
Total	9	9	8	9	9	9	9	9	2	9	9	9	9	8	8

✓ = criterion met; – = criterion not met

Table 8.2 Methodological quality of the quantitative studies

Downs and Black Checklist (1998)	Gross et al. (2015)	Hattori et al. (2011)	Kinney and Rentz (2005)	Pérez-Sáez et al. (2018)	Rusted et al. (2006)	Sauer et al. (2016)
Reporting	7/8	7/9	7/8	7/8	7/9	6/8
External validity	0/2	0/2	0/2	0/2	0/2	0/2
Internal validity (bias)	4/4	4/6	4/4	4/4	5/6	4/4
Internal validity (confounding)	1/2	4/6	1/2	1/2	4/6	1/2
Total	12/16 (75%) Medium	15/23 (65.21%) Fair	12/16 (75%) Medium	12/16 (75%) Medium	16/23 (69.57%) Medium	11/16 (68.75%) Medium

Score of the study/Score of the checklist after adaptations

Table 8.3 Clustering of the studies by main outcomes areas

Author (year)	Design	Art making	Combination view + make	Control condition	Programme evaluation	Cognition	Psychological aspects	Well-being	Social aspects
Belver et al. (2018)	Qualitative		x	None	x				
Burnside et al. (2017)	Qualitative		x	None	x				
Byrne and Mac Kinlay (2012)	Qualitative	x		None			x		
Camic et al. (2014)	Mixed methods		x	None		x		x	x
Camic et al. (2016)	Qualitative		x	None	x				
Eekelaar et al. (2012)	Mixed methods		x	None		x			
Flatt et al. (2015)	Mixed methods		x	None	x				
Gross et al. (2015)	Quantitative	x		None				x	
Hattori et al. (2011)	Quantitative	x		Calculation		x	x	x	
Hazzan et al. (2016)	Qualitative		x	None	x				
Kinney and Rentz (2005)	Quantitative	x		Traditional activity of the centre				x	

(Continued)

Table 8.3 (Continued)

Author (year)	Design	Art making	Combination view + make	Control condition	Programme evaluation	Cognition	Psychological aspects	Well-being	Social aspects
Pérez-Sáez et al. (2018)	Quantitative	x		None			x	x	
Roe et al. (2016)	Qualitative		x	None	x			x	
Rusted et al. (2006)	Quantitative	x		Activity groups (no emotional expression activities)		x	x	x	x
Sauer et al. (2016)	Quantitative	x		Traditional visual arts activities				x	
Schall et al. (2018)	Mixed methods		x	Waitlist-independent Museum tour			x	x	
Ullan et al. (2013)	Qualitative		x	None	x				
Windle et al. (2018)	Mixed methods		x	Social activities (not art related)	x			x	x
Wyatt and Liggett (2019)	Qualitative	x		None			x		
Young et al. (2015)	Mixed methods		x	None	x				
Total		8	12	6	8	5	6	10	3

2018) have used the Greater Cincinnati Chapter Well-being Observation Tool (GCWBT) (Kinney & Rentz, 2005) or an adapted version of this tool. The GCWBT (Kinney & Rentz, 2005) focuses on short and continuous observations of people with dementia while they participate in a visual art activity. Interviews and qualitative measures were also frequently included in the studies.

The interventions using art making, and art viewing with making are described later, although not all studies reported details of the intervention that would permit thorough comparisons. Lack of full descriptions is a recognised barrier to knowledge advancement in arts-based interventions (Hoffmann et al., 2014; Robb et al., 2018).

Art making (n = 8): Delivered by a facilitator with art training at a dementia care facility (long-term facility, hospital, day centre). People with all levels of dementia participated and most of the studies had included people with severe

Table 8.4 Study characteristics

Author (year)	Country	Design	Type of intervention	PwD	Age	Level of dementia
Belver et al. (2018)	Spain	Qualitative	Combination of art viewing and making	12: 9 female	75–92 (mean 84.4)	Mild to moderate
Burnside et al. (2017)	USA	Qualitative	Combination of art viewing and making	21: 48% male	60–84 (mean 76)	Mild
Byrne and MacKinlay (2012)	Australia	Qualitative	Art making	11	Not informed	Moderate to severe
Camic et al. (2014)	UK	Mixed methods	Combination of art viewing and making	12	58–94 (mean 78.3)	Mild to moderate
Camic et al. (2016)	UK	Qualitative	Combination of art viewing and making	12	58–94 (mean 78.3)	Mild to moderate
Eekelaar et al. (2012)	UK	Mixed methods	Combination of art viewing and making	6: 3 male	68–91 (mean 78.67)	Mild to moderate
Flatt et al. (2015)	USA	Mixed methods	Combination of art viewing and making	10: 5 male	6: 60 years or older	Early/mild
Gross et al. (2015)	USA	Quantitative	Art making	76: 63 female	Mean 84.28	Moderate to severe.
Hattori et al. (2011)	Japan	Quantitative	Art making	39: 21 female; 20 (IG)	mean 75.3 (IG) and 73.3 (CG)	Mild
Hazzan et al. (2016)	Canada	Qualitative	Combination of art viewing and making	8: 8 male	63–91 (mean 80)	Moderate to severe
Kinney and Rentz (2005)	USA	Quantitative	Art making	12: 7 female	65–85	Mild to severe
Pérez-Sáez et al. (2018)	Spain	Quantitative	Art making	30: 22 female	57–93 (mean 79.97)	Mild to severe
Roe et al. (2016)	UK	Qualitative	Combination of art viewing and making	17	Not informed	Not reported

(Continued)

Table 8.4 (Continued)

Author (year)	Country	Design	Type of intervention	PwD	Age	Level of dementia
Rusted et al. (2006)	UK	Quantitative	Art making	45: 31 female; 9 (IG) 38: 30 female; 10 (CG)	67–92	Mild to severe
Sauer et al. (2016)	USA	Quantitative	Art making		Not informed	Moderate to severe
Schall et al. (2018)	Germany	Mixed methods	Combination of art viewing and making	44: 23 female	51–93	Mild to moderate
Ullan et al. (2013)	Spain	Qualitative	Combination of art viewing and making	21: 13 female (workshop)	67–93	Mild to moderate
Windle et al. (2018)	UK	Mixed methods	Combination of art viewing and making	125: 73 female	mean 81.4	Mild to severe
Wyatt et al. (2018)	UK	Qualitative	Art making	8: 4 female (only results of 4 PwD were included)	over 65	Mild
Young et al. (2015)	UK	Mixed methods	Combination of art viewing and making	13: 11 female	60–94	Mild to moderate

CG (control group); IG (intervention group); PwD (people with dementia);

Table 8.5 Characteristics of the interventions

Author (year)	Setting	Delivery by	Description of intervention	Duration	Focus of the study	Principal findings
Belver et al. (2018)	Gallery and day centres	Art educator	Guided visits in small groups (3 or 4 PwD) and art-making workshops (collage, calligraphy, drawing and watercolour)	Six visits 60 to 90 min Making 90 min, 6 weeks	Participant's response to the activities in the programme	Positive effects on programme evaluation – engagement, interest, enjoyment and satisfaction. Additional positive results on well-being, psychological aspects and social aspects.
Burnside et al. (2017)	Gallery	Museum educator and artist (both trained in dementia)	Art viewing and making (5 or 6 dyads) in small groups (watercolour, clay, collage)	View 90 min Making 120 min, three classes	Impact of a museum-based experiential arts programme on PwD and carers	Positive effects on programme evaluation – enjoyment, socialisation, support of personhood and the dyad relationship
Byrne and MacKinlay (2012)	Long-term care facilities	Facilitators (chaplains or pastoral carers) and research assistant	Religious focus art making (11 PwD) in two groups (painting)	Making 60 min, 18 weeks	Art as spirituality mediator and impact of art in depression (person-centred art making)	No effects on psychological aspects. Additional positive results on social aspects, relationship, engagement, and support of personhood
Camic et al. (2014)	Galleries ($n = 2$)	Art educator and art professional	Art viewing and making (5 and 7 dyads) in small groups (painting, colouring, clay, collage, print making etc.)	Weekly viewing 60 min and making 60 min, 8 weeks	Explore the effects of art activities on PwD social and cognitive domains, QoL and ADL, and on carers' burden	Positive results on social aspects, cognition, dyad relationship and support of personhood. No effects ($p > 0.05$) on well-being, ADL and carers' burden

(Continued)

Table 8.5 (Continued)

Author (year)	Setting	Delivery by	Description of intervention	Duration	Focus of the study	Principal findings
Camic et al. (2016)	Galleries (n = 2)	Art educator and art professional	Art viewing and making (5 and 7 dyads) in small groups (painting, colouring, clay, collage, print making etc.)	Weekly viewing 60 min and making 60 min, 8 weeks	Impact of the gallery-based intervention on PwD and carers	Positive effects on programme evaluation. Additional positive results on psychological aspects, social aspects, cognition and dyad relationship
Eekelaar et al. (2012)	Gallery	Art therapist, art educator and researchers	Art viewing and making (6 dyads) in a group (painting)	Weekly viewing 30 min and making 60 min, 3 weeks	Investigate the association between art interventions and cognition (episodic memory and verbal fluency)	Positive effects on cognition – episodic memory and verbal fluency. Additional positive results on social aspects, psychological aspects, dyad relationship and support of personhood
Flatt et al. (2015)	Gallery	Trained facilitator (museum staff)	Guided visit and art-making activity (10 dyads) in small groups (photographic silkscreen technique)	Guided tour 60 min and making 120 min, once	Subjective experiences of PwD and carers that joined the art museum activity	Positive effects on programme evaluation – enjoyment and satisfaction. Additional positive results on cognition, social aspects and support of personhood

Gross et al. (2015)	Long-term care facilities (n = 4)	University student (psychology and art background)	Memories in the Making Programme. Art making (dyads) in groups (copy or freestyle painting and watercolour).	Weekly making 60 min, 12 weeks	Efficacy of the programme on improvements of well-being (interest, attention, pleasure, negative affect, sadness, self-esteem and normalcy)	Positive effects ($p < 0.05$) in some domains of well-being reported by facilitators during sessions (interest, attention, pleasure, self-esteem and normalcy); no effects ($p > 0.05$) on negative affect and sadness. No effects ($p > 0.05$) reported by staff outside sessions
Hattori et al. (2011)	Hospital	Research (1 artist and 3 ST)	Intervention group (5 PwD) – art therapy (colouring abstract patterns) or control group (4 or 5 PwD) (learning therapy using calculation)	Weekly 45 min sessions and daily 15 min at home, 12 weeks	Evaluate the usefulness of art therapy for PwD on cognitive functions (memory and orientation), psychological functions (mood and vitality/ apathy), QoL, behavioural impairment, ADL and carers' burden	Positive effects for intervention group on well-being ($p = 0.038$) and apathy ($p = 0.014$). There were no other significant differences

(Continued)

Table 8.5 (Continued)

Author (year)	Setting	Delivery by	Description of intervention	Duration	Focus of the study	Principal findings
Hazzan et al. (2016)	Hospital and gallery	Artist-instructors	'Artful Moments' pilot programme. Guided visits and art-making activity (up to 6 dyads) in small groups (mask making, painting, photography etc.)	Guided tour 60 min and making 60 min, 27 sessions in 11 months	Level of engagement PwD and impact of the programme on them	Positive effects on program evaluation – engagement, interest, socialisation, support of personhood and carer involvement
Kinney and Rentz (2005)	Day centres ($n = 2$)	Artist	Memories in the Making Programme. Intervention – art making (painting) vs control – traditional adult day centre activities (current events, word games, crafts) in groups (6 PwD)	Weekly making 40 min and control 40 min (participants join both activities)	Evaluation of the programme and contribution to PwD well-being (interest, sustained attention, pleasure, negative affect, sadness, self-esteem and normalcy)	Positive effects ($p < 0.05$) for intervention group in some domains of well-being (interest, sustained attention, pleasure, self-esteem and normalcy); no effects ($p > 0.05$) on negative affect and sadness

Pérez-Sáez et al. (2018)	National Reference Centre for Alzheimer's and Dementia care (CREA)	Facilitators (2 – professionals with experience in organising art workshops for PwD)	Art making in groups (6 to 10 PwD) (pottery)	Weekly making 45 min, 10 weeks	Assess the impact of the activity on PwD mood, self-esteem and well-being (interest, attention, pleasure, negative affect, sadness, self-esteem and normalcy)	Positive effects ($p < 0.05$) on psychological aspects and on some domains of well-being (interest, sustained attention, self-esteem and normalcy); no effects ($p > 0.05$) on pleasure, negative affect and sadness
Roe et al. (2016)	Galleries ($n = 2$)	Museum and gallery staff (4) and artist (2)	Art viewing and making in groups (up to 9 PwD) (drawing, print making etc.)	Guided tour 45 min and making 60 min, 6 sessions in 6 months	Benefits and impact on PwD well-being and feasibility of the sessions and programme	Positive effects on well-being and programme evaluation – socialisation, relationship, creativity and learning.
Rusted et al. (2006)	Day centres and care facilities ($n = 4$)	Art therapist or occupational therapist, and an assistant	Intervention group (up to 6 PwD) – art therapy (drawing and colouring) or control group (up to 6 PwD) (no emotional expression activities)	Weekly 60 min sessions, 40 weeks	Evaluate long-term effects on PwD cognition, depression, behaviour, mood, sociability and well-being	Positive effects ($p < 0.05$) for intervention group on well-being, social aspects and psychological aspects. No effects on cognition

(Continued)

Table 8.5 (Continued)

Author (year)	Setting	Delivery by	Description of intervention	Duration	Focus of the study	Principal findings
Sauer et al. (2016)	Long-term care facilities (n = 3)	Student volunteers (trained in OMA and basics of dementia)	Opening Minds through Art (OMA). Intervention (dyads) group (painting) vs control (dyads) group – traditional visual arts activities (e.g. colouring books, scrapbooking). Control is sub-sample of OMA	Weekly making 40 min, 12 weeks	Assess during OMA behaviours related to PwD well-being (social interest, engagement, pleasure) and ill-being (disengagement, negative affect, sadness, confusion)	Positive effects ($M = 8.81$, $SD = 1.6$; $p = 0.003$) for intervention group on total combined well-being (social interest, engagement, pleasure) and no effects ($p > 0.05$) in total combined ill-being (disengagement, negative affect, sadness, confusion)
Schall et al. (2018)	Gallery	Museum's qualified education staff (7)	ARTEMIS project. Guided tours and art making (3 to 5 dyads) in groups (painting, clay, collage and printing) or wait-list control group (independent visits to the museum)	Weekly guided tour 60 min and making 60 min, 6 weeks	Explore the impact of the activities in emotional PwD well-being, QoL and dementia related behavioural neuropsychiatric symptoms	Positive effects for intervention group on well-being ($t = -3.15$, $p < .05$) and psychological aspects (tNPI total = 2.43; $p = 0.029$)

Ullan et al. (2013)	State day centre	Art educator	Art viewing and making in groups (2 to 11 PwD) (cyanotype, painting and photographs)	Art viewing and making 60 to 90 min, four months	PwD participation in the programme, PwD response to the programme and contribution of the programme to their experience	Positive effects on programme evaluation – enjoyment, learning and support of personhood
Windle et al. (2018)	Residential care homes, a county hospital, community venues and galleries	Artist (2)	Guided tours and art making in groups (up to 15 PwD) (painting, collage, clay, iPad and printing) and control condition at baseline (unstructured social activity with no arts activities)	Weekly art viewing 60 min and making 60 min, 12 weeks	Evaluate PwD well-being (interest, attention, pleasure, normalcy, self-esteem, disengagement, sadness and negative affect), QoL, communication and PwD perceptions about the intervention	Across all sites there were positive effects ($p < 0.05$) for intervention compared to baseline on some domains of well-being (interest, attention, pleasure, self-esteem, negative affect and sadness) in at least in one of the time points. Positive effects ($p < 0.05$) on social aspects and proxy-reported QoL on follow-up

(Continued)

Table 8.5 (Continued)

Author (year)	Setting	Delivery by	Description of intervention	Duration	Focus of the study	Principal findings
Wyatt and Liggett (2019)	Local craft centre (gallery environment)	Researcher as practicing artist (1)	Art making in dyads (painting) PwD and carer painting alongside the researcher	Making 60 min, once	Investigate how PwD can express grief associated with dementia	Positive effects on psychological aspects – negative emotions were less profound at the end of the session
Young et al. (2015)	Gallery	Art educator	Art viewing and making in two groups (5 and 8 PwD) (drawing and colouring)	Weekly art viewing 60 min and making 60 min, 8 weeks	Identify the impact of the activities on PwD verbal fluency and lifetime memory reporting	Positive effects on cognition – verbal fluency (disfluency and semantic clustering) and reports of lifetime memories (when comparing the first with the last week)

ADL (activities of daily living); PwD (people with dementia); QoL (quality of life).

dementia. Usually, the family carers were not involved in the sessions. The art making was mainly painting, drawing and colouring. The length of sessions ranged from 40 to 60 minutes. Length of the study was variable, but most had at least a duration of 12 weeks.

Art viewing + making (n = 12): This was mostly delivered by art educators and museum staff at galleries. Most of the participants had mild to moderate dementia. Carers were often involved in the sessions. The most popular type of art making was painting, drawing, watercolour and colouring; however, most of the studies used a range of art activities. The length of the session was usually two hours. The studies also had a variable length, but typically the programme ran for eight weeks.

Discussion

The studies were very diverse in their design, which might be the reason for the inconsistent findings concerning the effects of the inventions. This has made it hard to generalise about the effects on participants of participatory visual arts. This review indicates that, overall, the use of visual participatory arts interventions appears to have positive effects on cognition, social and psychological well-being of people with dementia. Across all studies, the interventions were largely acceptable to participants and positively evaluated as enjoyable and engaging. However, the comparison of the data in sub-group analysis between the studies shows inconclusive results for specific effects on outcomes.

Attempts to cluster the interventions by tools used or by type of intervention show no clear trends in the effects of visual participatory arts in people with dementia. Cognition, for example, had positive effects in the studies of Camic et al. (2014), Eekelaar et al. (2012) and Young et al. (2015), while Hattori et al. (2011) and Rusted et al. (2006) found no significant effects on participants' cognition. Similar inconsistent results were observed in relation to the other main outcomes evaluated in this review, in some cases, even when the same tool for evaluation was used. While for cognition different measurement instruments were used, five of the studies evaluating well-being (Gross et al., 2015; Kinney & Rentz, 2005; Pérez-Sáez et al., 2018; Sauer et al., 2016; Windle et al., 2018) used adapted versions of the same tool, the Greater Cincinnati Chapter Well-being Observation Tool (GCWBT) (Kinney & Rentz, 2005). These studies showed some similarities with respect to the domain's 'interest' and 'attention', indicating positive effects in all five interventions.

With the use of the GCWBT, the domains of 'interest' and 'attention' showed the engagement of the participants during sessions. These were related to improvements of the participants' well-being during the sessions. However, they can also be related to other outcomes. Attention is connected to cognition (Kinney & Rentz, 2005; Windle et al., 2018) and may indicate that the use of participatory arts activities may increase cognitive stimulation of people with dementia (Windle et al., 2018). The participants also showed greater interest in other people during the activities (Gross et al., 2015; Kinney & Rentz, 2005; Pérez-Sáez et al., 2018; Sauer et al., 2016; Windle et al., 2018), and this could be related to social aspects, such as communication and building relationships with others (Sauer et al., 2016; Windle et al., 2018). Participants appeared to have more positive mood (Pérez-Sáez et al., 2018; Windle et al., 2018) during the activity and possibly increase in their self-esteem (Gross et al., 2015; Kinney & Rentz, 2005; Pérez-Sáez et al., 2018; Windle et al., 2018). The other domains of the GCWBT presented variable results between these five studies, with some showing no effects on the participants.

These differences in the effect of the domains of the GCWBT might be related to how observed behaviour is interpreted. It may be easier to notice if a participant is showing interest and sustaining attention to the arts activity rather than expressing non-verbal pride. Gross et al. (2015) say that the value of the visual art programmes can sometimes be very explicit to observers, who perceive positive effects during the activity. These effects cannot always be demonstrated quantitatively. This also seems to be true for other studies that used quantitative tools (Camic et al., 2014; Hattori et al., 2011; Kinney & Rentz, 2005; Pérez-Sáez et al., 2018; Rusted et al., 2006; Sauer et al., 2016; Windle et al., 2018). If we accept that eyewitnesses were reliably reporting what they see in the participants, it proves challenging to quantitatively assess the impact of these interventions, even more so when this may occur outside the sessions. It seems that using quantitative tools alone is insufficient for a comprehensive analysis; complementary qualitative approaches, such as participants questionnaires, are needed to have a better understanding of the effects of participatory visual arts (Beard, 2012; Windle et al., 2018; Zeilig et al., 2014).

Inconclusive results also emerged from the comparisons between interventions that used only art-making activities and interventions that combined art-viewing and art-making activities. The difference in the effects of the studies at first glance appeared to be related to the type of intervention, suggesting that using interventions with art-viewing and art-making activities might be more effective. Art-making evaluations involved more complex interventions and a greater range of outcomes, usually via quantitative tools. However, we cannot affirm that art-viewing and art-making interventions are more effective than art-making interventions alone. A possible reason for the inconsistencies found between study results is that the art interventions were extremely diverse and are also complex interventions (Windle et al., 2017; Windle et al., 2018). While diversity in art interventions is advantageous, permitting adaptation to settings and aims, this flexibility also makes it difficult to draw conclusions from comparative analyses.

In addition to the diversity of intervention characteristics shown in the studies, descriptions of the interventions and facilitators were generally not detailed and results were sometimes not clear. Moreover, none of the studies adequately addressed the optimal length of the intervention, nor why a specific type of art-making activity was included, such as whether it was based on a rationale or theory. Windle et al. (2017) and Deshmukh et al. (2018) faced the same challenge in their reviews. They have suggested that future research on visual arts should use the Template for Intervention Description and Replication (TIDieR) checklist (Hoffmann et al., 2014) to report the interventions. The use of reporting guidelines appears to be an effective way to summarise interventions and findings.

The comparison of the studies according to the type of intervention might give an indication of a description of what worked overall. However, the heterogeneity of these studies makes it hard to indicate with confidence why and how the interventions may affect participants in other forms of intervention. Therefore we can only report on which were the most common characteristics of the interventions.

Painting, drawing, watercolour and colouring were the most frequently used types of activities, although using more than one type of art activity was common (Belver et al., 2018; Burnside et al., 2017; Camic et al., 2016; Camic et al., 2014; Kinney & Rentz, 2005; Roe et al., 2016; Schall et al., 2018; Ullan et al., 2013; Windle et al., 2018). Studies that had positive effects on participants' interest and attention (Belver et al., 2018; Kinney & Rentz, 2005; Windle et al., 2018) usually employed more than one type of activity and for longer periods. As it might be difficult to maintain participants' interest across sessions, diversifying the activity could be a good strategy to keep people with dementia engaged in art interventions. All studies but one (Wyatt & Liggett, 2019) delivered the art sessions in groups, where people with dementia and carers or facilitators could be dyads to join the activity. The number of participants in each activity session was variable, with an average number of six people with dementia per session. Art-making activities lasted for about 60 minutes in most studies. Art-viewing activities usually also took 60 minutes of the time of the sessions. The range of the sessions was usually from eight to 12 weeks. Effects of the activity were usually only seen during the sessions, so this might be the reason why most studies favoured weekly 60-minute sessions as opposed to single sessions with the participants. It is difficult to sustain effects of psychosocial interventions if the maintenance of the sessions is not possible (Orrell et al., 2014). For this reason, it is important that visual art activities are provided regularly to people with dementia (Windle et al., 2018).

Interventions with an art-viewing component frequently involved a professional facilitator in art appreciation. Researchers and other professionals were often the facilitators in studies with art-making activities. In the latter case, the facilitator's role seemed to be to make the intervention pleasurable for the participants, making it relevant to them with a person-centred approach, rather than imparting expert knowledge (Belver et al., 2018; Byrne & MacKinlay, 2012; Gross et al., 2015; Hazzan et al., 2016; Sauer et al., 2016; Ullan et al., 2013; Wyatt & Liggett, 2019). It also seems to be important that all facilitators are supportive and engage in social exchange instead of focusing on the aesthetics of the piece (Byrne & MacKinlay, 2012).

The presence of carers in this context also appears to have a positive impact in the social relationships of people with dementia (Burnside et al., 2017; Camic et al., 2014; Flatt et al., 2015; Hazzan et al., 2016; Roe et al., 2016). Carers help to promote interest and engagement with the activity for the person with dementia (Hazzan et al., 2016). Hazzan et al. (2016) highlight that the presence of carers is of particular importance for participants with severe dementia, as the activity fosters communication between the dyad. This also aligns with findings from Windle et al. (2017) that enjoyable art activities are an excellent way to foster social aspects and relationships between people with dementia and carers. However, it is important that facilitators and carers let people with dementia to have autonomy in the art creation, stimulating their confidence, and not performing the activity for them (Windle et al., 2017).

The level of dementia did not appear to have an effect on the ability to participate and enjoy the activity (Ullan et al., 2013), though most of the participants in the studies had a mild to moderate level of dementia. Studies that included people with severe dementia usually had their sessions at the dementia care facilities, except for Hazzan et al. (2016) and Windle et al. (2018), which also had sessions in galleries. Differences between settings for the intervention delivery may explain the lack of association with the level dementia of the participants. One possible explanation is that participatory art activities are feasible to all levels of dementia and is independent of where it is performed, allowing the facilitator to offer person-centred interventions that meet the needs of people with dementia. We concur with the review by Windle et al. (2017); because of the small number of studies, it is not possible to say whether gallery environments are superior to dementia care facilities because of the small number of studies. It may be important for self-esteem and social status of people with dementia if they are included in cultural and social activities outside dementia care facilities (Belver et al., 2018; Burnside et al., 2017; Camic et al., 2016; Camic et al., 2014).

To summarise, interventions were associated with more positive outcomes if they met the following criteria:

- frequent sessions as the benefits only seem to last for the length of the session;
- facilitators to support participants in creating their own art but also to make it an enjoyable experience;
- variation in participatory art activities (e.g. painting, drawing, pottery) to maintain participants' engagement across the activity sessions;
- presence of carers whenever is possible during the activity to support the stimulation of social relationships, interest and engagement.

Limitations of the review

The search strategy created was comprehensive to include different types of participatory visual arts. This made the synthesis of the interventions a challenging task because of the differences in designs and outcomes of the interventions. The inadequate description of methods of the studies was also an obstacle for this review. We did not have consistent descriptions of all the interventions evaluated. Future research on visual arts should use reporting guidelines such as the TIDieR checklist (Hoffmann et al., 2014) to report the interventions (Deshmukh et al., 2018; Windle et al., 2017).

This review was limited to peer-reviewed English language articles, which may have led to other important studies not being included in this review. The tools chosen to quality assess the studies also might not have reflected the real quality of the studies included here. The CASP tool (Critical Appraisal Skills

Programme, 2017) was straightforward but provided little room to explore the effects of the studies. The Downs and Black (1998) checklist has a focus on randomised and non-randomised studies, making it more applicable to trials with medical interventions such as drugs, not psychosocial interventions. It was a delicate task to decide which questions should be removed to not compromise the validity of the tool, while still properly evaluating the studies.

Conclusion

This narrative synthesis systematic review has evaluated 20 articles that used participatory visual arts in research for people with dementia. The review of these studies suggests that participatory art activities are beneficial to the people with dementia, having positive effects on their cognition, psychological and social aspects. The studies evaluated here showed a great variety of art interventions, the focus of the studies and outcomes of interest. This made comparisons between studies challenging. Because of their heterogeneity, it is not possible to generalise broadly from the results but we have been able here to draw on the evidence to identify features of interventions that appear to be associated with positive outcomes. We cannot indicate with certainty how the interventions may affect the participants with dementia. We can only report on the most common characteristics of what has worked in the interventions. The review indicates that interventions associated with more positive outcomes provided different types of supported art activities in frequent sessions adopting an empowering approach and involving carers where possible. These interventions were able to maintain the participants engaged across the sessions and offered them enjoyable experiences with art creation.

The use of participatory visual arts in activities for people with dementia has many advantages. These activities can increase their overall well-being and positive mood during the activity sessions, as well as promoting social inclusion, self-esteem and independence. They are accessible to many people in different settings and they do not significantly increase the costs of healthcare. Our findings may be useful in the commissioning, design and implementation participatory visual arts interventions for people with dementia.

Acknowledgement

This chapter was originally published as a review article in Cavalcanti Barroso, A., Rai, H.K., Sousa, L., Orrell, M., & Schneider, J. (2022). Participatory visual arts activities for people with dementia: a review. *Perspectives in Public Health, 142*(3), 22–31. DOI:10.1177/1757913920948916

Note

1   The ⋆ is used as a wildcard symbol to broaden the search. It uses the word stems to retrieve variations of the term. E.g.: Paint⋆ -> painter, painting, painted, etc.

References

Beard, R.L. (2012). Art therapies and dementia care: A systematic review [Literature Review; Systematic Review]. *Dementia: The International Journal of Social Research and Practice, 11*(5), 633–656. https://doi.org/http://dx.doi.org/10.1177/1471301211421090

Belver, M.H., Ullán, A.M., Avila, N., Moreno, C., & Hernández, C. (2018). Art museums as a source of well-being for people with dementia: An experience in the Prado Museum. *Arts & Health, 10*(3), 213–226.

Burnside, L.D., Knecht, M.J., Hopley, E.K., & Logsdon, R.G. (2017). Here: Now – Conceptual model of the impact of an experiential arts program on persons with dementia and their care partners. *Dementia, 16*(1), 29–45. https://doi.org/10.1177/1471301215577220

Byrne, L., & MacKinlay, E. (2012). Seeking meaning: Making art and the experience of spirituality in dementia care. *Journal of Religion, Spirituality & Aging, 24*(1–2), 105–119. https://doi.org/http://dx.doi.org/10.1080/15528030.2012.633416

Camic, P.M., Baker, E.L., & Tischler, V. (2016). Theorizing how art gallery interventions impact people with dementia and their caregivers. *The Gerontologist, 56*(6), 1033–1041. https://doi.org/10.1093/geront/gnv063

Camic, P.M., Tischler, V., & Pearman, C.H. (2014). Viewing and making art together: a multi-session art-gallery-based intervention for people with dementia and their carers. *Aging & Mental Health, 18*(2), 161–168. https://doi.org/http://dx.doi.org/10.1080/13607863.2013.818101

Cavalcanti Barroso, A., Rai, H. K., Sousa, L., Orrell, M., & Schneider, J. (2022). Participatory visual arts activities for people with dementia: a review. *Perspectives in Public Health, 142*(3), 22–31. https://doi.org/10.1177/1757913920948916

Chancellor, B., Duncan, A., & Chatterjee, A. (2014). Art therapy for Alzheimer's disease and other dementias. *Journal of Alzheimer's Disease, 39*(1), 1–11.

Chung. (2004). Activity participation and well-being of people with dementia in long-term – Care settings. *OTJR: Occupation, Participation and Health, 24*(1), 22–31. https://doi.org/10.1177/153944920402400104

Chung, Ellis-Hill, C., & Coleman, P. (2017). Supporting activity engagement by family carers at home: maintenance of agency and personhood in dementia. *International Journal of Qualitative Studies on Health and Well-being, 12*(1), 1267316. https://doi.org/10.1080/17482631.2016.1267316

Cowl, A.L., & Gaugler, J.E. (2014). Efficacy of creative arts therapy in treatment of Alzheimer's disease and dementia: A systematic literature review [Literature Review; Systematic Review]. *Activities, Adaptation & Aging, 38*(4), 281–330. https://doi.org/http://dx.doi.org/10.1080/01924788.2014.966547

Critical Appraisal Skills Programme. (2017). *CASP qualitative checklist*. Retrieved from https://casp-uk.net/casp-tools-checklists/.

Deshmukh, S.R., Holmes, J., & Cardno, A. (2018). Art therapy for people with dementia. *Cochrane Database of Systematic Reviews, 9*.

Downs, S.H., & Black, N. (1998). The feasibility of creating a checklist for the assessment of the methodological quality both of randomised and non-randomised studies of health care interventions. *J Epidemiol Community Health, 52*(6), 377–384. www.ncbi.nlm.nih.gov/pubmed/9764259

Eekelaar, C., Camic, P.M., & Springham, N. (2012). Art galleries, episodic memory and verbal fluency in dementia: An exploratory study [Empirical Study; Quantitative Study].

Psychology of Aesthetics, Creativity, and the Arts, 6(3), 262–272. https://doi.org/http://dx.doi.org/10.1037/a0027499

Fancourt, D., & Finn, S. (2019). *What is the evidence on the role of the arts in improving health and well-being? A scoping review.* Copenhagen: WHO Regional Office for Europe. Retrieved from www.euro.who.int/en/publications/abstracts/what-is-the-evidence-on-the-role-of-the-arts-in-improving-health-and-well-being-a-scoping-review-2019

Flatt, J.D., Liptak, A., Oakley, M.A., Gogan, J., Varner, T., & Lingler, J.H. (2015). Subjective experiences of an art museum engagement activity for persons with early-stage Alzheimer's disease and their family caregivers [Research Support, N.I.H., Extramural]. *American Journal of Alzheimer's Disease & Other Dementias, 30*(4), 380–389. https://doi.org/http://dx.doi.org/10.1177/1533317514549953

Gillies, B., & Johnston, G. (2004). Identity loss and maintenance: Commonality of experience in cancer and dementia. *European Journal of Cancer Care, 13*(5), 436–442. https://doi.org/10.1111/j.1365-2354.2004.00550.x

Gross, S.M., Danilova, D., Vandehey, M.A., & Diekhoff, G.M. (2015). Creativity and dementia: does artistic activity affect well-being beyond the art class? *Dementia (London, England), 14*(1), 27–46. https://doi.org/http://dx.doi.org/10.1177/1471301213488899

Hattori, H., Hattori, C., Hokao, C., Mizushima, K., & Mase, T. (2011). Controlled study on the cognitive and psychological effect of coloring and drawing in mild Alzheimer's disease patients. *Geriatrics and Gerontology International, 11*(4), 431–437. https://doi.org/http://dx.doi.org/10.1111/j.1447-0594.2011.00698.x

Hazzan, A.A., Humphrey, J., Kilgour-Walsh, L., Moros, K.L., Murray, C., Stanners, S., . . . Papaioannou, A. (2016). Impact of the 'artful moments' intervention on persons with dementia and their care partners: A pilot study. *Canadian Geriatrics Journal, 19*(2), 1–8. https://doi.org/10.5770/cgj.19.220

Hoffmann, T.C., Glasziou, P.P., Boutron, I., Milne, R., Perera, R., Moher, D., . . . Johnston, M. (2014). Better reporting of interventions: Template for intervention description and replication (TIDieR) checklist and guide. *BMJ, 348*, g1687.

Kinney, J.M., & Rentz, C.A. (2005). Observed well-being among individuals with dementia: Memories in the Making, an art program, versus other structured activity. *American Journal of Alzheimer's Disease & Other Dementias, 20*(4), 220–227. http://ovidsp.ovid.com/ovidweb.cgi?T=JS&CSC=Y&NEWS=N&PAGE=fulltext&D=med5&AN=16136845; http://sfx.nottingham.ac.uk:80/sfx_local?genre=article&atitle=Observed+well-being+among+individuals+with+dementia%3A+Memories+in+the+Making%2C+an+art+program%2C+versus+o

MacPherson, S., Bird, M., Anderson, K., Davis, T., & Blair, A. (2009). An Art Gallery Access Programme for people with dementia: 'You do it for the moment'. *Aging & Mental Health, 13*(5), 744–752. https://doi.org/http://dx.doi.org/10.1080/13607860902918207

McDermott, O., Crellin, N., Ridder, H.M., & Orrell, M. (2013). Music therapy in dementia: A narrative synthesis systematic review. *International Journal of Geriatric Psychiatry, 28*(8), 781–794.

Noice, T., Noice, H., & Kramer, A.F. (2013). Participatory arts for older adults: A review of benefits and challenges. *The Gerontologist, 54*(5), 741–753.

Orrell, M., Aguirre, E., Spector, A., Hoare, Z., Woods, R.T., Streater, A., . . . Whitaker, C. (2014). Maintenance cognitive stimulation therapy for dementia: Single-blind, multicentre, pragmatic randomised controlled trial. *The British Journal of Psychiatry, 204*(6), 454–461.

Pérez-Sáez, E., Cabrero-Montes, E.M., Llorente-Cano, M., & González-Ingelmo, E. (2018). A pilot study on the impact of a pottery workshop on the well-being of people with dementia. *Dementia*, 1471301218814634.

Phinney, A., Chaudhury, H., & O'connor, D.L. (2007). Doing as much as I can do: The meaning of activity for people with dementia. *Aging & Mental Health, 11*(4), 384–393. https://doi.org/10.1080/13607860601086470

Popay, J., Roberts, H., Sowden, A., Petticrew, M., Arai, L., Rodgers, M., . . . Duffy, S. (2006). *Guidance on the conduct of narrative synthesis in systematic reviews* (Vol. 15).

Rentz, C.A. (2002). Memories in the Making©: Outcome-based evaluation of an art program for individuals with dementing illnesses. *American Journal of Alzheimer's Disease & Other Dementias®, 17*(3), 175–181.

Robb, S.L., Hanson-Abromeit, D., May, L., Hernandez-Ruiz, E., Allison, M., Beloat, A., . . . Oyedele, O.O. (2018). Reporting quality of music intervention research in healthcare: A systematic review. *Complementary Therapies in Medicine, 38*, 24–41.

Roe, B., McCormick, S., Lucas, T., Gallagher, W., Winn, A., & Elkin, S. (2016). Coffee, Cake & Culture: Evaluation of an art for health programme for older people in the community. *Dementia, 15*(4), 539–559. https://doi.org/10.1177/1471301214528927

Rusted, J., Sheppard, L., & Waller, D. (2006). A multi-centre randomized control group trial on the use of art therapy for older people with dementia. *Group Analysis, 39*(4), 517–536. https://doi.org/http://dx.doi.org/10.1177/0533316406071447

Sauer, P.E., Fopma-Loy, J., Kinney, J.M., & Lokon, E. (2016). "It makes me feel like myself": Person-centered versus traditional visual arts activities for people with dementia [Empirical Study; Qualitative Study]. *Dementia: The International Journal of Social Research and Practice, 15*(5), 895–912. https://doi.org/http://dx.doi.org/10.1177/1471301214543958

Schall, A., Tesky, V.A., Adams, A.-K., & Pantel, J. (2018). Art museum-based intervention to promote emotional well-being and improve quality of life in people with dementia: The ARTEMIS project. *Dementia, 17*(6), 728–743.

Ullan, A.M., Belver, M.H., Badia, M., Moreno, C., Garrido, E., Gomez-Isla, J., . . . Tejedor, L. (2013). Contributions of an artistic educational program for older people with early dementia: An exploratory qualitative study. *Dementia, 12*(4), 425–446. https://doi.org/http://dx.doi.org/10.1177/1471301211430650

Windle, G., Gregory, S., Howson-Griffiths, T., Newman, A., O'Brien, D., & Goulding, A. (2017). Exploring the theoretical foundations of visual art programmes for people living with dementia. *Dementia (London)*, 1471301217726613. https://doi.org/10.1177/1471301217726613

Windle, G., Joling, K., Howson-Griffiths, T., Woods, B., Jones, C., van de Ven, P., . . . Parkinson, C. (2018). The impact of a visual arts program on quality of life, communication, and well-being of people living with dementia: A mixed-methods longitudinal investigation. *International psychogeriatrics, 30*(3), 409–423.

Wyatt, M., & Liggett, S. (2019). The potential of painting: Unlocking disenfranchised grief for people living with dementia. *Illness, Crisis & Loss, 27*(1), 51–67.

Young, R., Tischler, V., Hulbert, S., & Camic, P.M. (2015). The impact of viewing and making art on verbal fluency and memory in people with dementia in an art gallery setting [Empirical Study; Interview; Quantitative Study]. *Psychology of Aesthetics, Creativity, and the Arts, 9*(4), 368–375. https://doi.org/http://dx.doi.org/10.1037/aca0000030

Zeilig, H., Killick, J., & Fox, C. (2014). The participative arts for people living with a dementia: a critical review. *International Journal of Ageing and Later Life, 9*(1), 7–34.

Chapter 9

Exergaming as meaningful activity for people with dementia

Evaluation of effect and implementation

Joeke van der Molen-van Santen, Marian Schoone-Harmsen, Carlijn Hendriks, Annemieke van Straten, Rose-Marie Dröes, Franka Meiland

Exergaming activities in the field of dementia

The importance of engaging in meaningful and pleasant activities for people with dementia is generally acknowledged. These activities can range from physical, creative or social activities and therewith contribute to physical, mental and/or social well-being (Heyn et al., 2004; Dröes et al., 2011; Nyman & Szymczynska, 2016). However, often, people with dementia are dependent on others to engage in these activities and many of them stop with preferred activities if they do not have the support needed to continue with them. As an alternative, and in an era where a 'tsunami' of demand for healthcare services is expected (Gauthier et al., 2021), increasingly new ways of electronically based care and support are developed, evaluated and implemented (Meiland et al., 2017). This also counts for meaningful and pleasant activities, such as exergaming.

Exergaming is defined as 'physical exercise interactively combined with cognitive stimulation in a gaming environment' (van Santen et al., 2018). Exergaming technology focuses on gaming exercises that are controlled by physical movements of the player. It is an innovative way of exercising that combines mental and physical stimulation. It has strong potential for people to start and continue with exercise activities in an enjoyable, safe way and subsequently promoting physical and mental well-being. Exergaming may tackle problems that people with dementia may encounter when performing regular and outdoors activities, like wandering, fall accidents and feelings of insecurity (Nyman, 2011). Within exergaming also the concept of 'serious games' is applied, which stands for games that are developed for other purposes than pleasure alone (Tong et al., 2017). Various types of exergaming exist such as virtual bowling (with competitions between individuals or residential care homes) (Dove & Astell, 2019), – tennis, dancing, games and interactive cycling. Previous research on exergaming showed that it provides older people with light to moderate physical activity and also in a more enjoyable way than traditional

DOI: 10.4324/9781003289005-12

exercise (Taylor et al., 2012; Peng et al., 2013; Graves et al., 2010; Fenney & Lee, 2010; Aarhus et al., 2011; Colombo et al., 2012). However, effects of exergaming were only described in a few studies (van Santen et al., 2018) and authors stressed the importance of larger and well-designed effect studies in this field.

Implementation of (eHealth) interventions proves to be challenging (Gitlin et al., 2015; Christie et al., 2018). Implementation refers to a set of planned, intentional activities that aim to put into practice evidence-informed policies and practices in real-world services.[1] The effectiveness of an intervention is highly influenced by the success of the implementation, for example the fit of the intervention into the organisation and to the expectations of care professionals, persons with dementia and their family members.

In this chapter, the investigation of the effectiveness of exergaming will be described, as well as issues with the implementation of exergaming. The type of exergaming we focus on here is *interactive cycling*: people with dementia cycle on a stationary bicycle (i.e. home trainer) in front of a screen where they see a route they selected. The faster they cycle, the faster they continue the route being played on the screen. There are various brands that offer this type of exergaming, such as Fietslabyrint, SilverFit and PraxFit.

How did we design the study?

Our study encompassed a cluster randomised controlled trial (c-RCT) among people with dementia who visited day-care centres in the Netherlands. Twenty day-care centres participated with in total 112 couples of people with dementia and their informal carers. Eleven centres were randomly assigned to the

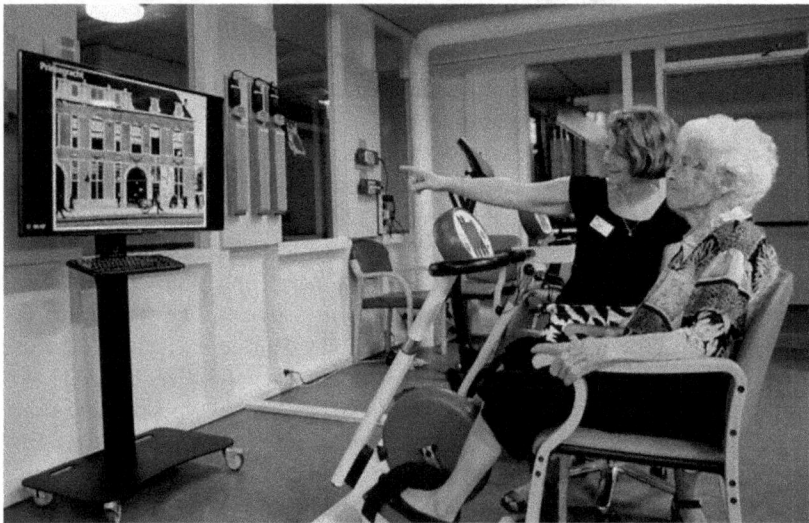

Figure 9.1 A person doing exergaming (interactive cycling)

group that offered exergaming (73 couples) and nine centres (39 couples) were assigned to the group that offered day-care activities as usual (including movement activities) but without exergaming.

We investigated whether:

1) people with dementia visiting day-care centres with exergaming are more physically active and have better mobility than people with dementia visiting day-care centres without exergaming;
2) exergaming has more effect on the physical, cognitive, emotional and social functioning and quality of life of people with dementia and on the burden, quality of life and positive care experiences of informal caregivers than usual activities in day-care centres.

Assessments with questionnaires and performance tests took place at the start of the intervention and after three and six months. For people with dementia these included among others: registration of physical activities during one week (in minutes), mobility (Short Physical Performance Battery, SPPB; Guralnik et al., 1994), cognition (Mini Mental State Examination, MMSE; Cockrell & Folstein, 1988, and Trail Making Test-TMT; Ashendorf et al., 2008), social functioning (Behavior Observation Scale for Intramural Psychogeriatrics subscale 1, GIP; Verstraten et al., 1987) and various questions from The Older Persons and Informal Caregivers Survey Minimum DataSet (TOPICS-MDS; Van den Brink et al., 2015). Additionally among family caregivers, subjective burden and stress were assessed with the Short Sense of Competence Questionnaire (SSCQ; Vernooij-Dassen et al., 1999) and the NeuroPsychiatric Inventory (NPI-Q-emotional distress; Cummings et al., 1994) respectively, and also positive experiences of caregiving were assessed (PES; De Boer et al., 2012). See for more details van Santen et al., 2020.

Alongside the c-RCT, we conducted a process evaluation to find out how exergaming could be successfully applied for people with dementia. To this end, at the start of the study, we administered the Measurement Instrument for Determinants of Innovations (MIDI; Fleuren et al., 2014) to the participating organisations in the exergaming group. On the basis of the outcomes of the MIDI, we have made recommendations to the organisations to alter some critical issues to improve the implementation of exergaming, for instance to involve volunteers, interns or family to support and stimulate the persons with dementia during the exercises when there was limited availability of staff; to direct the care organisations to discuss technical issues with the equipment with the supplier; to use the information materials offered by the research team to inform and gain approval from higher management; to find another location for the exergaming bike, for example closer to the living rooms. The MIDI was again used after six months. At that time also semi-structured interviews were held to gain more in-depth insight into factors influencing implementation success. The interviews were held with one organisation that succeeded well in implementing the exergaming intervention and one organisation that was least successful in this.

The day-care centres in the exergaming group either already provided interactive cycling exergames or they had to buy or lease one of the following systems: DiFiets (now part of SilverFit), Fietslabyrint, PraxFit or SilverFit Mile. When participating in the study, they received a discount for the purchase of one of these systems. Although various brands of equipment were used in the participating day-care centres, these did not vary significantly regarding their functionalities. The costs ranged from €1,500 to 4,700.

During a one-hour meeting, the staff (e.g. physiotherapists, activity coordinator) of the day-care centre received instructions about offering exergaming (e.g. five times per week as part of their regular activity programme and to encourage research participants to take part at least twice per week for six months). Besides exergaming, persons with dementia could also join the regular activity programme of the day-care centre.

In the non-exergaming, usual activity (control) group, five days per week a varied activity programme was offered, such as arts and crafts, music and physical exercise such as walking outdoors.

Main findings of our exergaming study

With regard to baseline characteristics, there were no statistically significant differences between the exergaming and control group (van Santen et al., 2020). In the exergaming group, the mean (SD) age of people with dementia was 79.0 (6.0) years, and in the control group, this was 79.0 (7.0) years. There were 37 (51%) male persons with dementia participating in exergaming group, and 23 (57%) in the control group. Most common dementia types were Alzheimer's Disease (25 (34%) exergaming group, 12 (31%) control group), followed by Vascular Dementia (6 (8%) exergaming group, three (8%) control group). The mean age (SD) of informal caregivers in the exergaming group was 65.0 (13.0) years and 67.0 (12.0) years in the control group. There were 54 (74%) female informal caregivers in the exergaming group and 29 (74%) in the control group.

During the intervention period on average, exergaming was done for about 30 minutes a week in total. Although at post-test participants in the exergaming group tended to be more physically active (the primary study outcome) than participants in the control group, this difference was not statistically significant. Also, on mobility, we did not find (statistically significant) differences between the two groups. We did find positive effects of exergaming on some of the secondary outcomes, that is after six months we saw improvements in the persons with dementia on cognition (MMSE): $r = 2.30$, 95% confidence interval (CI): 0.65, 3.96, $P = 0.007$ and (TMT-part A): $r = -28.98$, 95% CI: -54.89, -3.08, $P = 0.029$) and social functioning (GIP): $r = -1.86$, 95% CI: -3.56, -0.17, $P = 0.031$). Additionally, in informal caregivers, we found positive effects on the distress caused by neuropsychiatric symptoms of the person with dementia (NPI-Q total distress: $r = -3.30$, 95% CI: -6.57, -0.03,

P = 0.048) and on the sense of competence of the carers (SSCQ: r = 2.78, 95% CI: 0.85, 4.71, P = 0.005).

With regard to the implementation of exergaming, all stakeholders experienced a variety of benefits and enablers for optimal use, but they also mentioned barriers and tips and tricks to improve implementation. Nearly all of the participants with dementia and care professionals were positive about the exergaming cycling activity and equipment. They wanted to recommend it to others because it offers a fun and varied activity, physical activity is positive and useful, it is nice to cycle in a known neighbourhood, and it is easy to talk about what you see.

According to the care professionals, the most enabling factors were that exergaming gives a routine and incentive for exercise, leads to social contact, provides a meaningful way to spend the time and makes people feel better after this activity.

Main barriers mentioned by the professional stakeholders were absence of clear procedures for use and lack of information on exergaming, little directly visible effects, amount of time and money to be invested as well as the work-related adjustments that needed to be made by the care professionals. Also, the professionals involved experienced little support from their management and peers, and they received little feedback from within their organisation on their efforts. Other important barriers mentioned by care professionals were: there is less time for other stimulating activities (i.e. going outside), the equipment takes up a lot of space and is not suited for persons with advanced dementia or physical impairments.

Points mentioned by persons with dementia and other stakeholders to consider were: the equipment is too big to set up in your own home; it must be well tuned to the physical abilities of the user; with exergaming, you miss the outdoor effects (wind, slopes); there is now a limited number of routes and sometimes the system is not working well because of technical problems.

What can we conclude and how to proceed?

In this project, we assessed the effectiveness of exergaming through interactive cycling in dementia by comparing people with dementia attending day-care centres providing exergaming compared to people attending day-care centres offering usual care without exergaming. In addition, we performed a process evaluation to gain insight in factors influencing the success of implementation of exergaming in the day-care centres. Our results show positive effects for people with dementia participating in exergaming and for their informal carers. However, these effects were found on secondary outcome measures (cognitive and social functioning among people with dementia and competence and distress among family carers) only, not on the primary outcome's physical activity level and mobility. This could be caused by the low frequency of exergaming: it was performed for only 30 minutes a week, which may not be enough to have impact on the selected primary outcomes, although there was a tendency for the exergaming group to be physically more active than the non-exergaming group. Another reason may be that our study sample was smaller than power calculations suggested for demonstrating small to moderate effects. However, other studies on exergaming, some of whom also were based on smaller samples, did find positive effects of exergaming on physical functioning (balance), besides effects on cognitive, emotional and social functioning and QoL (Mura et al., 2018; Zhao et al., 2020).

Regarding the implementation of exergaming in the different participating care organisations there were similarities and differences in the type of care organisation, population, type of exergaming (cycling) equipment, place and access of the equipment, number of participants, experience with the exergames, intensity of the use (although five times a week was recommended), way in which the exercises were offered etc.

On the basis of the users' feedback, some important lessons were learned regarding the exergaming activity: the equipment and activity is experienced as fun, easy to use and has a variety of applications. The more the offered exercises and activities are part of the organisation's vision and strategy, the better. It should not be the responsibility of one person (i.e. the physiotherapist) alone. The activity should be offered tailored to each participant. Furthermore, when introducing exergaming some organisational challenges must be met: capacity, time and money to buy and set up the equipment, finding a suitable place and ensuring the support of management and colleagues. On the basis of these findings, a factsheet was developed with tips and recommendations for successful implementation of exergaming for people with dementia (van Santen et al., 2019). The recommendations in this factsheet may help to make an implementation plan. As is known from literature, implementation of effective interventions is not done without effort; it requires a well-designed plan (Nilsen, 2015).

The findings of our study need to be interpreted with caution, because of the earlier mentioned study limitations, such as underpowered study and the many drop-outs in the study, and also the large number of outcome measures. With regard to research into exergames for people with dementia, we recommend larger randomised controlled studies, to try to offer exergaming at least three to five days a week with a duration of 20–30 minutes per session to the study participants and to study exergaming also in other settings (at home, in residential care settings). If these future studies show positive results on physical outcomes, in addition to cognitive, social and emotional outcomes, this may help care organisations to adopt exergaming as structural part of their care programmes, and will interest healthcare insurance and funding organisations to invest in exergames, which will also promote further implementation of exergaming.

On the basis of the positive effects, tendencies and experiences resulting from our research, the lack of negative effects or adverse events linked to the exergaming intervention, and the high users' appreciation of the intervention, we recommend care organisations to use exergaming and to include our implementation recommendations. When offering exergaming to persons with dementia, this should be done in a person–centred manner, which means, for example with an appropriate duration and difficulty of exercises, choosing games or routes familiar and appealing to the user, offering the exercise at a time that fits the daily routine and offering adequate support during the exercises.

Box 9.1   Case report 'Thomas keeps cycling because he enjoyed the route so much'

Eighty-year-old Thomas has been diagnosed with Alzheimer's disease and currently lives at home with his partner, Emma. He was headmaster of an elementary school for many years and very sporty in his spare time. Over time, he gradually deteriorated. He could not stay at home alone anymore. During the night he was often very restless and awake. During the day he often fell asleep. Emma tried to go out with Thomas as much as possible to increase his activity level during the day and to restore his sleep-wake cycle, but at a certain point it was decided that it was best for him to visit a day-care centre a few days a week. For Emma, this offered some time of relaxation, enabling her to cope better with the care of her partner.

At the day-care centre Thomas regularly goes for a walk with the walking group in the morning. In the afternoon he uses the SilverFit Mile to cycle a long distance. Each time he chooses a different route. Sometimes other visitors stand next to him, and they talk about the route. The route motivates Thomas to keep cycling.

> 'I really see a smile on his face. Today he cycled more than half an hour. When his partner came to pick him up, we really had to ask him to stop cycling. He kept on cycling because he enjoys the route so much.' – Founder and supervisor of the day-care centre

During the COVID-19 pandemic, Thomas could not attend the day-care centre for several weeks because of the lockdown measures. During this period, he was inactive at home and as a result his physical and mental condition deteriorated. However, when he returned to day-care after the lockdown, Emma noticed that he became more active again. She also noticed Thomas was more alert when he had cycled. That is why they had a stationary bicycle installed at their home, but Thomas hardly ever used it. It turned out that a home trainer without routes and interactive cycling was not inviting and motivating enough for him.

Emma stressed the transformation Thomas had gone through since visiting the day-care centre. She remarked that he would fall asleep while she was talking to him. But now he stayed awake and responded. 'That's very important to me. He had such difficulty sleeping at night, but now he's sleeping much better. Also, when he gets back from the day-care centre, he doesn't fall asleep anymore, he's fitter and more energized'.

Note

1   www.implementation.eu

References

Aarhus, R., Grönvall, E., Larsen, S.B., & Wollsen, S. (2011). Turning training into play: Embodied gaming, seniors, physical training and motivation. *Gerontechnology*, *10*(2), 110–120.

Ashendorf, L., Jefferson, A.L., O'Connor, M.K., Chaisson, C., Green, R.C., & Stern, R.A. (2008) Trail Making Test errors in normal aging, mild cognitive impairment, and dementia. *Archives of Clinical Neuropsychology*, *23*(2), 129–137 https://doi.org/10.1016/j.acn.2007.11.005

Christie, H.L., Bartels, S.L., Boots, L.M.M., Tange, H.J., Verhey, F.J.J., & de Vugt, M.E. (2018). A systematic review on the implementation of eHealth interventions for informal caregivers of people with dementia. *Internet Interventions*, *7*(13), 51–59. https://doi: 10.1016/j.invent.2018.07.002.

Cockrell, J., & Folstein, M.F. (1988). Mini-mental state examination (MMSE). *Psychopharmacology Bulletin*, *24*(4), 689–92.

Colombo, M., Marelli, E., Vaccaro, R., Valle, E., Colombani, S., Polesel, E., Garolfi, S., Fossi, S., & Guaita, A. (2012). Virtual reality for persons with dementia: An exergaming experience. In *ISARC. Proceedings of the International Symposium on Automation and Robotics in Construction* (Vol. 29, p. 1). IAARC Publications.

Cummings, J.L., Mega, M., Gray, K., Rosenberg-Thompson, S., Carusi, D.A., & Gornbein, J. The Neuropsychiatric Inventory: Comprehensive assessment of psychopathology in dementia. *Neurology 1994*, *44*(12), 2308–2314. 10.1212/wnl.44.12.2308.

De Boer, A.H., Oudijk, D., van Groenou, M.I.B., & Timmermans, J.M. (2012). Positive experiences through informal care: Construction of a scale. *Tijdschrift voor Gerontologie en Geriatrie*, *43*(5), 243–254.

Dove, E., & Astell, A. (2019). The Kinect Project: Group motion-based gaming for people living with dementia. *Dementia*, *18*(6), 2189–2205. https://doi.org/10.1177/1471301217743575.

Dröes, R.M., van der Roest, H.G., Van Mierlo, L.D., & Meiland, F.J.M. (2011). Memory problems in dementia: Adaptation and coping strategies and psychosocial treatments. *Expert Reviews Neurotherapeutics*, *11*(12), 1769–1782. 10.1586/ern.11.167.

Fenney, A., & Lee, T.D. (2010). Exploring spared capacity in persons with dementia: What WiiTM can learn. *Activities, Adaptation & Aging*, *34*(4), 303–313. https://doi.org/10.1080/01924788.2010.525736

Fleuren, M.A.H., Paulussen, T.G.W.M., Van Dommelen P., & Van Buuren S. (2014). Towards a measurement instrument for determinants of innovations. *International Journal for Quality in Health Care, 26*(5), 501–510. 10.1093/intqhc/mzu060.

Gauthier, S., Rosa-Neto, P., Morais, J.A., & Webster, C. (2021). *World Alzheimer Report 2021: Journey through the diagnosis of dementia.* London: Alzheimer's Disease International.

Gitlin, L.N., Marx, K., Stanley, I.H., Hodgson, N. (2015). Translating evidence-based dementia caregiving interventions into practice: State-of-the-science and next steps. *The Gerontologist, 55*, 210–226. https://doi: 10.1093/geront/gnu123.

Graves, L.E., Ridgers, N.D., Williams, K., Stratton, G., & Atkinson, G.T. (2010). The physiological cost and enjoyment of Wii Fit in adolescents, young adults, and older adults. *Journal of Physical Activity & Health, 7*(3), 393–401.

Guralnik, J.M., Simonsick, E.M., Ferrucci, L., Glynn, R.J., Berkman, L.F., Blazer, D.G., Scherr, P.A., & Wallace, R.B. (1994). A short physical performance battery assessing lower extremity function: Association with self-reported disability and prediction of mortality and nursing home admission. *Journal of Gerontology, 49*(2), M85–M94. https://doi: 10.1093/geronj/49.2.m85.

Heyn, P., Abreu, B.C., & Ottenbacher, K.J. (2004). The effects of exercise training on elderly persons with cognitive impairment and dementia: A meta-analysis. *Archives of Physical Medicine and Rehabilitation, 85*(10), 1694–1704. 10.1016/j.apmr.2004.03.019.

Meiland, F., Innes, A., Mountain, G., Robinson, L., van der Roest, H., García-Casal, J.A., Gove, D., Thyrian, J.R., Evans, S., Dröes, R.M., Kelly, F., Kurz, A., Casey, D., Szcześniak, D., Dening, T., Craven, M.P., Span, M., Felzmann, H., Tsolaki, M., & Franco-Martin, M. (2017). Technologies to support community-dwelling persons with dementia: A position paper on issues regarding development, usability, effectiveness and cost-effectiveness, deployment, and ethics. *JMIR Rehabilitation and Assistive Technologies, 4*(1), e1. https://rehab.jmir.org/2017/1/e1/

Mura, G., Carta, M.G., Sancassiani, F., Machado, S., & Prosperini, L. (2018). Active exergames to improve cognitive functioning in neurological disabilities: A systematic review and meta-analysis. *European Journal of Physical and Rehabilitation Medicine, 54*(3), 450–462. 10.23736/S1973-9087.17.04680-9.

Nilsen, P. (2015). Making sense of implementation theories, models and frameworks. *Implementation Science, 10*, 53 https://doi.org/10.1186/s13012-015-0242-0.

Nyman, S.R. (2011). Psychosocial issues in engaging older people with physical activity interventions for the prevention of falls. *Canadian Journal on Aging, 30*(1), 45–55. https://doi.org/10.1017/S0714980810000759

Nyman, S.R., & Szymczynska, P. (2016). Meaningful activities for improving the wellbeing of people with dementia: beyond mere pleasure to meeting fundamental psychological needs. *Perspectives in Public Health, 136*(2), 99–107. 10.1177/1757913915626193.

Peng, W., Crouse, J.C., & Lin, J.H. (2013). Using active video games for physical activity promotion: A systematic review of the current state of research. *Health Education & Behavior, 40*(2), 171–192. https://doi.org/10.1177/1090198112444956

Taylor, L.M., Maddison, R., Pfaeffli, L.A., Rawstorn, J.C., Gant, N., & Kerse, N.M. (2012). Activity and energy expenditure in older people playing active video games. *Archives of Physical Medicine and Rehabilitation, 93*(12), 2281–2286. https://doi.org/10.1016/j.apmr.2012.03.034

Tong, T., Chan, J.H., & Chignell, M. (2017). *Serious Games for Dementia.* In Proceedings of the 26th International Conference on World Wide Web Companion (WWW'17

Companion). International World Wide Web Conferences Steering Committee, Republic and Canton of Geneva, CHE, 1111–1115. https://doi.org/10.1145/3041021.3054930

Van den Brink, D., Lutomski, J.E., Qin, L., den Elzen, W.P., Kempen, G.I., Krabbe, P.F., Steyerberg, E.W., Muntinga, M., Moll van Charante, E.P., Bleijenberg, N., Olde Rikkert, M.G.M., & Melis, R.J.F. (2015). TOPICS-MDS: a versatile resource for generating scientific and social knowledge for elderly care. *Tijdschrift voor Gerontologie en Geriatrie*, *46*(2), 78–91. https://doi.org/10.1007/s12439-015-0127-3

Van Santen, J., Dröes, R.M., Holstege, M., Henkemans, O.B., van Rijn, A., de Vries, R., van Straten, A., & Meiland, F. (2018). Effects of exergaming in people with dementia: Results of a systematic literature review. *Journal of Alzheimer's Disease*, *63*(2), 741–760. https://doi.org/10.3233/JAD-170667

Van Santen, J., Dröes, R.M., Schoone, M., Blanson Henkemans, O.A., Bosmans, J.E., van Bommel, S., . . . Meiland, F. (2019). *FACTSHEET Exergaming for people with dementia: Come and join us! Recommendations to promote successful implementation* [in Dutch: FACTSHEET Exergaming voor mensen met dementie: beweeg je mee? Adviezen ter bevordering van succesvolle implementatie]. Amsterdam: VU Medisch Centrum.

Van Santen, J., Dröes, R.M., Twisk, J.W.R., Blanson Henkemans, O.A., Van Straten, A., & Meiland, F.J.M. (2020). Effects of Exergaming on Cognitive and Social Functioning of People with Dementia: A Randomized Controlled Trial. *Journal of the American Medical Directors Association*, *21*(12), 1958–1967. https://doi.org/10.1016/j.jamda.2020.04.018

Vernooij-Dassen, M.J.F.J., Felling, A.J.A., Brummelkamp, E., Dauzenberg, M.G., van den Bos, G.A., & Grol R. (1999). Assessment of caregiver's competence in dealing with the burden of caregiving for a dementia patient: A Short Sense of Competence (SSCQ) suitable for clinical practice. *Journal of the American Geriatrics Society*, *47*(2), 256–257. https://doi.org/10.1111/j.1532-5415.1999.tb04588.x

Verstraten, P.F.J., & van Eekelen, C.W.J.M. (1987). *Manual for the GIP: Behavioural Observation Scale for Intramural Psychogeriatrics*. Deventer, The Netherlands: Van Loghum Slaterus.

Zhao, Y., Feng, H., Wu, X., Du, Y., Yang, X., Hu, M., Ning, H., Liao, L., Chen, H., & Zhao, Y. (2020). Effectiveness of exergaming in improving cognitive and physical function in people with mild cognitive impairment or dementia: Systematic review. *JMIR Serious Games*, *30*(2), e16841. https://doi: 10.2196/16841.

Chapter 10

Development and evaluation of FindMyApps

Fulfilling the needs and wishes of
people with dementia to maintain
Social Health[1]

*Kim Beentjes, Yvonne Kerkhof, David Neal,
Gianna Kohl, Steve Course, Lucas Vroemen,
Maud JL Graff, Rose-Marie Dröes*

Introduction

In the Netherlands, 70% of people with dementia live at home. The majority
of them are cared for by informal carers of which 52% feel fairly to heavily
burdened and 12% overburdened (Heide et al., 2018). People with dementia often want to continue to participate in self-management and meaningful
(social) activities. Over the past decade, many apps have been developed that
offer solutions to fulfil such needs. But which ones are suitable for people with
dementia? And how do you find usable apps in the 'forest' of apps that suits
personal interests? To simplify the search process for suitable apps, researchers from Saxion University, Amsterdam UMC, and Radboudumc developed a
person-centred tablet program called FindMyApps, in co-creation with people
with dementia, informal carers, professionals and ICT experts from the software company EuMediaNet.

Involving people with dementia in technology research

There are many ways to involve people with dementia in research, to ensure that
the results are relevant to the target group (Miah et al., 2019). Their involvement
can vary from informants and advisors to co-designers and co-decision makers.
In the design phase, one can think of involving people with dementia in setting
the research priorities, design of the protocol and composing a lay summary. In
the phase of preparation for the research execution they can be involved in fun-
draising, composing information brochures, informed consent forms and ethical
review. During the execution of the research they could be involved in the project group, reporting and informing study participants. Finally, they can also play
an important role in disseminating and communicating research findings.

DOI: 10.4324/9781003289005-13

Although patient and public involvement is recommended to increase the impact and relevance of health research (Miah et al., 2019), several considerations can be made when involving people with dementia in research of which researchers need to be aware of (Wang et al., 2019). For example, participation of the person with dementia may increase carer burden and lead to stress in the person with dementia, for example when a prototype does not work optimally; participation is restricted to persons who can express themselves verbally; it may be difficult to manage a continuity of information with the person with dementia; it can be time-consuming for the researcher and therefore expensive to execute; as sample sizes are often small and sometimes biased, also because of high drop-out rates, findings may be difficult to generalise; the duration of sessions is usually short; and researchers could influence what people with dementia say and do.

In the development of technology, a distinction is made between participatory design and user-centred design as far as the involvement of future users is concerned. *Participatory design* (also called co-design) attempts to actively involve all stakeholders (e.g. end users, care professionals and experts, researchers, software developers and designers) in the design process to help ensure the result meets their needs and is usable, user-friendly and efficient. In *user-centred design*, the development process starts with an exploration of people's experiences and needs on the basis of which a new product is proposed and developed. In this approach, the future users are thus completely central in the development, from the initial idea to final product. In the development of the FindMyApps program a participatory design was applied, although much energy was put into exploring the needs of the target group regarding the intended product, concept development and user requirements.

The FindMyApps project

The FindMyApps program consists of an app with a selection tool and training for carers to teach the person with dementia how to use the tablet and FindMyApps app. The FindMyApps selection tool, initially a web application which was later developed into a native app, can be used on tablets with an Android or iOS operating system. The app gives access to a database containing pre-selected apps ('FindMyApps-app library'), focusing on self-management and meaningful (social) activities, that have all been assessed on dementia-friendliness. The criteria to include apps in this library were based on research with people with dementia and carers (Joddrell et al., 2016). FindMyApps makes it easier to find dementia-friendly apps, which fit the needs, wishes and abilities of the person with dementia.

The training for carers is based on the 'error-less learning' method and includes written and oral instructions on how to implement this method, such as using a stepwise approach, encouraging the person with dementia not to make guesses about how to perform an activity, and repeating steps frequently

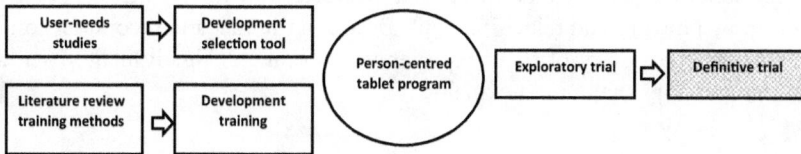

Figure 10.1 The process of development and evaluation of FindMyApps

while preventing mistakes (Clare & Jones, 2008). The aim of the FindMyApps program is to promote self-management in daily life and having satisfying meaningful and social activities. FindMyApps also aims to relieve some of the burden on carers.

As this person–centred tablet program can be viewed as a complex intervention, the Medical Research Council (MRC) framework for the development and evaluation of complex interventions was used to define the problems/needs the programme aims at, to model the intervention, and to prepare and execute the evaluation in exploratory pilot studies and a definitive trial (see Fig.10.1; Campbell et al., 2007).

Development of the prototype

The development process started with a study to identify user needs in the domains of self-management and meaningful activities and to get insight into user requirements for a tool for selecting usable apps in these domains (Kerkhof et al., 2017).

User needs studies

Eight focus groups with people with Mild Cognitive Impairment (MCI) or mild dementia and informal carers were conducted. In study 1 needs for self-management support and meaningful activities were identified in two focus groups with people with dementia ($n = 8$, age range 60–82 years) and two with carers ($n = 10$; age range 62–79 years). In study 2 the needs, wishes and abilities regarding the use of apps were explored in, again, two focus groups with five people with dementia (age range 59–95) and two with five carers (age range 39–79). For study two, participants were selected that had some experience with the use of a tablet or smartphone.

Study 1: To gain insight into the target group's relevant self-management activities and other meaningful activities, the methodology of the Occupational History Performance Interview (OPHI-II-NL) was applied (Baaijen et al., 2008), which focuses on the identification of meaningful activities in the past, present and future.

Study 2: In the first and second sessions insight was gained into the current use and types of apps, the choices made in selecting certain kind of apps, and the experiences of participants with new apps selected by the researchers (Word puzzle apps, a history and television app). Between the first and second sessions participants kept a diary of their experiences (advantages/disadvantages) with new apps and apps they used normally.

Identification of meaningful and self-management activities (study 1)

Most of the mentioned needs and wishes for *self-management* were related to 'memory support' such as maintaining daily structure, finding the way and memory training. Other frequently cited needs for self-management support were related to 'maintaining freedom of movement'. For example, participants reported feelings of sadness because their driver's license had been taken away, or because cycling was no longer possible. This was perceived as a loss of self-management and meaningful activities. It is worth noting that people with dementia felt the need for maintaining autonomy and respect, for example when memory loss or communication problems affected having normal conversations. Examples of apps that may be supportive in these areas of self-management are: the Clock aid for maintaining daily structure; Navigation apps like *Blokje Om* for finding the way and maintaining freedom of movement; the Diaro App for language and communication support; and memory training apps, such as Clevermind.

The most frequently mentioned *meaningful activity* in the past and present was 'being socially active', for example having regular and good contact with family members. Being socially active also appears to be a motivating factor to engage in other meaningful activities, for example those that take place at the meeting centre or day-care centre, such as shuffleboard and handicrafts, as well as various types of sports that have been practiced in the past, such as football. This implies that apps that support people with being socially active (e.g. Skype, WhatsApp) or apps for meaningful activities with a social component, such as playing games (e.g. Wordfeud) or playing sports together (e.g. football or tennis) are desirable for people with dementia.

Furthermore, the study showed that activities performed in the past can provide relevant information for preferred activities in the present, and therefore for suitable apps. For example, career-related activities such as iHandy carpenter for a carpenter who still likes to repair furniture, and Art Gallery apps for an art specialist who still likes to visit a museum.

Identification of functional and technical requirements of apps (study 2)

The majority of user requirements identified in these sessions addressed needs and wishes related to the technical selection criteria of apps. Most of them were in line with requirements for interfaces described in the literature, such as providing a simple and intuitive use and help tutorial; minimising the use of clutter (no advertising); using a calm interface and background (less text); readable letters and sizes and clear pictures and photos. New requirements were: as little typing as possible to navigate within the apps; language and settings in the apps must be configurable in the native language.

During the focus groups we observed that persons with dementia generally chose apps for familiar games from the past, that is the non-digital version of checkers or solitaire, not only out of personal interest but also because of familiarity with the operation of these games. Nonetheless, research shows that novel games should not be avoided as they can be easy to use and playable (Astell et al., 2016). This was confirmed in our study: persons with dementia were enthusiastic about apps that offered the possibility of learning new games. However, we also found that despite varying degrees of performance, persons with dementia needed support to operate the tablet and apps.

Participatory development of selection tool

To ensure the usability of the FindMyApps selection tool, the users (people with dementia and carers) were invited to test whether the prototypes harmonised with their needs, wishes and abilities in three short iterative rounds, so called 'sprints' (Kerkhof et al., 2019).

On the basis of the Scrum method (Stellman & Greene, 2015) and user-participatory method (Span et al., 2013), four phases represented one sprint:

- Phase I: Design, collecting data on needs, wishes and abilities of users regarding the desired design;
- Phase II: Development, converting these user requirements in mock-ups;
- Phase III: Usability tests, testing to ensure that the tool meets the user requirements;
- Phase IV: Discover usability issues to improve the tool and discover needs for further development (adapting or creation of new user requirements).

The progression from one sprint to another was conducted as an iterative process, that is returning to the phase of design and development based on feedback or new information collected during a sprint. This provided the opportunity to optimise the tool constantly according to the needs, wishes and abilities of users. We gained an understanding of issues regarding usefulness (e.g. meaningful content of (sub)categories for apps in domains of self-management and meaningful activities), as well as issues to increase user-friendliness (e.g. intuitive design with instructive navigation support). The three sprints were conducted over a nine-month period (Figure 10.2).

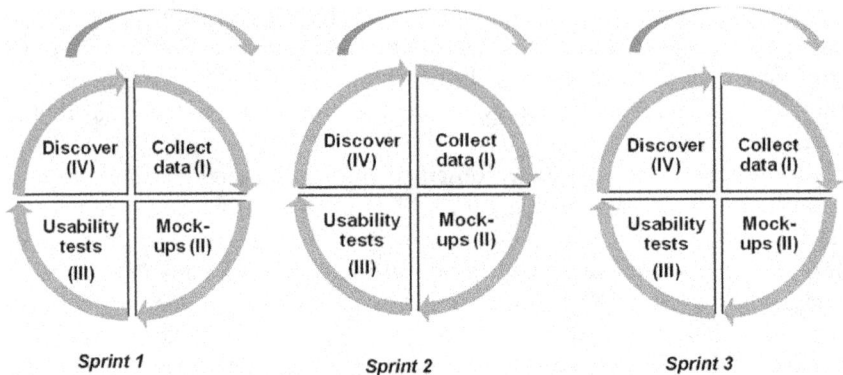

Figure 10.2 Development of the FindMyApps selection tool in three sprints

Phases I and II: Design and development

Major principles of the tool were established on the basis of the scientific literature (Martin et al., 2013), our previous study (Kerkhof et al., 2017) and best practices (Joddrell et al., 2016) and the intended functionalities in FindMyApps. The developers and designers from the software company translated these principles into a programme of requirements. Mock-ups were created and tested to assess whether they met the requirements. A cognitive walkthrough took place within the second ($n = 4$) and third sprint ($n = 5$) in which both researchers and experts performed a series of assignments aimed at identifying usability problems in the tool that could impede successful completion of a task (Nijland, 2011). After integrating all feedback from a sprint and redesigning the tool to address the usability issues, the next phases started, that is usability testing with potential users and discovering new usability issues.

Phases III and IV: Usability testing and discovering usability issues

Both usability tests involved the participation of four persons with mild dementia or MCI (total eight persons: one female, seven males; mean age 78.6, range 72–86). Five informal carers participated in sprint 1 and three in sprint 2 (four males, four females; mean age 73.1, range 58–82).

During the tests the 'scenario-based testing' method was applied (Nijland, 2011). The scenarios concerned realistic assignments of how users may carry out tasks in a specific context with the tool. An example is: *Which activity do you prefer? Try to find an app for that.* After each assignment, questions were posed to identify usability issues regarding content and design of the FindMyApps tool.

Prototype ready for piloting

The development process resulted in a workable FindMyApps tool with an unambiguous routing for finding apps, requiring minimal effort from the target group to master. User experiences generated important insights into useful content and user-friendly design of the tool. They told us that combining many options for main and subcategories on one screen was not desirable. We therefore decided to incorporate more pages with fewer possible options, supported by a clear and simple navigation. Furthermore, they provided relevant information on suitable dementia-friendly icons, a suitable supply of apps within subcategories, and the use of clear and short explanations of the content of apps. In addition, they clarified how to best formulate the personal settings and help instructions. A major insight was that user-interface elements, such as pages and interactive buttons, had to be simple and logically integrated to support users in intuitively operating and understanding the tool.

Feasibility testing of the prototype

After the development of the FindMyApps selection tool the feasibility, implementation and mechanisms of impact of FindMyApps were tested in an exploratory, small-scale pilot randomised controlled trial (RCT) with a mixed-methods design (Kerkhof et al., 2020). Stratified by cohabiting with their carer, 20 persons with mild dementia/carer dyads were randomly assigned to the FindMyApps group ($n = 10$), receiving the FindMyApps training and tool, or a control condition ($n = 10$), receiving a short tablet training. Participants in both groups were given a written manual with the information explained. In the control group this also included a list of websites that suggested useful apps for people with dementia/MCI.

Mean age of the people with dementia in the FindMyApps group was 68.9 years (50–87) and in the control group 76 years (72–81). Mean age of the informal carers in the FindMyApps group was 63 years (47–79) and in the control group 61 years (40–71).

Measurements were conducted at baseline (T0) and after three months of using the tablet (T1). Standard questionnaires were used regarding self-management, meaningful activities, self-efficacy, perceived autonomy and quality of life of persons with dementia, and sense of competence, positive care experience and quality of life of informal carers and post-test semi-structured interviews. During the intervention period a helpdesk was available for participants.

Qualitative results indicated that the FindMyApps intervention has the potential to improve self-management abilities and engagement in meaningful activities of people with dementia. The FindMyApps tool was mostly perceived as useful and easy to use. Persons with dementia found apps through the tool which they used regularly.

'Icons are fine. They are recognisable' (PwD5).

'There are [apps] in there that are very useful, you know, in my case with dementia' (PwD13).

'It is very user-friendly. It is not difficult at all. I am not at all technical with computers and tablets, but even I understand this' (IC5).

'You notice that the initiative of the person with dementia decreases and it's very useful and nice that FindMyApps gives new ideas for spending spare time' (IC13).

Persons with dementia and carers were positive about the FindMyApps training and the support they received. However, one informal carer indicated that one training session provided by the researcher at the start was insufficient to effectively support the person with dementia. Persons with dementia were generally able to learn how to use the tablet and tool, though they regularly needed support from carers, for example with downloading new apps. Previous experience using a tablet made the training easier for persons with dementia.

'For me, it was a revelation that people with mild dementia could learn new things, I thought this was not possible anymore. So, I taught her the FindMyApps tool and tablet in accordance with this [errorless learning] method and I hope this will also work out for the long term' (IC14).

'I think he managed very well, of course we practice on a regular basis, but he was already very experienced using a computer and a tablet' (IC5).

No significant differences were found on the quantitative outcome measures used for the persons with dementia. However, medium positive effect sizes on self-management and social and domestic activities showed that FindMyApps has potential to positively influence the person with dementia's self-management and engagement in meaningful activities. No effects were found on the carer outcomes measures. Regarding positive care experience a significant difference in favour of the control group was found.

Recommendations to improve the intervention were adding demonstrational videos for tool and tablet use to support informal carers in the training, and adding short explanatory descriptions of activities on the (sub)category buttons. Recommendations for future effectiveness studies concerned using shorter questionnaires for people with dementia and a required sample size of 88 participants per group (experimental/control), including a dropout rate of 37.5% (as occurred in the feasibility study), based on a power calculation to detect a medium effect.

Pilot trial

After the first small-scale feasibility study the FindMyApps selection tool and research procedures were improved, and a second, larger, pilot study was conducted to explore again the feasibility of the FindMyApps intervention compared to usual tablet use and the trial procedures as preparation for a definitive effectiveness trial. Again a two-arm, non-blinded, RCT was applied, with a process evaluation alongside (Beentjes et al., 2020a,b).

Fifty-nine participant dyads consisting of a person diagnosed with mild dementia or MCI and their informal carer were initially included and randomised into the experimental (n = 29) and control group (n = 31), stratified by diagnosis (dementia/MCI) and whether or not they cohabited with their carer. Before the baseline measurement, four people with dementia and one carer dropped out resulting in 27 persons with dementia/MCI and 28 carers participating in the FindMyApps intervention and 28 persons with dementia/MCI and 30 carers in the control group. Measurements were conducted at baseline (T0) and after three months of using the tablet (T1) on the same outcomes measures as in the previous study (Kerkhof et al., 2020); however, shorter questionnaires were used for persons with dementia. The intervention for the experimental and control group did not differ from the previous study. An important exception was that during the training videos were shown on how to use the tablet (in both groups) and how to use the FindMyApps selection tool (experimental group only), which remained viewable on the FindMyApps project website to support users during the intervention period. Also, a helpdesk was available during the intervention period.

As in the first pilot study, after three months (T1), no significant differences on measures of self-management, social participation and engagement in activities, self-efficacy, experienced autonomy or quality of life of the person with dementia/MCI were observed between the experimental and control group. Additionally, no significant differences were observed for the carers' positive care experience, sense of competence or quality of life. However, small positive effect sizes showed tendencies in favour of the FindMyApps group for self-management and social participation and positive care experiences of carers. These trends were in line with the results of the first pilot study into FindMyApps (see section 'Feasibility testing of the prototype'). It was therefore suggested that the program has potential to positively influence self-management and social participation in people with dementia and may positively impact carers as well, but that a larger, sufficiently powered study would be needed to properly investigate the effectiveness.

In the process evaluation, semi-structured interviews were held with 20 participant dyads (10 FindMyApps group, 10 control group) to trace contextual, implementation and mechanism of impact factors that could have influenced the trial outcomes.

Findings regarding *contextual factors* were that people sometimes experienced technical problems, such as apps being unavailable and FindMyApps being temporarily offline.

Regarding *implementation*, some participants noted that the training was insufficient. The demonstration videos were little used. Nevertheless, the support of people with dementia/MCI by the carers and the errorless learning method were generally rated as helpful. In addition, results showed that persons with dementia/MCI needed help searching and downloading apps.

> Searching independently [for apps] was not possible.
>
> [IC19, experimental group]

> She [caregiver] has to help me. I couldn't do it myself.
>
> [PwD/MCI28, experimental group]

With respect to *mechanisms of impact*, although dyads reported that they did not use FindMyApps regularly, they did regularly use the apps they found through FindMyApps. When these apps were downloaded, FindMyApps was not used for a while until they wished to find new apps. This suggests that FindMyApps may be a useful tool to find apps, confirming previous findings (Kerkhof et al., 2020).

> We spent whole evenings with music playing, singing along with old songs from the past via the dementia and memories app.
>
> [PwD/MCI28, FindMyApps-group]

The frequency of use of FindMyApps though may increase if the app library is regularly updated. Regarding learnability, it proved important that participants were motivated to learn how to use a tablet and FindMyApps. Overall the process evaluation demonstrated that the FindMyApps selection tool was usable for people with dementia/MCI and positively valued by those who used it regularly (Beentjes et al., 2020b).

Design of the definitive trial

Following the feasibility and pilot studies, a definitive RCT was set up, following a similar method to the pilot (Neal et al., 2021). This study is actively recruiting at time of writing, with a target of $n = 150$ dyads (75 experimental/75 control). The primary objective is to evaluate the effectiveness of FindMyApps, compared to usual care (tablet use without FindMyApps), with respect to the ability to self-manage and social participation of the person with dementia, and sense of competence of carers.

We will also evaluate the cost-effectiveness of FindMyApps. As in the pilot study, a process evaluation will be conducted, in line with the MRC guidance for process evaluation (Moore et al., 2015). People with dementia have been involved in the design and execution of this definitive trial in three important ways. First, based on feedback from participants in the pilot studies, the intervention and protocol were both revised. From the SSIs conducted, we learned that the FindMyApps web app was sometimes slow to react. We resolved this issue by creating a more stable and reactive native app. Many participants found interviews for the baseline and follow-up measurements too long. We there-fore reviewed the instruments used and chose a selection which should be less burdensome.

Seeing the value of participants' feedback from the pilot studies, the second way of including participants in the definitive trial is to continue to conduct SSIs. Many participants provide insightful information about their experiences, so this remains very valuable to us. It also seems valuable for participants, many of whom are happy to contribute in a more meaningful way than simply as a subject receiving an intervention and providing data.

Finally, we have established a Sounding Board. The primary governance of this study flows from the Project Group, which comprises researchers from collaborat-ing institutions. The Sounding Board provides complementary input, to support decision-making with respect to pragmatic issues. There are no fixed members of the Sounding Board but those invited to participate each time include former study participants (people with dementia and informal caregivers), as well as vol-unteers and professionals who work with people with dementia. Topics discussed have included safety measures with respect to COVID-19, and approaches to recruiting participants. Input of people with dementia is shaping the way we conduct the research, to meet the needs and expectations of all involved.

Concluding remarks

In this study into the development and evaluation of FindMyApps, in addition to researchers, professional and technological designers, people with dementia and carers were intensively and successfully involved in all phases of the research, sometimes as informants or advisors to guide and support decision-making, sometimes as test subjects and finally as ambassadors for the recruitment of new study participants in the pilot and definitive trial. This participatory process resulted in a user-friendly, usable and well-accepted program, which is now being further evaluated on its effectiveness and cost-effectiveness in a larger scale RCT of which the results are expected in 2023.

The findings of the two pilot studies into the FindMyApps program are in line with the study of Joddrell et al. (2016), who concluded that touch screen technology is usable for people with dementia, and offers potential for meaningful occupation, fun, entertainment and independent activities. Whether FindMyApps will encourage the use of apps for self-management and social participation and consequently improve the social health of people with dementia will become clear from the definitive trial.

Acknowledgements

The FindMyApps project was set up by Saxion University of Applied Sci-ences in collaboration with VU University medical center, Radboudumc and EuMediaNet in the Netherlands, thereafter has been part of INDUCT and will be finalised in DISTINCT, which received funding from both the

European Union's Horizon 2020 research and innovation programme under Marie Sklodowska-Curie grant agreement No. 676265 and No. 813196. The study was co-funded by the Foundation for Support VCVGZ and Stichting Hofje Codde en Van Beresteyn.

Note

1   Parts of this chapter were previously published in Kerkhof et al. (2017). Selecting apps for people with mild dementia: Identifying user requirements for apps enabling meaningful activities and self-management. *Journal of Rehabilitation and Assistive Technologies Engineering,* 4:2055668317710593; Kerkhof et al. (2019). User-participatory development of FindMyApps; a tool to help people with mild dementia find supportive apps for self-management and meaningful activities. *Digital Health,* 5, 1–19. https://doi.org/10.1177/2055207618822942; Kerkhof et al. (2020). Randomised controlled feasibility study of FindMyApps: First evaluation of a tablet-based intervention to promote self-management and meaningful activities in people with mild dementia. *Disabil Rehabil Assist Technol.* 1–15. https://doi.org/10.1080/17483107.2020.1765420. Publisher Taylor & Francis Ltd, www.tandfonline.com reprinted by permission of the publisher; Beentjes et al. (2020a). Impact of the FindMyApps Program on People with Mild Cognitive Impairment or Dementia and their Caregivers; an Exploratory Randomized Controlled Trial. *Disability and Rehabilitation: Assistive Technology.* https://doi.org/https://doi.org/10.1080/17483107.2020.1842918; and Beentjes et al. (2020b). Process Evaluation of the FindMyApps Program Trial among People with Dementia or MCI and their Caregivers based on the MRC Guidance. *Gerontechnology,* 20(5), 1–15. https://doi.org/10.4017/gt.2020.20.005.11

References

Astell, A.J., Joddrell, P., Groenewoud, H., de Lange, J., Goumans, M., Cordia, A., et al. (2016). Does familiarity affect the enjoyment of touchscreen games for people with dementia? *International journal of medical informatics,* 91, e1–e8.

Baaijen, R., Boon, J., & Tichelaar, E. (2008). *De Nederlandse samenvattende handleiding van de OPHI-II (versie 2.1.) Occupational Performance History Interview-II NL.* The Netherlands: Amsterdam: Hogeschool van Amsterdam, Expertise Centrum Ergotherapie.

Beentjes, K.M., Kerkhof, Y.J.F., Neal, D.P., Ettema, T.P., Koppelle, M.A., Meiland, F.J.M., . . . Dröes, R.M. (2020b). Process evaluation of the FindMyApps program trial among people with dementia or MCI and their caregivers based on the MRC guidance. *Gerontechnology,* 20(5), 1–15. https://doi.org/10.4017/gt.2020.20.005.11

Beentjes, K.M., Neal, D.P., Kerkhof, Y.J.F., Broeder, C., Moeridjan, Z.D.J., Ettema, T.P., . . . Dröes, R.M. (2020a). Impact of the FindMyApps program on people with mild cognitive impairment or dementia and their caregivers; an exploratory randomized controlled trial. *Disability and Rehabilitation: Assistive Technology.* https://doi.org/https://doi.org/10.1080/17483107.2020.1842918

Campbell, N.C., Murray, E., Darbyshire, J., Emery, J., Farmer, A., Griffiths, F., et al. (2007). Designing and evaluating complex interventions to improve health care. *British Medical Journal,* 334, 455–459.

Clare, L., & Jones, R.S.P. (2008). Errorless learning in the rehabilitation of memory impairment: A critical review. *Neuropsychology Review,* 18(1):1–23.

Heide, I., Buuse, S., & Francke, A.L. (2018). *Dementiemonitor Mantelzorg 2018: mantelzorgers over ondersteuning, zorg, belasting en de impact van mantelzorg op hun leven*. Utrecht, The Netherlands: Nivel.

Joddrell, P., Hernandez, A., O'Neil-Watts, S., Moore, E., Davenport, E., & Astell, A.J. (2016). *AcToDementia, app selection framework. Guidance manual*. Sheffield: Centre for Assistive Technology and Connected Healthcare (CATCH) at the University of Sheffield.

Kerkhof, Y., Pelgrum-Keurhorst, M., Mangiaracina, F., Bergsma, A., Vrauwdeunt, G., Graff, M., & Dröes, R.M. (2019). User-participatory development of FindMyApps; a tool to help people with mild dementia find supportive apps for self-management and meaningful activities. *Digital Health, 5*, 1–19. https://doi.org/10.1177/2055207618822942

Kerkhof, Y.J.F., Bergsma, A., Graff, M.J.L., & Dröes, R.M. (2017). Selecting apps for people with mild dementia: Identifying user requirements for apps enabling meaningful activities and self-management. *Journal of Rehabilitation and Assistive Technologies Engineering, 4*, 2055668317710593.

Kerkhof, Y.J.F., Kohl, G., Veijer, M., Mangiaracina, F., Bergsma, A., Graff, M., et al. (2020). Randomised controlled feasibility study of FindMyApps: First evaluation of a tablet-based intervention to promote self-management and meaningful activities in people with mild dementia. *Disability and Rehabilitation: Assistive Technology*, 1–15. https://doi.org/10.1080/17483107.2020.1765420

Martin, F., Turner, A., Wallace, L.M., Bradbury, N. (2013). Conceptualisation of self-management intervention for people with early stage dementia. *European Journal of Ageing, 10*(2), 75–87.

Miah, J., Dawes, P., Edwards, S., Leroi, I., Starling, B., & Parsons, S. (2019). Patient and public involvement in dementia research in the European Union: A scoping review. *BMC Geriatrics, 19*(1), 220. https://doi.org/10.1186/s12877-019-1217-9

Moore, G., Audrey, S., Barker, M., Bond, L. (external link), Bonell, C., Hardeman, W., . . . Baird, J (2015). Process evaluation of complex interventions: A summary of Medical Research Council guidance. In D.A. Richards & R. Hahlberg (Eds.), *Complex interventions in health: An overview of research methods* (pp. 222–231). Milton Park, Abingdon, Oxon: Routledge.

Neal, D.P., Kerkhof, Y.J.F., Ettema, T.P, Muller, M., Bosmans, J.E., Finnema, E.J., Graff, M.J.L., Dijkstra, K., Stek, M.L., & Dröes, R.M. (2021). Evaluation of FindMyApps: protocol for a randomized controlled trial of the effectiveness and cost-effectiveness of a tablet-based intervention to improve self-management and social participation of community-dwelling people with mild dementia, compared to usual tablet use. *BMC Geriatrics, 21*, 138. https://doi.org/10.1186/s12877-021-02038-8

Nijland, N. (2011). *Grounding eHealth: towards a holistic framework for sustainable eHealth technologies*. Enschede: University of Twente.

Span, M., Hettinga, M., Vernooij-Dassen, M., Eefsting, J., & Smits, C. (2013). Involving people with dementia in the development of supportive IT applications: A systematic review. *Ageing Research Reviews, 12*(2), 535–551.

Stellman, A., & Greene, J. (2015). *Learning Agile, understanding Scrum, XP, Lean and Kanban*. Sebastopol: O'Reilly.

Wang, G., Marradi, C., Albayrak, A., & van der Cammen, T.J.M. (2019). Co-designing with people with dementia: A scoping review of involving people with dementia in design research. *Maturitas, 127*, 55–63, ISSN 0378–5122, https://doi.org/10.1016/j.maturitas.2019.06.003.

Chapter 11

Internet-based interventions for family carers of people with dementia

Anne Margriet Pot, Kieren Egan, Katrin Seeher

Introduction

Globally, families represent the cornerstone of care and support for people living with dementia, especially in low- and middle-income countries (LMICs) where resources and access to services are scarce (WHO, 2017; WHO, 2021; Wimo et al., 2018). This comes often at a high personal and financial cost to carers, who may feel stressed or report significant health issues. Providing evidence-based training to family or informal carers will not only lead to better outcomes for carers but also benefit the over 55 million people currently living with dementia worldwide (WHO, 2021).

In response to the growing challenge posed by dementia, the Member States of the World Health Organization (WHO) adopted the global action plan on the public health response to dementia 2017–2025 in May 2017 (WHO, 2017). The plan recognises the important role that informal carers play and calls on Member States to provide carers with training and support in order to reduce the burden and negative toll that caregiving can have on carers' physical health and well-being. The global dementia action plan aims to ensure that 75% of countries provide support and training for dementia carers by 2025.

For over three decades, research has been conducted into personal interventions for carers of people with dementia, delivered either face-to-face or by telephone. The approach of such interventions varies widely and originally focused on one or more of the following: coping strategies, behavioural management techniques and the provision of social support. The theoretical basis for such interventions predominantly builds on stress models such as Pearlin's stress process model (Pearlin et al., 1990; Raina et al., 2004).

Early systematic review work (Selwood et al., 2007) identified that not all face-to-face studies with carers demonstrated improvements (such as group behavioural therapy and supportive therapy). However, the authors identified that higher dose interventions, delivering six or more sessions, demonstrated efficacy for individual behavioural management therapy. In addition, individual and group interventions focused on coping strategies established good evidence for improving distress and depression.

DOI: 10.4324/9781003289005-14

Nowadays, interventions are commonly designed as 'multi-component interventions' (Schulz et al., 2020). This means that 'one' intervention includes a range of components such as information sharing, coping and communication skills training, alongside social supports (e.g. balancing theoretical material with practical and 'actionable' insights or interactive elements, including human supports such as a 'coach'). Different techniques are often integrated within interventions such as Cognitive Behavioural Therapy (CBT) or meditation. Such approaches have been shown to independently improve depression, anxiety, burden, stress and dysfunctional thoughts among carers (Collins & Kishita, 2019; Kwon et al., 2017; Schulz et al., 2020).

There is a strong and increasing research interest to develop more accessible interventions to support carers of people living with dementia (Wiegelmann et al., 2021), particularly in LMICs. While technology-focused efforts began with a dependency on specific hardware (e.g. specialised computer networks/ CD-ROM based solutions), over time such innovations have become web-based, and this is an increasingly popular approach for training and support programmes for carers of people living with dementia (Blom et al., 2015; Egan et al., 2018; Kajiyama et al., 2013).

From the perspective of carers, web-based training programmes may have several advantages when compared with face-to-face interventions. For example, they may reach carers in remote areas that cannot be reached otherwise. They will save time for carers who are often already time constrained due to the care they provide and other roles and tasks in life. Carers do not have to leave the person living with dementia unattended. Moreover, not needing to attend a mental health institution in person may be perceived as less stigmatising. Where carers have continued access to web-based support, they also have the freedom to revisit materials at a time of their convenience/need, which holds value considering the progressive nature of dementia. Further, since the global COVID-19 pandemic has exerted more pressure on carers (Altieri & Santangelo, 2021; Budnick et al., 2021), an added value of web-based training is to deliver support when critically needed and avoid the unnecessary risk of contracting infections outside the home.

From a system's perspective, self-help interventions present a universal advantage in that face-to-face interventions are often resource intense, with respect to human and financial resources. In lower income settings, health professionals often lack the knowledge and abilities to provide face-to-face skills training and support programmes for carers. In addition, in high- and low-resource settings alike, economic pressures favour financially sustainable models of delivery (Winblad et al., 2016).

There are now many published systematic reviews that echo the plausibility of web-based or online skills training and support programmes for carers of people living with dementia (Egan et al., 2018; Etxeberria et al., 2021). Such programmes and interventions, that have been tested across many high-income countries but rarely in LMICs, have the potential to reduce carers' psychological distress, improve mental health, and be cost-effective.

Studies demonstrate a wide variety of intervention programmes for carers of people with dementia. However, unfortunately, the quality of these studies is often poor. For example, there is a lack of sufficiently powered randomised controlled trials and details about interventions are often lacking. In one review, only half of the online programmes were described in enough detail to understand which components they included (Egan et al., 2018). Of the programmes that provided at least some description of the content, the following themes were covered: understanding dementia, improving communication skills, arranging help and support, coping with carer stress, dealing with functional decline and with behaviour changes of the person with dementia, and preparation for the future.

Most programmes (with sufficient information) use a variety of techniques ranging from psychoeducation, behavioural analysis, relaxation, behavioural activation, cognitive reframing and improvement of communication skills, problem-solving/decision-making skills, to time-management. The programmes also vary in the delivery approach, for example through written text, videos, (interactive) exercises and quizzes/assessments, a forum and/or videoconferencing. Moreover, there are different ways in which the programmes are personalised, for example by involving a therapist/psychologist, nurse or peer carer (Egan et al., 2018).

Benefits are not universal. It remains unclear whether specific subgroups of carers may benefit more than others. There is a drive to undertake studies with larger sample sizes and longer intervention exposures. There is also a need to move from efficacy research towards implementation research. For example, a recent systematic review suggests that despite much research being undertaken, implementation readiness remains low and existing work has not been delivered in terms of accessible solutions to carers (Christie et al., 2019). In addition, programmes often are not described in sufficient detail: information is lacking on the underlying theoretical model, the content, the psychological techniques used and the way in which personalisation has (or has not) been integrated in the programme. As a result, less scientific progress has been made than hoped for.

iSupport: WHO training and support programme for carers of people living with dementia

Since skills training and support for carers of people living with dementia are urgently needed worldwide, WHO has developed iSupport (WHO, 2019). iSupport aims to teach carers to provide better care, for a longer period of time, thus allowing the person living with dementia to live in the community for longer, while at the same time preventing or reducing detrimental consequences on carers' health and well-being.

iSupport is based on the latest evidence, described in detail, freely accessible and available for scaling worldwide, online, in hardcopy and shortened poster format. There is an opportunity to co-ordinate excellence in research in multiple country settings, for example to: improve the overall reporting, share the background theory and components of the intervention, and better understand the differential impact of iSupport for example in subgroups of carers. iSupport has been developed in collaboration with an international expert group and Alzheimer's Disease International and reflects the needs of carers of people living with dementia.

The following describes iSupport in detail, the translation and adaptation process to tailor iSupport to a specific cultural setting or group of carers, and findings from preliminary research on its effectiveness.

iSupport consists of 23 sessions in total, covering five modules: (a) what is dementia (one session); (b) being a carer (four sessions); (c) caring for me (three sessions); (d) providing everyday care (five sessions) and (e) dealing with changing behaviour (ten sessions). All sessions follow the same structure. They start with a summary of why the specific session is important, how it will help and what the carer will learn. The summary is followed by new information, examples and activities with instant feedback to internalise knowledge and develop carer skills. Carers can take all sessions from start to finish or choose the sessions that are most relevant to their own situation. For more information on iSupport, see www.iSupportforDementia.org.

The iSupport content is deeply grounded in Kitwood's model of personhood. It conceptualises care provision as an interaction between the person with dementia and the carer based on the individual's needs, personality and ability. Behaviour changes that occur in dementia are not only a reflection of deteriorating brain functioning but also the result of a person's personality, coping mechanisms, personal history, health status and the social/physical environment. iSupport integrates all these elements into interactive exercises for carers that are grounded in therapeutic techniques that have proven beneficial in the context of dementia caregiving, such as CBT, psychoeducation, relaxation, behavioural activation, cognitive reframing and some problem-solving elements (Pot et al., 2019).

WHO is promoting a broad use of iSupport. The programme has been developed initially as a self-help tool because face-to-face training programmes might be difficult to implement in LMICs where prerequisites for sustainable delivery are often lacking. In addition, iSupport might be used by groups of carers, with or without the guidance of a volunteer or healthcare worker, or by healthcare workers themselves (WHO, 2019). Although iSupport is originally developed as an online tool, there is also a hardcopy manual available for areas challenged with aspects of the digital divide (e.g. limited Internet bandwidth or low digital literacy) (Pot et al., 2019; WHO, 2019). In response to the breakdown of carer support services during the COVID-19 pandemic, an additional Lite version has been developed. This Lite version consists of posters with easy read tips based on, and referring to iSupport, covering topics such as Reaching out to others for help and Ensuring that the person with dementia continues to receive care (WHO, 2020).

Translation, adaptation and implementation of iSupport worldwide

To implement iSupport in a specific setting, the programme needs to be translated and adapted to the context and culture of that setting and the specific group of carers, for ecological validity (Gearing et al., 2013). Currently, implementations of iSupport at various states are ongoing in over 30 countries worldwide. This ranges from initial planning stages to the completion of pilot Randomised Controlled Trials (RCTs) with published results (Baruah et al., 2021; Mehta et al., 2018; Teles et al., 2020; Teles et al., 2021; Xiao et al., 2021). Together, these implementation projects cover over 30 different languages, including all official WHO languages (i.e. Arabic, Chinese, English, French, Russian and Spanish). WHO provides a standardised guide for translation and adaptation to ensure that local versions of iSupport are accurate and in line with the generic version, while at the same time appropriate for local target groups of carers. The guide describes the actual changes that might be (in)appropriate, such as specific words, names and links to local Alzheimer's organisations and care and support services. Translations and adaptations for different settings have been described (Baruah et al., 2021; Oliveira et al., 2020; Teles et al., 2021; Teles et al., 2021; Xiao et al., 2021).

The first adaptation was made for the Indian context (Baruah et al., 2021; Baruah et al., 2020). The adaptation process was guided by a heuristic framework (Barrera & Castro, 2006), and included a literature review and focus group discussions with family carers and health professionals, content modifications based on WHO's adaptation guide, online user testing with face-to-face interviews followed by final modifications to the intervention. The modifications ranged from words, names, references to resources and case descriptions to audio files. Overall, the online programme was developed in a way to cater particularly for low Internet bandwidth in India. Preliminary data showed that carers who participated in the adaptation process were satisfied with the changes, although the translation to different Indian languages was suggested.

The second country adaptation has been documented for Portugal (Teles et al., 2021). In collaboration with the national Alzheimer Association, the adaptation process was carried out in five steps, including a needs assessment, content translation and technical accuracy check, cultural adaptation, expert panel appraisal and fidelity check. The study revealed the complexity of translating and adapting a generic training programme such as iSupport to a specific cultural setting, including the involvement of a multidisciplinary team, which comprised a translator, professionals and experts in ageing, dementia and caregiver support. Translations were carried out in a 'sense to sense', rather than in a 'word to word' (literal) approach, requiring a solid understanding of idioms, grammar and conventions in the cultural context of the source language. The translation and adaptation process also resulted in small improvements of the generic English version of iSupport. On the basis of the initial findings of a mixed-methods study (Teles et al., 2021), involving two focus groups ($n = 15$)

and 15 usability test sessions with carers and health professionals, the usability of iSupport was rated as excellent. Participants perceived iSupport as trustworthy, and were satisfied with the content, 'look and feel' and easiness of use. The feedback and personalisation features of the programme were valued.

The third country adaptation explored the best way to adapt and deliver iSupport to the Australian context (Xiao et al., 2021). Two focus groups with family and other unpaid carers ($n = 16$) and two focus groups with care staff ($n = 20$) were conducted using semi-structured interviews. Prior to participation, participants were given access to iSupport, and asked to review the programme. Topics covered in the interviews were accessibility, appropriateness, acceptability, user-friendliness, and barriers and enablers for using the programme. Thematic data analysis (Xiao et al., 2021) revealed that participants perceived iSupport as an opportunity for an online one-stop shop to meet their needs for education and managing care services. They wanted an integrated carer network attached to iSupport, to share and translate dementia care knowledge into everyday care and socialise with others. Discussions showed the need to have a systematic approach to promote the programme among family carers, in rural and remote regions in particular. Lastly, challenges regarding time constraints using a programme such as iSupport were discussed. Suggestions were made to facilitate the feasibility of the programme, for example by enabling searching of sessions based on carers' needs.

Adaptation of iSupport has also been reported for the Brazilian context (Oliveira et al., 2020). After professional translation of the programme, the Brazilian-Portuguese content was discussed and checked for relevance, clarity and accuracy by a multidisciplinary team of researchers. In the next step, the translation was discussed and checked within 16 focus groups ($n = 48$) with family carers of people living with dementia and health and social care professionals from different geographic regions in Brazil. Representatives of the Brazilian Ministry of Health and Alzheimer's Associations also contributed to this assessment. In general, participants were positive about the programme in terms of content and relevance to the Brazilian context. They helped to refine the text and examples and suggested a few changes. Thus, with the input from the different groups of participants, iSupport was successfully culturally adapted for the Brazilian setting. Meanwhile, adaptation of iSupport is continuing, for carers in other countries, such as Greece (Efthymiou et al., 2022), and subpopulations, such as Chinese-Australian carers (Xiao et al., 2022).

Research on the feasibility and effectiveness of iSupport

Although a beneficial impact of Internet-based interventions has been found in Western countries, it cannot be assumed that Internet-based interventions are equally feasible and effective in LMICs settings. For this reason, the feasibility and effectiveness of iSupport were tested in a pilot RCT in India (Baruah et al., 2021), recruiting carers nationwide over a period of 15 months (2017–2018) who were aged 18 years and older, caring for a family member with dementia for at least six months, living in India and had regular access to the Internet. To confirm the dementia diagnosis, the AD8 Dementia Screening Interview (AD8 ≥ 2) was used.

In total, 151 carers were recruited and split into two groups to test whether those completing iSupport online (i.e. intervention group) would feel less burdened and less depressed compared to carers reading a control caregiving e-book (i.e. control group). For those who completed the study ($n = 55$), no significant difference between both groups regarding carer burden and depression was found. Carers in the iSupport group did have more positive attitudes towards people with dementia at the end of the study.

Several challenges likely influenced the outcomes of the study and also had implications for future work in this area. For example, recruitment for the study proved challenging, leading to smaller than expected samples. In addition, the study faced very high attrition rates in both study arms, which reduced samples further. Small samples make it statistically difficult to detect differences between groups. In addition, a lot of carers did not complete the recommended minimum number of online iSupport sessions. This suggests that for the involved carers in India, completing an online carer training and participating in a research study in addition to their normal daily workload and carer responsibilities may be very challenging.

Interestingly, the study attracted an unusual group of carers. Compared to more typical carer populations for whom iSupport was originally developed and later culturally adapted in India, there were more men, more non-spousal carers in this efficacy study. Furthermore, almost all carers in this study had completed college or university. This could mean that the content needed to be more contextualised for the needs of this particular group of carers. In addition, very stressed carers who might have benefitted the most from completing an online carer training and support programme might have dropped out or chosen not to participate in the first place due to time constraints, workload and feelings of being overwhelmed.

Meanwhile, in other countries and regions studies on the impact of iSupport on the mental health and well-being of carers of people with dementia have been initiated. Results from a pilot RCT in Portugal (N = 42) suggest a beneficial impact on carers' symptoms of anxiety and their satisfaction with access to information or health services (Teles et al., 2022). No impact was found on other outcomes, including burden, depression and self-efficacy. In addition, the user satisfaction of people completing the generic online iSupport course available on www.iSupportforDementia.org is being monitored. For the first 51 people who completed the online course (as of August 2022), overall user satisfaction with the online training was high: 82% of users strongly agreed that the content was relevant for building their skills as carers; 72% of users strongly agreed that the lessons were useful and suitable; 69% of users strongly agreed that the included exercises are interesting and useful. The majority of users access iSupport on their laptop (63%) and from home (67%). Perceived barriers to accessing iSupport include time required to complete all lessons

(61% of users), internet bandwidth/speed (26% of users) and complexity of the intervention (7%). Users of iSupport reported self-rated improvements for the following symptoms: depression (18%), anxiety (31%), relationship with the care recipient (54%), stress (61%) and confidence (69%). These findings are preliminary and do not reflect the views or feedback of users who have not completed the online training (yet).

Ongoing iSupport work shows that web-based interventions for carers of people with dementia especially in LMICs require further consideration. Recruitment challenges as well as low uptake of, and adherence to, the intervention limit the evidence. Yet, studies like the ones presented here help us better understand which barriers carers face and as a result how future studies can tailor iSupport better to carers' needs. For example, carers might still be less familiar with receiving training and support via the Internet and less computer- and Internet-savvy than the general population. They might be using smartphones rather than computers or tablets and might have less stable Internet connectivity. Additional research is required to further improve translation, adaptation and implementation of the iSupport programme in India.

Conclusion

There is an urgent global need for accessible, usable, effective and scalable skills training and support programmes for carers of people with dementia, particularly in LMICs. WHO's iSupport is filling this gap by providing such a programme, accessible for translation and cultural adaptation worldwide. First steps have been undertaken to support the systematic and culturally fair translation and adaptation of the programme in several countries.

However, while web-based or online programmes for dementia carers such as iSupport seem to be promising, the scaling of these programmes remains challenging and is a common issue for digital health solutions (Greenhalgh et al., 2017). In fact, the findings of a first efficacy study from India highlight the need to understand carers' individual situation better and tailor support programmes even more to their specific needs. Going forward, iSupport could be improved by adding a mobile phone application to offer more flexibility to users, including an interactive or moderated chat function or more audio-visual materials to the online programme to increase its appeal. To assist carers who wish to use more traditional ways of learning, WHO has released the iSupport hardcopy manual, which presents the entire iSupport content in book format. Further robust cultural adaptations and high-quality research investigating the effectiveness of iSupport across different settings and for different groups of carers are required.

Finally, in the context of the ongoing COVID-19 pandemic, digital support services such as iSupport are more important than ever and present a real opportunity to build back better, which will help to reach the global target set by WHO that 75% of countries will provide support and training programmes for carers and families of people with dementia by 2025.

Acknowledgements/Conflicts of interest

The authors declare no conflicts of interest. The authors alone are responsible for the views expressed in this article and they do not necessarily represent the views, decisions or policies of the institutions with which they are affiliated.

List of abbreviations

CBT   Cognitive Behavioural Therapy
LMICs   Low- and middle-income countries
RCT   Randomised controlled trial
WHO   World Health Organization

References

Altieri, M., & Santangelo, G. (2021). The psychological impact of COVID-19 pandemic and lockdown on caregivers of people with dementia. *The American Journal of Geriatric Psychiatry: Official Journal of the American Association for Geriatric Psychiatry, 29*(1), 27–34. doi:10.1016/j.jagp.2020.10.009

Barrera, M., & Castro, F.G. (2006). A heuristic framework for the cultural adaptation of interventions. *Clinical Psychology: Science and Practice, 13*(4), 311–316. doi:10.1111/j.1468-2850.2006.00043.x

Baruah, U., Loganathan, S., Shivakumar, P., Pot, A.M., Mehta, K.M., Gallagher-Thompson, D., . . . Varghese, M. (2021). Adaptation of an online training and support program for caregivers of people with dementia to Indian cultural setting. *Asian Journal of Psychiatry, 59*, 102624. doi:10.1016/j.ajp.2021.102624

Baruah, U., Shivakumar, P., Loganathan, S., Pot, A.M., Mehta, K.M., Gallagher-Thompson, D., . . . Varghese, M. (2020). Perspectives on components of an online training and support program for dementia family caregivers in India: A focus group study. *Clinical Gerontologist, 43*(5), 518–532. doi:10.1080/07317115.2020.1725703

Baruah, U., Varghese, M., Loganathan, S., Mehta, K.M., Gallagher-Thompson, D., Zandi, D., . . . Pot, A.M. (2021). Feasibility and preliminary effectiveness of an online training and support program for caregivers of people with dementia in India: A randomized controlled trial. *International Journal of Geriatric Psychiatry, 36*(4), 606–617. doi:10.1002/gps.5502

Blom, M.M., Zarit, S.H., Groot Zwaaftink, R.B.M., Cuijpers, P., & Pot, A.M. (2015). Effectiveness of an internet intervention for family caregivers of people with dementia: Results of a randomized controlled trial. *Plos One, 10*(2), e0116622. doi:10.1371/journal.pone.0116622

Budnick, A., Hering, C., Eggert, S., Teubner, C., Suhr, R., Kuhlmey, A., & Gellert, P. (2021). Informal caregivers during the COVID-19 pandemic perceive additional burden: Findings from an ad-hoc survey in Germany. *BMC Health Services Research, 21*(1), 353. doi:10.1186/s12913-021-06359-7

Christie, H.L., Martin, J.L., Connor, J., Tange, H.J., Verhey, F.R.J., de Vugt, M.E., & Orrell, M. (2019). eHealth interventions to support caregivers of people with dementia may be proven effective, but are they implementation-ready? *Internet Interventions, 18*, 100260. doi:10.1016/j.invent.2019.100260

Collins, R.N., & Kishita, N. (2019). The effectiveness of mindfulness- and acceptance-based interventions for informal caregivers of people with dementia: A meta-analysis. *Gerontologist, 59*(4), e363–e379. doi:10.1093/geront/gny024

Egan, K.J., Pinto-Bruno, A.C., Bighelli, I., Berg-Weger, M., van Straten, A., Albanese, E., & Pot, A.M. (2018). Online training and support programs designed to improve mental health and reduce burden among caregivers of people with dementia: A systematic review. *Journal of the American Medical Directors Association, 19*(3), 200–206 e201. doi:10.1016/j.jamda.2017.10.023

Efthymiou, A., Karpathiou, N., Dimakopoulou, E., Zoi, P., Karagianni, C., Lavdas, M., Mastroyiannakis, A., Sioti, E., Zampetakis, I., & Sakka, P. (2022). Cultural Adaptation and Piloting of iSupport Dementia in Greece. *Studies in health technology and informatics, 289*, 184–187. https://doi.org/10.3233/SHTI210890

Etxeberria, I., Salaberria, K., & Gorostiaga, A. (2021). Online support for family caregivers of people with dementia: A systematic review and meta-analysis of RCTs and quasi-experimental studies. *Aging and Mental Health, 25*(7), 1165–1180. doi:10.1080/13607863.2020.1758900

Gearing, R.E., Schwalbe, C.S., MacKenzie, M.J., Brewer, K.B., Ibrahim, R.W., Olimat, H.S., . . . Al-Krenawi, A. (2013). Adaptation and translation of mental health interventions in Middle Eastern Arab countries: A systematic review of barriers to and strategies for effective treatment implementation. *International Journal of Social Psychiatry, 59*(7), 671–681. doi:10.1177/0020764012452349

Greenhalgh, T., Wherton, J., Papoutsi, C., Lynch, J., Hughes, G., A'Court, C., . . . Shaw, S. (2017). Beyond adoption: A new framework for theorizing and evaluating nonadoption, abandonment, and challenges to the scale-up, spread, and sustainability of health and care technologies. *Journal of Medical Internet Research, 19*(11), e367. doi:10.2196/jmir.8775

Kajiyama, B., Thompson, L., Eto-Iwase, T., Yamashita, M., Mario, J., Tzuang, M., & Gallagher-Thompson, D. (2013). Exploring the effectiveness of an internet-based program for reducing caregiver distress using the icare stress management e-training program. *Aging & Mental Health, 17.* doi:10.1080/13607863.2013.775641

Kwon, O.Y., Ahn, H.S., Kim, H.J., & Park, K.W. (2017). Effectiveness of Cognitive behavioral therapy for caregivers of people with dementia: A systematic review and meta-analysis. *Journal of Clinical Neurology, 13*(4), 394–404. doi:10.3988/jcn.2017.13.4.394

Mehta, K.M., Gallagher-Thompson, D., Varghese, M., Loganathan, S., Baruah, U., Seeher, K., . . . Pot, A.M. (2018). iSupport, an online training and support program for caregivers of people with dementia: Study protocol for a randomized controlled trial in India. *Trials, 19*(1), 271. doi:10.1186/s13063-018-2604-9

Messina, A., Amati, R., Albanese, E., & Fiordelli, M. (2022). Help-Seeking in Informal Family Caregivers of People with Dementia: A Qualitative Study with iSupport as a Case in Point. *International journal of environmental research and public health, 19*(12), 7504. https://doi.org/10.3390/ijerph19127504

Oliveira, D., Jacinto, A.F., Gratao, A.C.M., Ottaviani, A.C., Ferreira, C.R., Monteiro, D.Q., . . . Pavarini, S.C.I. (2020). Translation and cultural adaptation of iSupport in Brazil. *Alzheimer's & Dementia, 16*(S7). doi:10.1002/alz.038917

Pearlin, L.I., Mullan, J.T., Semple, S.J., & Skaff, M.M. (1990). Caregiving and the stress process: an overview of concepts and their measures. *Gerontologist, 30*(5), 583–594. doi:10.1093/geront/30.5.583

Pot, A.M., Gallagher-Thompson, D., Xiao, L.D., Willemse, B.M., Rosier, I., Mehta, K.M., . . . iSupport development, t. (2019). iSupport: a WHO global online intervention for informal caregivers of people with dementia. *World Psychiatry, 18*(3), 365–366. doi:10.1002/wps.20684

Raina, P., O'Donnell, M., Schwellnus, H., Rosenbaum, P., King, G., Brehaut, J., . . . Wood, E. (2004). Caregiving process and caregiver burden: conceptual models to guide research and practice. *BMC Pediatrics, 4*, 1. doi:10.1186/1471-2431-4-1

Schulz, R., Beach, S.R., Czaja, S.J., Martire, L.M., & Monin, J.K. (2020). Family caregiving for older adults. *Annual Review of Psychology*, *71*(1), 635–659. doi:10.1146/annurev-psych-010419-050754

Selwood, A., Johnston, K., Katona, C., Lyketsos, C., & Livingston, G. (2007). Systematic review of the effect of psychological interventions on family caregivers of people with dementia. *Journal of Affective Disorders*, *101*(1–3), 75–89. doi:10.1016/j.jad.2006.10.025

Teles, S., Ferreira, A., & Paúl, C. (2022). Feasibility of an online training and support program for dementia carers: results from a mixed-methods pilot randomized controlled trial. *BMC geriatrics*, *22*(1), 173. https://doi.org/10.1186/s12877-022-02831-z

Teles, S., Ferreira, A., Seeher, K., Freel, S., & Paul, C. (2020). Online training and support program (iSupport) for informal dementia caregivers: Protocol for an intervention study in Portugal. *BMC Geriatr*, *20*(1), 10. doi:10.1186/s12877-019-1364-z

Teles, S., Napolskij, M.S., Paul, C., Ferreira, A., & Seeher, K. (2021). Training and support for caregivers of people with dementia: The process of culturally adapting the World Health Organization iSupport programme to Portugal. *Dementia (London)*, *20*(2), 672–697. doi:10.1177/1471301220910333

Teles, S., Paul, C., Lima, P., Chilro, R., & Ferreira, A. (2021). User feedback and usability testing of an online training and support program for dementia carers. *Internet Interventions*, *25*, 100412. doi:10.1016/j.invent.2021.100412

WHO. (2017). Global action plan on the public health response to dementia 2017–2025. Retrieved from World Health Organization https://apps.who.int/iris/handle/10665/259615

WHO. (2019). *iSupport for dementia: Training and support manual for carers of people with dementia*. Geneva: World Health Organization.

WHO. (2020). *iSupport*. Retrieved from www.iSupportforDementia.org

WHO. (2021). *Global status report on the public health response to dementia (Publication no. https://apps.who.int/iris/handle/10665/344701.)*. Retrieved from https://apps.who.int/iris/handle/10665/344701 License: CC BY-NC-SA 3.0 IGO

Wiegelmann, H., Speller, S., Verhaert, L.M., Schirra-Weirich, L., & Wolf-Ostermann, K. (2021). Psychosocial interventions to support the mental health of informal caregivers of persons living with dementia – A systematic literature review. *BMC Geriatrics*, *21*(1), 94. doi:10.1186/s12877-021-02020-4

Wimo, A., Gauthier, S., & Prince, M. (2018). *Global estimates of informal care*. London: Alzheimer's Disease International (ADI).

Winblad, B., Amouyel, P., Andrieu, S., Ballard, C., Brayne, C., Brodaty, H., . . . Zetterberg, H. (2016). Defeating Alzheimer's disease and other dementias: a priority for European science and society. *Lancet Neurology*, *15*(5), 455–532. doi:10.1016/S1474-4422(16)00062-4

Xiao, L.D., McKechnie, S., Jeffers, L., De Bellis, A., Beattie, E., Low, L.F., . . . Pot, A.M. (2021). Stakeholders' perspectives on adapting the World Health Organization iSupport for Dementia in Australia. *Dementia (London)*, *20*(5), 1536–1552. doi:10.1177/1471301220954675

Xiao, L. D., Ye, M., Zhou, Y., Rita Chang, H. C., Brodaty, H., Ratcliffe, J., Brijnath, B., & Ullah, S. (2022b). Cultural adaptation of World Health Organization iSupport for Dementia program for Chinese-Australian caregivers. *Dementia (London, England)*, *21*(6), 2035–2052. https://doi.org/10.1177/14713012221110003

Part 4

Implementation of technology in dementia care

Chapter 12

Implementing eHealth interventions in dementia care

Lessons learned

Hannah Christie, Lizzy M. M. Boots, Huibert J. Tange,
Frans R. J. Verhey, Marjolein de Vugt

The promise of eHealth for people with dementia and their carers

eHealth interventions are '*treatments, typically behaviourally based, that are operationalized and transformed for delivery via the Internet*'. eHealth interventions can take the form of a web-based course, accessed via desktop; they can also be smartphone or tablet applications aimed at providing support through the expertise of peers.

In general, the advantages of eHealth interventions include easy personalisation, fast delivery and real-time feedback (Kaplan & Stone, 2013). In the context of today's ageing population and society's increasing reliance on informal caregiving, eHealth interventions are especially suitable. In this regard, benefits include the potential of eHealth to widen service access to more remote areas, lower thresholds to participation, improve service efficiency and reduce costs (Janssen et al., 2013). eHealth interventions can also offer dementia-specific advantages, as they can be adapted to the progressing stages of dementia, offer caregivers psychoeducation without requiring them to leave the person with dementia home alone and provide support without facing the stigma often present with a dementia diagnosis. For example, carers can seek anonymous, online peer support and avoid anxieties around discussing personal issues in local, less anonymous peer support settings, if they so wish.

For these reasons, eHealth has become an integral part of many dementia policy plans. In its *eHealth Action Plan 2012–2020*, the European Commission advocated developing more eHealth services, in line with their proposed 'citizen-centric' system of care, which increases socio-economic inclusion and patient empowerment. The Council of the European Union also called for discussions on the use of eHealth and other interventions to support people with dementia and their caregivers. Such policy plans have created an impetus for change, resulting in the allocation of considerable funds for the development and testing of eHealth interventions. The subsequent research has produced evidence of the effectiveness of these interventions in improving a wide range of outcomes for caregivers of people with dementia, including increased

DOI: 10.4324/9781003289005-16

self-efficacy and dementia caregiving knowledge, as well as the reduction of symptoms of depression and anxiety (Boots et al., 2014). Also, these studies have demonstrated that the addition of a coach or other form of person-to-person interaction, also known as the 'blended' aspect of an intervention, significantly enhances outcomes for caregivers of people with dementia. Interventions that are tailored to the individual and multicomponent interventions (interventions with two or more intervention components) were shown to be more effective than both untailored and single-component interventions.

The implementation challenge

Previous research into psychosocial interventions to support informal caregivers of people with dementia has shown that less than 3% of evidence-based interventions are implemented into practice (Gitlin et al., 2015). Here, implementation refers to '*the process of putting to use or integrating evidence-based interventions within a setting*' (Rabin et al., 2008). In large part, this is due to a lack of information on barriers and facilitators to their implementation and translation into clinical practice.

Specifically regarding eHealth interventions, previous research has shown that, like psychosocial interventions in general, its implementation into routine practice has proven challenging (Mair et al., 2012). Again, studies point to a lack of insight into eHealth interventions' contextual determinants and process changes as important factors in the slow implementation of many eHealth interventions (van Gemert-Pijnen & Span, 2016). Common implementation issues for eHealth interventions include sparse evidence of their demonstrable effects on improving outcomes for healthcare organisations, sceptical attitudes from care professionals, insufficient coordination and management of the eHealth intervention, and lack of involvement of end users in the eHealth development (Scheibner et al., 2021). Moreover, eHealth bypasses traditional care delivery structures. Care organisations and governing bodies have reported that this significantly complicates the implementation of the interventions, as these existing structures and norms are difficult to adapt to adequately integrate eHealth. There is little public awareness and confidence in eHealth, insufficient legal clarity (in particular concerning data security and reimbursement) and high eHealth start-up costs (European Parliament and the Council of the European Union, 2016).

Previous research on the effectiveness of eHealth interventions for caregivers of people with dementia has pinpointed a number of implementation barriers specific to the dementia caregiving target population. For instance, the older age of many dementia caregivers is a barrier. Their declining motor, cognitive and perceptive abilities, as well as the rapidly changing technological market, have been described as age-related barriers (Wildenbos et al., 2018). On the other hand, many older adults do show high levels of digital literacy (Arcury et al., 2020). In any case, there has been very little systematic, theory-based implementation research regarding the implementation of these eHealth interventions for dementia.

Thus, eHealth interventions show promise as a potential solution for various issues associated with dementia caregiving. However, more research was needed on how to best implement these promising eHealth solutions in dementia care. Hence, we carried out a variety of studies using a wide range of methods, to explore barriers and facilitators to the implementation of eHealth in dementia care. This resulted in a number of lessons learned.

Lessons learned

Our research took into account the viewpoints of stakeholders from a broad range of sectors, such as clinicians, dementia case managers, policy makers, research funders, healthcare organisations managers, municipality officials, industry representatives and health insurers, as well as people with dementia and their caregivers. Involving people with dementia and their caregivers was especially important, and the incorporation of their perspectives and opinions was safeguarded through regular in-person meetings with the European Working Group for People with Dementia (EWGPWD), and two consultations with dementia client panels, in Nottingham and in Maastricht. In order to bring this wide range of viewpoints to light, this these studies also made use of a variety of mainly qualitative research methodologies. These included systematic literature review, qualitative surveys, semi-structured qualitative interviews, inductive and deductive thematic analysis, stakeholder analysis, multiple case study analysis and business model analysis.

Consider whether all effective eHealth interventions for caregivers of people with dementia should be implemented into practice

We followed up on 12 eHealth interventions for caregivers of people with dementia that had been included in a previous systematic review exploring their effectiveness in improving caregiver outcomes (Christie et al., 2019). With this follow-up, we were able to shed light on what had happened to promising, evidence-based eHealth interventions after their effectiveness trials. A first important finding was that ten out of 12 included interventions were no longer available to use. The long-term implementation of the two still available interventions was achieved through long-term aid from an external funding body. This underscored the fact that, in contrast to other industries (such as the pharmaceutical industry), there is no clear pathway to acquire the funding necessary to market and implement effective eHealth interventions for dementia caregivers into practice. To accomplish this, policy makers and funding bodies should pay more attention to the sustainable and long-term implementation of evidence-based eHealth interventions for dementia carers. This raises an important question: *Should* researchers endeavour to implement all effective eHealth interventions for caregivers of people with dementia into practice?

This discontinuation of evidence-based eHealth interventions constitutes a squandering of vast sums of public money, research resources and a failure to achieve anticipated benefits for the intended users. Indeed, although the premise of this chapter seems based on the assumption that all evidence-based eHealth interventions should be implemented into practice, some consideration is needed. A good product is not the same as good clinical practice. Some research has even pointed to adverse effects for users following unsuccessful eHealth implementations (Han et al., 2005). Our research indicated that an intervention may be effective in a research context, but without additional information on whether it can sustainably be integrated into the broader healthcare organisation and policy context, it is very difficult for decision makers to know which interventions will be not only effective, but efficacious. It is also important to note that it is likely that at least some of the interventions reviewed by us were never meant to be implemented into practice, but rather to acquire knowledge on the topic of eHealth for caregivers of people with dementia. It is true that gathering evidence on the effectiveness of the interventions and their mechanisms is a worthwhile goal in itself, and perhaps not all effective interventions can or should be implemented at all.

Moreover, when considering whether all effective eHealth interventions for caregivers of people with dementia should be implemented, there are a number of ethical considerations that must be taken into account. First, there is a potentially changing relationship between care provider, care professional and caregiver. For this reason, implementation research is even more important, so we can gain insight into how this could change care and whom these changes would affect. Second, there are indubitably important privacy and security concerns associated with eHealth. Especially when examining eHealth interventions with commercial interests, this is an important consideration to weigh against potential benefits for caregivers. These benefits include the potential to alleviate social isolation and encourage the pursuit of meaningful activities. Some eHealth might predominantly benefit users of higher socio-economic status and perpetuate inequalities, as it requires advanced verbal and technological skills, informed access to care services, and specific hardware and software. As a result, the benefits of eHealth do not seem to reach everyone equally. However, other research has pushed back at these claims, and pointed to the emergence and uptake of mobile phone interventions as a mediating factor in making eHealth more accessible throughout society (Glasgow et al., 2014).

So, how will we know which effective eHealth interventions should be implemented, to best benefit those caregivers of people with dementia who wish to use these technologies? Incorporating checkpoints throughout the research process could be one way to assess whether continued implementation makes sense for the eHealth intervention in question. These checkpoints, installed at various crucial decision moments throughout the implementation process, should demarcate distinct *go* or *no-go* moments, where the utility of continuing with the implementation of the intervention is decided. The Centre for eHealth Research and Disease Management (CeHRes) roadmap provides a relevant example of a suitable framework for the incorporation of regular checks with stakeholders and potential markets, to ensure optimally adapted eHealth implementation in dementia care (van Gemert-Pijnen & Span, 2016). In this regard, it is also important to consider what, exactly, constitutes successful implementation. From a research perspective, an eHealth intervention is successful if it makes a difference in caregiver outcomes. From a commercial perspective, an eHealth intervention is successful if it makes money. Moreover, commercially developed interventions often supply clients with what they like, while academically developed strive to offer clients what they need. These academically developed interventions are based on empirical research and supported with evidence, often both in terms of improving outcomes and in terms of cost-effectiveness, while commercially developed interventions are seldom evidence-based. This is in contrast to the pharmaceutical industry, where evidence-based is the norm. As both medicine and eHealth are medical devices, it would make sense for them to meet similar norms. In terms of lesson learned, we suggest merging these perspectives and considering both kinds of success continuously throughout the development and implementation process at predefined checkpoints, incorporating perspectives from a variety of fields and backgrounds, and making use of alternative, flexible research designs. This could result in more interventions that are evidence-based, commercially viable and easier to implement in practice.

Form 'innovation clusters' from the start

These checkpoints should be established from the very start, and the decision-making regarding these checkpoints should involve a carefully selected and expansive group of stakeholders, in order to include the perspectives off all sectors involved in the implementation cycle of an intervention. Recent INDUCT research has emphasised the importance involving people with dementia and their caregivers in the co-design of technology-based interventions (Rai et al., 2020). Co-design entails '*the collective creativity as it is applied across the whole span of a design process*' and specifically refers to integrating the creativity of both designers and people not trained in design to cooperate on the design development process (Sanders & Stappers, 2008). The benefits of involving people with dementia and caregivers in co-design include the development of technologies that are better suited to their needs and that facilitate the pursuit of meaningful activities after a dementia diagnosis (Leorin et al., 2019). In addition to this feasible and necessary involvement of people with dementia and their caregivers in co-design, our research has also emphasised the importance of involving representatives from the organisational healthcare context.

This finding is based on several studies we have conducted on the eHealth intervention 'Partner in Balance' a blended care intervention to support caregivers of people with dementia. These studies included an implementation strategy paper (Christie et al., 2020) and two implementation studies in the municipality context (Christie et al., 2021). The qualitative interviews with over 25 stakeholders in these studies has resulted in the following 'lesson learned': We suggest forming so-called 'innovation clusters' from the start of eHealth interventions' development, consisting of a technology developer, research team, intervention provider, health insurer/other funders and people with dementia and their carers. The formation of this innovation cluster can also be seen as a part of co-design, in that it involves the perspectives of non-designers in the development process. Involving these different elements of an innovation cluster can inform a more efficient study design, geared at providing stakeholders with the data they need to make informed decisions on future long-term implementation. The inclusion and utilisation of a range of intersectoral and interdisciplinary perspectives in the innovation cluster are crucial.

Construct flexible and intersectoral research designs

In medical (so also eHealth) research, the standard method of measuring an intervention's effectiveness has long been the Randomised Controlled Trial (RCT). While the RCT is an established and proven method to gain insight into eHealth effectiveness, it is time and resource-intensive and often results in a lack of important, qualitative implementation data (Vernooij-Dassen & Moniz-Cook, 2014). Conversely, this time and resource intensiveness makes it unattractive for commercial enterprises to provide evidence of the effectiveness of their interventions. Moreover, eHealth technologies change quickly and eHealth research should not be years behind on the market. Staying up-to-date with technological advancements is difficult due to the expansive time frame of typical RCT-based effectiveness studies. One way of developing eHealth interventions that are suitable to implementation when proven effective is by using more flexible research designs, such as designs that can more easily adapt and evaluate the intervention based on iterative feedback. In combination with the proposed input from co-design through innovation clusters, these novel research designs can result in technologically innovative eHealth interventions for caregivers of people with dementia that can be more easily evaluated for specific dementia caregiving contexts, and adapted to these contextual needs. Moreover, our previously described follow-up study indicated that these alternative, flexible designs could facilitate the implementation of more technologically up-to-date interventions and avoid the longer duration of traditional evaluation methods (Christie et al., 2019).

As a result, our lessons learned include the suggestion to gain inspiration for methods to evaluate the addition of new functionalities to the eHealth interventions from industry, where many commercial platforms use real-time evaluations to gain feedback from users. These can include pop-ups, which ask the user to rate their experiences, or the launch of different versions of the same functionality in order to assess which of the two versions is more successful. The inclusion of these methods into research designs can help achieve continuous monitoring and evaluation of eHealth interventions for caregivers of people with dementia. Of course, also here it is important to remember that commercial evaluations are more targeted at the attractiveness of an intervention (what people like), over its effectiveness (what people need).

Create self-efficacy and ownership within implementing organisations

Having an effective eHealth intervention for caregivers of people with dementia – even one that has the necessary infrastructural implementation components in place – is not sufficient to guarantee successful implementation. Much depends on the attitudes of the implementing individuals towards the eHealth intervention. In our evaluation of the implementation of eHealth interventions Partner in Balance and Myinlife in the municipality context, we found that a sense of ownership of the municipality implementers towards the successful implementation of the interventions was a significant determinant of successful implementation (Christie et al., 2021). It also suggested increasing the self-efficacy of the implementers, within both the municipality and the external implementing organisation, for instance through incorporating role play exercises into Partner in Balance coach trainings. As in previous sections of this chapter, our evaluation underscored the importance of monitoring and evaluating the implementation to increase implementer motivation and self-efficacy. On the basis of our interview and usage data findings from these municipality implementation evaluations, we suggest that this monitoring and evaluating of the interventions can be implemented in two ways. First, setting and achieving implementation goals by monitoring progress could increase motivation and self-efficacy in the organisation's implementing professionals. Second, by building functionalities into the eHealth intervention for organisational management to evaluate implementation (such as local use statistics), the management of the implementing organisations can better justify the resources spent on the eHealth implementation and increase their ownership of implementation successes and failures. As a result, we suggest that interventions create self-efficacy and ownership in implementing organisations through monitoring and motivating, for both implementing professionals and organisational management.

Even in eHealth, human interaction remains essential

A recurring theme in the results of our review is the necessity of continued human interactions in the implementation of eHealth interventions for caregivers of people with dementia, starting from our systematic review of implementation determinants in eHealth for caregivers of people with dementia (Christie et al., 2018). There is often an underlying assumption that eHealth implies a reduction of human contact and increased distance. However, our findings from the Myinlife (an online platform to help caregivers of people with dementia organise informal care) process evaluation (Dam et al., 2019) provided additional support to the existing literature asserting that blended eHealth interventions for caregivers of people with dementia are more effective at improving outcomes for caregivers of people with dementia than non-blended interventions (Boots et al., 2014). Our study showed that the caregivers required more personal guidance to optimally use Myinlife, despite it being a 'stand-alone' eHealth intervention. Furthermore, findings from our previously described Partner in Balance and Myinlife implementation studies in the municipality context raised the question of whether the blended aspect of eHealth might result in increased effectiveness due to not only the effect of the intervention itself on caregiver outcomes, but also due to its potential effect of increasing engagement among implementers through the human contact. Here, we observed not only that the Partner in Balance intervention required more hours to implement in the municipality context than Myinlife, but also that it was more often successfully implemented. Hence, it is possible that including a blended aspect of the intervention increases ownership of the intervention in implementers. By necessitating the integration of the intervention into an organisational context, the implementers could become more familiar with the intervention, and more invested in its implementation.

The above is in line with findings from our business model study (Christie et al., 2021). In this study, we investigated eHealth interventions for caregivers of people with dementia that were already being used in practice, and explored how their implementation lessons could be applied to facilitate the implementation of their counterparts originating from the academic research context. One of our main findings was that many of the successful eHealth interventions for caregivers of people with dementia reported community creation and management as one of their most important value propositions. This referred to forming and maintaining a community of intervention users, who are in contact with each other through the intervention. Furthermore, our interviews with Partner in Balance stakeholders (Christie et al., 2020) described the importance of creating a community around the implementing coaches. As a result, strategies were formulated to make sure that bonds were formed between coaches and structures were put in place for sustainability. Indeed, previous research has mentioned the potential of blended interventions to increase adherence in eHealth interventions (Wentzel et al., 2016), further emphasising the need to keep incorporating human interaction into eHealth. Hence, here our most important lesson learned was to formulate strategies for sustained human interaction and engagement with the eHealth intervention over time.

Conclusions

Our implementation research took an intersectoral approach in investigating the implementation of eHealth interventions for dementia. The overarching implications of this research were that future developers of eHealth interventions for caregivers of people with dementia should aim to: (1) consider whether all effective eHealth interventions dementia should be implemented into practice, with the use of checkpoints; (2) form 'innovation clusters' from the start; (3) construct flexible and intersectoral research designs; (4) create self-efficacy and ownership within implementing organisations and (5) incorporate human interaction into the eHealth implementation. These lessons will help realise the development and implementation of evidence-based eHealth interventions for dementia that are better adapted to their financial and organisational contexts. This can potentially lead to a more effective spending of research resources, allowing these interventions to make a difference to individuals and healthcare systems at large.

References

Arcury, T.A., Sandberg, J.C., Melius, K.P., Quandt, S.A., Leng, X., Latulipe, C., . . . Bertoni, A.G. (2020). Older adult internet use and eHealth literacy. *Journal of Applied Gerontology, 39*(2), 141–150.

Boots, L., de Vugt, M.E., Van Knippenberg, R., Kempen, G., & Verhey, F. (2014). A systematic review of Internet-based supportive interventions for caregivers of patients with dementia. *International journal of geriatric psychiatry, 29*(4), 331–344.

Christie, H., Boots, L., Hermans, I., Govers, M., Tange, H., Verhey, F., & de Vugt, M. (2021). Business models of eHealth interventions to support informal caregivers of people with dementia in the Netherlands: Case study analysis. *JMIR Aging, 4*(2), e24724.

Christie, H., Boots, L., Tange, H., Verhey, F., & de Vugt, M. (2021). Implementations of evidence-based eHealth interventions for caregivers of people with dementia in municipality contexts (Myinlife and Partner in Balance): Evaluation study. *JMIR Aging, 4*(1), e21629.

Christie, H., Martin, J., Connor, J., Tange, H., Verhey, F., de Vugt, M., & Orrell, M. (2019). eHealth interventions to support caregivers of people with dementia may be proven effective, but are they implementation-ready? *Internet Interventions, 18*, 100260.

Christie, H.L., Bartels, S.L., Boots, L.M., Tange, H.J., Verhey, F.R., & de Vugt, M.E. (2018). A systematic review on the implementation of eHealth interventions for informal caregivers of people with dementia. *Internet Interventions, 13*, 51–59.

Christie, H.L., Boots, L.M.M., Peetoom, K., Tange, H.J., Verhey, F.R.J., & de Vugt, M.E. (2020). Developing a plan for the sustainable implementation of an electronic health intervention (Partner in Balance) to support caregivers of people with dementia: Case study. *JMIR aging, 3*(1), e18624.

Dam, A.E., Christie, H.L., Smeets, C.M., van Boxtel, M.P., Verhey, F.R., & de Vugt, M.E. (2019). Process evaluation of a social support platform 'Inlife' for caregivers of people with dementia. *Internet Interventions, 15*, 18–27.

European Parliament and the Council of the European Union. (2016). *Regulation EU 2016/679 of the European Parliament and of the council of 27 April 2016.* Luxembourg: Official Journal of the European Union.

Gitlin, L.N., Marx, K., Stanley, I.H., & Hodgson, N. (2015). Translating evidence-based dementia caregiving interventions into practice: State-of-the-science and next steps. *The Gerontologist*, *55*(2), 210–226.

Glasgow, R.E., Phillips, S.M., & Sanchez, M.A. (2014). Implementation science approaches for integrating eHealth research into practice and policy. *International Journal of Medical Informatics*, *83*(7), e1–e11.

Han, Y.Y., Carcillo, J.A., Venkataraman, S.T., Clark, R.S., Watson, R.S., Nguyen, T.C., . . . Orr, R.A. (2005). Unexpected increased mortality after implementation of a commercially sold computerized physician order entry system. *Pediatrics*, *116*(6), 1506–1512.

Janssen, R., Hettinga, M., Visser, S., Menko, R., Prins, H., Krediet, I., . . . Bodenstaff, L. (2013). Innovation routes and evidence guidelines for eHealth small and medium-sized Enterprises. *International Journal of Advanced Life Sciences*, *5*.

Kaplan, R.M., & Stone, A.A. (2013). Bringing the laboratory and clinic to the community: mobile technologies for health promotion and disease prevention. *Annual Review of Psychology*, *64*, 471–498.

Leorin, C., Stella, E., Nugent, C., Cleland, I., & Paggetti, C. (2019). The value of including people with dementia in the co-design of personalized eHealth technologies. *Dementia and Geriatric Cognitive Disorders*, *47*(3), 164–175.

Mair, F.S., May, C., O'Donnell, C., Finch, T., Sullivan, F., & Murray, E. (2012). Factors that promote or inhibit the implementation of e-health systems: An explanatory systematic review. *Bulletin of the World Health Organization*, *90*, 357–364.

Rabin, B.A., Brownson, R.C., Haire-Joshu, D., Kreuter, M.W., & Weaver, N.L. (2008). A glossary for dissemination and implementation research in health. *Journal of Public Health Management and Practice*, *14*(2), 117–123.

Rai, H.K., Barroso, A.C., Yates, L., Schneider, J., & Orrell, M. (2020). Involvement of people with dementia in the development of technology-based interventions: Narrative synthesis review and best practice guidelines. *Journal of Medical Internet Research*, *22*(12), e17531.

Sanders, E.B.-N., & Stappers, P.J. (2008). Co-creation and the new landscapes of design. *Co-design*, *4*(1), 5–18.

Scheibner, J., Sleigh, J., Ienca, M., & Vayena, E. (2021). Benefits, challenges, and contributors to success for national eHealth systems implementation: A scoping review. *Journal of the American Medical Informatics Association*, *28*(9), 2039–2049.

van Gemert-Pijnen, L., & Span, M. (2016). CeHRes roadmap to improve dementia care. In *Handbook of smart homes, health care and well-being* (pp. 1–11). New York: Springer.

Vernooij-Dassen, M., & Moniz-Cook, E. (2014). Raising the standard of applied dementia care research: Addressing the implementation error. *Aging & Mental Health*, *18*(7), 809–814.

Wentzel, J., van der Vaart, R., Bohlmeijer, E.T., & van Gemert-Pijnen, J.E. (2016). Mixing online and face-to-face therapy: How to benefit from blended care in mental health care. *JMIR Mental Health*, *3*(1), e9.

Wildenbos, G.A., Peute, L., & Jaspers, M. (2018). Aging barriers influencing mobile health usability for older adults: A literature based framework (MOLD-US). *International journal of Medical Informatics*, *114*, 66–75.

Chapter 13

Implementation and usefulness of cognitive stimulation computer-based GRADIOR software

Angie A. Diaz-Baquero, Eider Irazoki,
Leslie María Contreras Somoza, José Miguel
Toribio-Guzmán, Esther Parra, María Victoria
Perea Bartolomé, Henriëtte G. van der Roest,
Manuel A. Franco Martín

Background

Applying technology in the field of cognitive interventions looks promising, as it makes interventions more accessible and more cost-effective than traditional cognitive interventions (Gooding et al., 2015; Maldonado, 2016). The interest generated by this approach has prompted the development of computer-based cognitive intervention programs for people with cognitive impairment and dementia. Most of this software contains exercises to improve multiple cognitive domains (Lobbia et al., 2019) and is aimed at any disorder involving cognitive impairment. This type of intervention is also used to prevent cognitive decline in healthy people.

One of the major challenges faced by these programs is to achieve good interaction between the system and people with dementia, which is eventually made easier through the use of touchscreen devices (Joddrell & Astell, 2016). An additional significant concern is age-related visual or motor difficulties, which can, nevertheless, be overcome by using simple intervention programs without too many accessories (Meiland et al., 2017).

Another key feature is the customisation of the content and parameters of the sessions to the cognitive profile and wishes of the technology's users. Flexible and appropriate software needs to be developed for people with dementia. A further challenge is Internet connectivity to make remote access possible regardless of location. This could potentially improve the availability of treatment for people living in rural areas, where Internet connections could be a drawback due to lack of accessibility in such areas (Irazoki et al., 2020).

Computerised programs are designed to be enjoyable, including a wealth of exercises aimed at promoting engagement, while they may also include neurocognitive assessment tools, physical exercises and individualised and group cognitive training.

DOI: 10.4324/9781003289005-17

Currently, the scientific literature offers studies evaluating the effectiveness, usability and user experience of cognitive training programs that are commonly used by people with MCI and mild dementia. However, few studies describe and specify the methodological design followed during the development process of these programs.

The foregoing raises a context of great interest that deserves to be taken into consideration. Recently, a systematic review carried out by Diaz-Baquero et al. (2021) pointed out a few studies describing the methodological design followed in the development of Computerized Cognitive Training (CCT) programs. According to the results, the user-centred methodological design was the most frequently used, this design being mainly characterised by including end users from the beginning of the development of these tools (Diaz-Baquero et al., 2021). Although ISO9241–210 (2019) proposes a series of criteria for the development of these programs, the systematic review provided by Diaz-Baquero et al. (2021) established that the development of these programs does not always meet these minimum criteria. The main findings of this systematic review for each criterion are specified later:

1 *Specify the context*: All the studies included specified the needs and interests of the users and application environment of the program based on population observation exercises and a review of the literature.
2 *User requirements*: Only half of the studies included user perspective. Indeed, many of them disregarded most of the minimum requirements for the development of these technologies: the development of intuitive and familiar interfaces, programs adapted to motor and cognitive difficulties, cognitive exercises with an intermediate level of difficulty and adapted to the cognitive level of the patient, exercises with ecological validity.
3 *Assessment of usability and user experience*: Usability is a key feature for the implementation of these tools in the real world (Irazoki et al., 2021). Most of the programs focused on including a touch screen, clear instructions, a graphic interface and exercises adapted to the target population. Users also positively evaluated most of the exercises and mentioned the benefits obtained at the cognitive, physical and social levels. The foregoing represents a subjective perspective associated with user experience that may positively or negatively influence possible adherence to a CCT program.

GRADIOR. A cognitive rehabilitation program

GRADIOR is a neuropsychological rehabilitation program that allows cognitive evaluation using different neuropsychological tests aimed at obtaining a cognitive profile for each user (Góngora Alonso et al., 2019; Toribio-Guzmán et al., 2018). Likewise, it includes a variety of cognitive training exercises associated with different cognitive functions, including orientation, attention, memory, language, calculus, executive function, perception and reasoning.

Regarding its technical requirements, GRADIOR software is compatible with a Windows operating system and can be used on computers with touch screens, mouse or keyboard. The system requirements are RAM (2–4 GB recommended), graphics card (RAM) (256 MB–1 GB) and Microsoft Office 2003 or later versions. Microsoft Visual Studio is employed as an integrated development framework for the implementation of GRADIOR, and the Visual Basic. NET. SQL Server is the database management system.

GRADIOR has been developed to design and manage personalised cognitive rehabilitation treatments, save patients' clinical features, overview results and adapt exercise difficulty to the patient's cognitive level. The current version includes eight different moduli (orientation, memory, attention, calculus, executive function, perception, language and reasoning) for clients to follow (Franco-Martin et al., 2020). The GRADIOR platform has four functions:

a) Clinical Management, which provides an overview of the user accounts of all the patients who are under treatment by a specific therapist;
b) Clinical History Management, where sociodemographic, personal and clinical data, medication and cognitive test results are stored;
c) Treatment management, which allows the therapists to design personalised treatment plans based on the user's cognitive profile, selecting the most suitable exercises according to the cognitive modality to be trained (e.g. memory), the level of difficulty and display mode of the exercises, and the duration of the treatment. The therapist can continually change, adjust and personalise the intervention plan according to the user's evolution.
d) Report Manager, which allows the therapist to obtain reports of a general or specific nature (modality, sub-modality and level). This facilitates the adaptation of the intervention plan.

Usability and user experience

Older adults often lack experience with technology or technological skills (Contreras-Somoza et al., 2020), and they may also struggle due to cognitive decline or age (Pirhonen et al., 2020). Their difficulties increase if they are affected by cognitive impairment, so a technology that does not fit in well with this population may cause negative feelings and discourage them from using it (Smeenk et al., 2018).

Usability encompasses the level at which users can use a system/product/service with: (a) Effectiveness: precision and completeness for achieving specific objectives; (b) Efficiency: resources employed to obtain those results; (c) Satisfaction: the degree of expectations and needs are met (ISO9241–210, 2019). User experience involves users' emotions, preferences, beliefs, perceptions and behaviours before, during or after using a system/product/service (ISO9241–210, 2019). A recent systematic review considered user experience as part of usability, because usability encompasses both subjective and objective aspects (Contreras-Somoza et al., 2021).

In the case of GRADIOR, studies on its usability and user experience have been carried out since its first versions. GRADIOR was integrated with physical activities into the Long-Lasting Memories (LLM) platform, the physical training can also improve cognition in the elderly (González-Palau et al., 2013). Older adults with MCI, people with dementia (PwD) and healthy elderly perceived LLM as beneficial and satisfactory, even users who needed explanations to connect and hold the devices properly (González-Palau et al., 2013). Similar results were found in other studies. However, PwD were identified as needing more help with physical training devices, although the perception of usability increased after performing more sessions (Góngora Alonso et al., 2020; Toribio Guzmán, 2015).

A further step was taken by integrating GRADIOR into ehcoBUTLER (Contreras-Somoza et al., 2020), which is an Information and Communication Technology with a cognitive (GRADIOR), social, emotional, healthy lifestyle, free time and leisure module. Potential users (people with MCI) and stakeholders (formal/informal caregivers and administration/management staff) showed acceptability, and considered it ergonomic, useful and interesting (Contreras-Somoza et al., 2020). It was concluded that the acceptability of cognitive programs could be optimised by complementing them with other functions such as social ones (Contreras-Somoza et al., 2020).

In GRADIOR 4.5, the objective was to better satisfy the needs and preferences of users and therapists. The program was upgraded by adding new features to the interface, improving exercises with familiar and realistic images, and revamping the logo (Irazoki et al., 2021; J. M Toribio Guzmán et al., 2017). It should be noted that previous research tended to use surveys or questionnaires as part of their methodology. A recent study used focus groups to assess usability and user experience in the elderly with MCI, dementia and healthcare professionals (Irazoki et al., 2021).

No experience with the technology is required to run GRADIOR 4.5, so learning to use the program is quite simple. As expected with any program or technology, during the first 3–4 days, users should be supported in using the tool. Usually, older adults do not have much experience with digital devices and may experience fear of using computers (Góngora Alonso et al., 2020). In our experience, most users can use GRADIOR 4.5 autonomously under minimal supervision of therapists.

Using GRADIOR 4.5 was considered satisfactory, fun, entertaining and a chance to be active, learn and expand the user's social circle. It was also perceived to improve memory and attention. Likewise, older people's willingness to access the program from home showed motivation and commitment. Moreover, failure to get all the exercises right did not discourage older people from trying again (Irazoki et al., 2021).

Interface design is important for a cognitive intervention program's usability and user experience. GRADIOR's interface is considered attractive and appropriate (Irazoki et al., 2021). However, the program could be improved by avoiding interference with auditory and visual instructions and specific tasks and moving stimuli to more intuitive locations. Replacing feedback messages with more positive ones and simplifying access to the program could also be helpful.

Another essential feature of GRADIOR 4.5 is its PC-only availability and the high-speed Internet connection it requires. Internet availability and the price of this type of intervention were identified as the main barriers to older adults' use of technology (McCausland & Falk, 2012). Nevertheless, the use of it would be more influenced by a lack of confidence in handling technology than by the price of the devices (Vaportzis et al., 2017). Interestingly, some users of GRADIOR were willing to pay a small quantity of money for the computer program, which suggests that they might value the perceived benefits above the cost of technology (Mitzner et al., 2010).

GRADIOR effectiveness

Effectiveness usually consists of the number of tasks completed and the number of errors made by the participants. Efficiency consists of the time they spent completing the tasks, the number of unnecessary actions and the help they received from the moderator (Contreras-Somoza et al., 2021). Regularly, they are measured through questionnaires, scales, interviews, observation of participants' behaviour, the time spent and the number of tasks they performed freely at home, or attendance if they use the program in a centre (Contreras-Somoza et al., 2021).

Lastly, Cavallo and Angilletta (2018) indicated a cognitive improvement in Alzheimer's patients after using a structured CCT program for 12 weeks, an effect that was maintained even six months later. Other studies have indicated an improvement in working memory after five (Vermeij et al., 2016) and seven weeks (Hyer et al., 2016) of training in adults with MCI. Flak et al. (2019) highlighted the improvement in working memory after a personalised training programme compared to a non-personalised one in people with MCI. Nevertheless, Yang et al. (2019) took a more conservative approach with their findings, mentioning the maintenance of working memory in people with MCI. Hwang et al. (2015) mentioned an improvement in delayed memory, recent memory and visual recognition in a patient with Alzheimer's. Peretz et al. (2011) underlined improvements in visuospatial working memory, learning and attention. Improvements in executive control have also been reported in older adults (Shatil et al., 2014), as well as an enhancement in processing speed, hand-eye coordination, denomination and visuospatial processing (Shatil, 2013), executive functioning (Barban et al., 2016) and global cognition (Bahar-Fuchs et al., 2017). Regarding psychological factors, some studies have indicated a reduction of anxiety in people with MCI and mild dementia (Gaitán et al., 2013).

The findings of some of these studies need to be taken with caution due to two important limitations: sample size and short intervention periods (Lee et al., 2018). A systematic review conducted by García-Casal et al. (2017) indicated an acceptable methodological quality of those studies whose objective was to evaluate the effectiveness of these programs.

The effectiveness of GRADIOR has been little studied, and most of the studies about it are focused on usability and user experience (Góngora Alonso et al., 2019; Irazoki et al., 2021). Recently, a single-blind multicentre randomised clinical trial (RCT) was carried out by the authors. The main objective of this RCT was to evaluate the effectiveness of GRADIOR in people with MCI and mild dementia at four and 12 months of cognitive training with a follow-up period of 16 and 24 months (Vanova et al., 2018). The RCT included conducting assessments and then CCT sessions with GRADIOR. The evaluations consisted of the application of a series of clinical, cognitive, social and emotional scales, which made up the application protocol. Regarding the intervention plan, two and three CCT sessions were carried out weekly, lasting 30 minutes.

This RCT is based on a final sample of 62 and 23 users who managed to reach four and 12 months, respectively. The RCT highlighted better visual reasoning at four months for the experimental group (EG) (GRADIOR) and the maintenance of slight improvements at four and 12 months compared to the control group (CG). The EG improved slightly in sustained attention and semantic fluency at four months. After a long-lasting intervention with GRADIOR, the EG showed a slight improvement in processing speed, divided attention, alternation, cognitive flexibility, inhibitory control, phonological fluency, working memory and visual recognition at 12 months compared to four months. Visuoconstructive praxis was maintained at four and 12 months in the EG, whereas the performance of the CG dropped, especially at 12 months. Finally, as a significant outcome of the interaction, the EG improved their mood and sustained attention at 12 months compared to the CG (Diaz-Baquero et al., 2022a).

Our study showed the importance of providing long-lasting CCT programs, since efficacy was more marked at eight months than at four months of intervention. Some studies have recommended trials with long intervention periods (Lee et al., 2018), which could be consistent with the natural course of dementia and its association with a long neurodegenerative process.

This RCT presented a limitation that has been continuously pointed out by previous studies, which is the small size of the sample (Klimova & Maresova, 2017). The RCT was originally intended to recruit a higher number of people; however, this was not possible due to the outbreak of COVID-19 and subsequent lockdown, which forced the treatment and recruitment process to be stopped in many cases.

Adherence to GRADIOR

Adherence has been commonly applied and studied at the pharmacology level, analysing it in association with various medications and assessing its influence on the improvement or maintenance of health (WHO, 2019). However, there are few studies on adherence to CCT programs (Turunen et al., 2019). The aforementioned RCT afforded the possibility to study the rate of adherence to the CCT GRADIOR program, which was found to be 83% (Diaz-Baquero et al., 2022b). This datum involves a higher percentage than that determined in other studies; for example Sjösten et al. (2007) established 66% as the percentage or cut-off point to consider whether a person is an adherent or not.

Although there are hardly any data regarding predictors of adherence to CCT programs, Diaz-Baquero et al. (2022b) mentioned how good executive functioning is associated with functions such as attention, working memory, phonological verbal fluency, numerical reasoning and cognitive flexibility helped to predict adherence to the CCT program in people with MCI and mild dementia.

Conclusions

Computer programs seem to be a promising strategy for enhancing the cognitive function of older people as they are more accessible and cost-effective in comparison to traditional cognitive interventions. There is a wide range of different cognitive software programs to treat people with MCI and dementia. This variety of programs allows professionals and end users to choose the most suitable for every user.

The user-centred methodological design was the most used for the development of these programs, posing an interesting perspective because it includes the active participation of the user from the beginning to the end of the development process. However, few programs have used this methodology considering the wide variety of programs on the market.

Usability and user experience provide a broader view for the design of cognitive intervention technologies according to the target population, since they consider their skills, needs and feelings. In the case of GRADIOR, the assessment of usability and user experience has revealed high acceptability, usability and good user experience. Few sessions are needed to learn how to use GRADIOR 4.5 and, consequently, the tool is considered intuitive and easy to use for people with cognitive impairment. Using GRADIOR 4.5 was considered a positive experience for both users and professionals. However, access to the program needs to be gradually improved by involving user experience in the program. Thus, technologies can be employed as part of a cognitive rehabilitation intervention for people with MCI and dementia.

In terms of efficacy and effectiveness, GRADIOR showed better outcomes at 12 months, suggesting that it would be recommendable to provide these kinds of treatments for long periods of time. Although its effects are mainly on processing speed, divided attention, alternation, cognitive flexibility, inhibitory control, phonological fluency, working memory and visual recognition, GRADIOR also showed a significant impact on mood and sustained attention in the EG with respect to the CG.

The determinants of adherence to GRADIOR were good executive functioning associated with functions like attention, working memory, phonological verbal fluency, numerical reasoning and cognitive flexibility.

References

Bahar-Fuchs, A., Webb, S., Bartsch, L., Clare, L., Rebok, G., Cherbuin, N., & Anstey, K.J. (2017). Tailored and adaptive computerized cognitive training in older adults at risk for dementia: A randomized controlled trial. *Journal of Alzheimer's Disease*, *60*(3), 889–911. doi: 10.3233/JAD-170404

Barban, F., Annicchiarico, R., Pantelopoulos, S., Federici, A., Perri, R., Fadda, L., . . . Caltagirone, C. (2016). Protecting cognition from aging and Alzheimer's disease: A computerized cognitive training combined with reminiscence therapy. *International Journal of Geriatric Psychiatry*, *31*(4), 340–348. doi: 10.1002/gps.4328

Cavallo, M., & Angilletta, C. (2018). Long-lasting neuropsychological effects of a computerized cognitive training in patients affected by early stage Alzheimer's disease: Are they stable over time? *Journal of Applied Gerontology*, *38*(7), 1035–1044. doi: 10.1177/0733464817750276

Contreras-Somoza, L.M., Irazoki, E., Castilla, D., Botella, C., Toribio-Guzmán, J.M., Parra-Vidales, E., . . . Franco-Martín, M.Á. (2020). Study on the acceptability of an ICT platform for older adults with mild cognitive impairment. *Journal of Medical Systems*, *44*(120), 1–12. doi: 10.1007/s10916-020-01566-x

Contreras-Somoza, L.M., Irazoki, E., Toribio-Guzmán, J.M., de la Torre-Díez, I., Diaz-Baquero, A.A., Parra-Vidales, E., . . . Franco-Martín, M.A. (2021). Usability and User Experience of cognitive intervention technologies for elderly people with MCI or dementia: A systematic review. *Frontiers in Psychology*, *12*, 1–15. doi: 10.3389/fpsyg.2021.636116

Diaz-Baquero, A.A., Dröes, R.-M., Perea Bartolomé, M.V., Irazoki, E., Toribio-Guzmán, J.M., Franco-Martín, M.A., & van der Roest, H. (2021). Methodological designs applied in the development of computer-based training programs for the cognitive rehabilitation in people with mild cognitive impairment (MCI) and mild dementia. Systematic review. *Journal of Clinical Medicine*, *10*(6), 1222.

Diaz-Baquero, A.A., Franco-Martín, M.A., Parra Vidales, E., Toribio-Guzmán, J.M., Bueno-Aguado, Y., Martínez Abad, F., . . . van der Roest, H.G. (2022a). The Effectiveness of GRADIOR: A neuropsychological rehabilitation program for people with mild cognitive impairment and mild dementia. Results of a randomized controlled trial after 4 and 12 months of treatment. *Journal of Alzheimer's Disease*. doi: 10.3233/JAD-215350

Diaz-Baquero, A.A., Perea Bartolomé, M.V., Toribio-Guzmán, J.M., Martínez Abad, F., Parra Vidales, E., Bueno-Aguado, Y., . . . Franco-Martín, M.A. (2022b). Determinants of adherence to a "GRADIOR" computer-based cognitive training program in people with mild cognitive impairment (MCI) and mild dementia. *Journal of Clinical Medicine*. doi: 10.3233/JAD-215350

Flak, M.M., Hol, H.R., Hernes, S.S., Chang, L., Engvig, A., Bjuland, K.J., . . . Løhaugen, G. (2019). Adaptive computerized working memory training in patients with mild cognitive impairment. A randomized double-blind active controlled trial. *Frontiers in Psychology*, *10*(807). doi: 10.3389/fpsyg.2019.00807

Franco-Martin, M.A., Diaz-Baquero, A.A., Bueno-Aguado, Y., Cid-Bartolomé, M.T., Parra Vidales, E., Perea Bartolomé, M.V., . . . van der Roest, H.G. (2020). Computer-based cognitive rehabilitation program GRADIOR for mild dementia and mild cognitive impairment: New features. *BMC Journal: BMC Medical Informatics and Decision Making, 20*(274). doi: 10.1186/s12911-020-01293-w

Gaitán, A., Garolera, M., Cerulla, N., Chico, G., Rodriguez-Querol, M., & Canela-Soler, J. (2013). Efficacy of an adjunctive computer-based cognitive training program in amnestic mild cognitive impairment and Alzheimer's disease: A single-blind, randomized clinical trial. *International Journal of Geriatric Psychiatry, 28*(1), 91–99. doi: 10.1002/gps.3794

García-Casal, J.A., Loizeau, A., Csipke, E., Franco-Martín, M., Perea-Bartolomé, M.V., & Orrell, M. (2017). Computer-based cognitive interventions for people living with dementia: a systematic literature review and meta-analysis. *Aging and Mental Health, 21*(5), 1–14. doi: 10.1080/13607863.2015.1132677

Góngora Alonso, S., Fumero Vargas, G., Morón Nozaleda, L., Sainz de Abajo, B., de la Torre Díez, I., & Franco, M. (2020). Usability analysis of a system for cognitive rehabilitation, "Gradior", in a Spanish Region. *Telemedicine and e-Health, 26*(5), 671–682. doi: 10.1089/tmj.2019.0084

Góngora Alonso, S., Toribio Guzmán, J.M., Sainz de Abajo, B., Muñoz Sánchez, J.L., Martín, M.F., & de la Torre Díez, I. (2019). Usability evaluation of the eHealth Long Lasting Memories program in Spanish elderly people. *Health Informatics Journal,* 1460458219889501. doi: 10.1177/1460458219889501

González-Palau, F., Franco, M., Toribio, J.M., Losada, R., Parra, E., & Bamidis, P. (2013). Designing a computer-based rehabilitation solution for older adults: The importance of testing usability. *PsychNology Journal, 11*(2), 119–136.

Gooding, A.L., Choi, J., Fiszdon, J.M., Wilkins, K., Kirwin, P.D., van Dyck, C.H., . . . Rivera Mindt, M. (2015). Comparing three methods of computerised cognitive training for older adults with subclinical cognitive decline. *Neuropsychological Rehabilitation, 26*(5–6), 810–821. doi: 10.1080/09602011.2015.1118389

Hwang, J.H., Cha, H.G., Cho, Y.S., Kim, T.S., & Cho, H.S. (2015). The effects of computer-assisted cognitive rehabilitation on Alzheimer's dementia patients memories. *Journal of Physical Therapy Science, 27*(9), 2921–2923. doi: 10.1589/jpts.27.2921

Hyer, L., Scott, C., Atkinson, M.M., Mullen, C.M., Lee, A., Johnson, A., & McKenzie, L.C. (2016). Cognitive training program to improve working memory in older adults with MCI. *Clinical Gerontologist, 39*(5), 410–427. doi: 10.1080/07317115.2015.1120257

Irazoki, E., Contreras-Somoza, L.M., Toribio-Guzmán, J.M., Jenaro-Río, C., van der Roest, H., & Franco-Martín, M.A. (2020). Technologies for cognitive training and cognitive rehabilitation for people with mild cognitive impairment and dementia. A systematic review. *Frontiers in Psychology, 11*, 648. doi: 10.3389/fpsyg.2020.00648

Irazoki, E., Sánchez-Gómez, M.C., Contreras-Somoza, L.M., Toribio-Guzmán, J.M., Martín-Cilleros, M.V., Verdugo-Castro, S., . . . Franco-Martín, M.A. (2021). A qualitative study of the cognitive rehabilitation program GRADIOR for people with cognitive impairment: Outcomes of the focus group methodology. *Journal of Clinical Medicine, 10*(4), 859. doi: 10.3390/jcm10040859

ISO9241–210. (2019). Ergonomics of human-system interaction – Part 210. In I. c. office (Ed.), *INTERNATIONAL STANDARD: Human-centred design for interactive systems.* Switzerland. Retrieved from https://richardcornish.s3.amazonaws.com/static/pdfs/iso-9241-210.pdf.

Joddrell, P., & Astell, A.J. (2016). Studies involving people with dementia and touchscreen technology: A literature review. *JMIR Rehabilitation and Assistive Technologies, 3*(2). doi: 10.2196/rehab.5788

Klimova, B., & Maresova, P. (2017). Computer-based training programs for older people with mild cognitive impairment and/or dementia. *Frontiers in Human Neuroscience*, *11*(262). doi: 10.3389/fnhum.2017.00262

Lee, G.J., Bang, H.J., Lee, K.M., Kong, H.H., Seo, H.S., Oh, M., & Bang, M. (2018). A comparison of the effects between 2 computerized cognitive training programs, Bettercog and COMCOG, on elderly patients with MCI and mild dementia: A single-blind randomized controlled study. *Medicine (Baltimore)*, *97*(45), e13007. doi: 10.1097/MD.0000000000013007

Lobbia, A., Carbone, E., Faggian, S., Gardini, S., Piras, F., Spector, A., & Borella, E. (2019). The efficacy of cognitive stimulation therapy (CST) for people with mild-to-moderate dementia: A review. *European Psychologist*, *24*(3), 257–277. doi: 10.1027/1016-9040/a000342

Maldonado, P.M. (2016). Introducción de nuevas tecnologías y APPs en patologías geriátricas y enfermedades neurodegenerativas. *Neurama, Revista Electrónica de Psicogerontología*, *3*, 12–26.

McCausland, L., & Falk, N.L. (2012). From dinner table to digital tablet: technology's potential for reducing loneliness in older adults. *Journal of Psychosocial Nursing and Mental Health Services*, *50*(5), 22–26. doi: 10.3928/02793695-20120410-01

Meiland, F., Innes, A., Mountain, G., Robinson, L., van der Roest, H., García-Casal, J.A., ... Franco-Martin, M. (2017). Technologies to support community-dwelling persons with dementia: A position paper on issues regarding development, usability, effectiveness and cost-effectiveness, deployment, and ethics. *JMIR Rehabilitation and Assistive Technologies*, *4*(e1). doi: 10.2196/rehab.6376

Mitzner, T.L., Boron, J.B., Fausset, C.B., Adams, A.E., Charness, N., Czaja, S.J., ... Sharit, J. (2010). Older adults talk technology: Technology usage and attitudes. *Computers in Human Behavior*, *26*(6), 1710–1721. doi: 10.1016/j.chb.2010.06.020.Older

Peretz, C., Korczyn, A.D., Shatil, E., Aharonson, V., Birnboim, S., & Giladi, N. (2011). Computer-based, personalized cognitive training versus classical computer games: A randomized double-blind prospective trial of cognitive stimulation. *Neuroepidemiology*, *36*(2), 91–99. doi: 10.1159/000323950

Pirhonen, J., Lolich, L., Tuominen, K., Jolanki, O., & Timonen, V. (2020). "These devices have not been made for older people's needs" – Older adults' perceptions of digital technologies in Finland and Ireland. *Technology in Society*, *62*, 101287. doi: 10.1016/j.techsoc.2020.101287

Shatil, E. (2013). Does combined cognitive training and physical activity training enhance cognitive abilities more than either alone? A four-condition randomized controlled trial among healthy older adults. *Frontiers in Aging Neuroscience*, *5*, 8. doi: 10.3389/fnagi.2013.00008

Shatil, E., Mikulecká, J., Bellotti, F., & Bureš, V. (2014). Novel television-based cognitive training improves working memory and executive function. *PLoS One*, *9*(7), e101472. doi: doi:10.1371/journal.pone.0101472

Sjösten, N.M., Salonoja, M., Piirtola, M., J, V.T., Isoaho, R., Hyttinen, H.K., ... Kivelä, S.L. (2007). A multifactorial fall prevention programme in the community-dwelling aged: predictors of adherence. *European Journal of Public Health*, *17*(5), 464–470. doi: 10.1093/eurpub/ckl272

Smeenk, W., Sturm, J., & Eggen, B. (2018). Empathic handover: how would you feel? Handing over dementia experiences and feelings in empathic co-design. *CoDesign*, *14*(4), 259–274. doi: 10.1080/15710882.2017.1301960

Toribio-Guzmán, J.M., Parra Vidales, E., Viñas Rodríguez, M.J., Bueno Aguado, Y., Cid Bartolomé, M.T., & Franco-Martín, M.A. (2018). Rehabilitación cognitiva por ordenador en personas mayores: Programa gradior. *Ediciones Universidad de Salamanca, 24*, 61–75. doi: http://dx.doi.org/10.14201/aula2018246175

Toribio Guzmán, J.M. (2015). *Long Lasting Memories, una plataforma TIC integrada contra el deterioro cognitivo relacionado con la edad: Estudio de usabilidad.* Salamanca: Universidad de Salamanca.

Toribio Guzmán, J.M., García-Holgado, A., Soto Pérez, F., García-Peñalvo, F.J., & Franco Martín, M. (2017). Usability evaluation of a private social network on mental health for relatives. *Journal of Medical Systems, 41*(9). doi: 10.1007/s10916-017-0780-x

Turunen, M., Hokkanen, L., Bäckman, L., Stigsdotter-Neely, A., Hänninen, T., Paajanen, T., . . . Ngandu, T. (2019). Computer-based cognitive training for older adults: Determinants of adherence. *PLoS One, 14*(7), e0219541–e0219541. doi: 10.1371/journal.pone.0219541

Vanova, M., Irazoki, E., García-Casal, J.A., Martínez-Abad, F., Botella, C., Shiells, K.R., & Franco-Martín, M.A. (2018). The effectiveness of ICT-based neurocognitive and psychosocial rehabilitation programmes in people with mild dementia and mild cognitive impairment using GRADIOR and ehcobutler: study protocol for a randomised controlled trial. *Trials, 19*(1), 100–100. doi: 10.1186/s13063-017-2371-z

Vaportzis, E., Giatsi Clausen, M., & Gow, A.J. (2017). Older adults perceptions of technology and barriers to interacting with tablet computers: A focus group study. *Frontiers in Psychology, 8*. doi: 10.3389/fpsyg.2017.01687

Vermeij, A., Claassen, J.A., Dautzenberg, P.L., & Kessels, R.P. (2016). Transfer and maintenance effects of online working-memory training in normal ageing and mild cognitive impairment. *Neuropsychological Rehabilitation, 26*(5–6), 783–809. doi: 10.1080/09602011.2015.1048694

WHO. (2019). *Coronavirus disease 2019 (COVID-19) situation report – 67.* Geneva: World Health Organization.

Yang, H.L., Chu, H., Kao, C.C., Chiu, H.L., Tseng, I.J., Tseng, P., & Chou, K.R. (2019). Development and effectiveness of virtual interactive working memory training for older people with mild cognitive impairment: A single-blind randomised controlled trial. *Age and Ageing, 48*(4), 519–525. doi: 10.1093/ageing/afz029

Chapter 14

The role of Electronic Patient Records (EPR) for planning and delivering dementia care in nursing homes

Kate Shiells, Olga Štěpánková, Angie A. Diaz-Baquero, Vladmíra Dostálová, Iva Holmerová

Introduction

Nursing homes face a multitude of challenges, such as providing care for individuals with a wide range of needs, specifically those living with dementia, and organisational issues, including high staff turnover and low employee morale (Gibson & Barsade, 2003). They also often experience fragmented community care with a lack of multidisciplinary collaboration across services which is required to plan and deliver optimal care for people with dementia living in nursing homes (Fossey, 2008; Minkman et al., 2009). However, this chapter focuses specifically on the challenge faced by nursing homes in the form of documentation, a task frequently described as a burden by those working in the sector (Fournier et al., 2006). This can be attributed to a rise in the demands for documentation, which have come about from 'increasing regulatory scrutiny and soaring public awareness' (Fournier et al., 2006). Furthermore, nursing home staff have expressed resistance towards documentation because they do not see its value (Edelstein, 1990). Staff may also experience difficulties with articulating the nursing process in written format (Hanesbo et al., 1999).

Documentation practices in nursing homes

Documentation used in nursing homes will usually reflect the different stages of the nursing process (Forster, 2003a). Documentation plays an important role in the care of people living in nursing homes, particularly for those with dementia, as emphasised by Alzheimer's Disease International (2013), who describe assessment and care planning as one of the four main 'apparatus' of long-term care. The first stage in the nursing process, assessment, involves collecting information relating to a person's physical, psychological and social needs (Forster, 2003b). Assessment may take place in a direct or proxy manner, such as through observations or discussions with relatives. Various tools may be used in the assessment process, for

DOI: 10.4324/9781003289005-18

example the Resident Assessment Instrument-Minimum Data Set (Hutchinson et al., 2010). However, assessment is often a time-consuming process for staff, and in addition can be a potentially stressful activity for the person with dementia (Forster, 2003b).

Information gathered during the assessment process is then used to formulate a care plan (Dellefield, 2006). Care plans have been described as 'prescriptions for nursing care' (Forster, 2003c) and act as a reference for nurses to facilitate continuity of care, as well as record care provided (Ballantyne, 2016). Care plans are also 'dynamic documents' that should be updated regularly as part of the evaluation process (Forster, 2003c). An essential characteristic of the care plan is that it should be fully personalised to reflect the individual (Jeon et al., 2013), such as information relating to the maintenance of physical health and the most appropriate physical and social environment (Nasso & Celia, 2007). Plans should include goals which maximise individuals' current abilities and minimise their deterioration (Nasso & Celia, 2007). This personalised approach has been influenced by the work of Carl Rogers and later Tom Kitwood (Brooker, 2003). Kitwood challenged the medical model of care focused on treatment of disease, which had led to care plans purely focused around routines and organisational needs (Fazio et al., 2018). Instead, he emphasised the importance of maintaining selfhood, and respecting each person's needs whilst trying to view the world through their perspective (Fazio et al., 2018). In this way, as far as possible, care planning should also be participatory (Forster, 2003c).

An area of care planning that has been found to be poor for people with dementia is the recording of neuropsychiatric symptoms (Jeon et al., 2013). This is an important aspect as systematic documentation can provide an insight into the triggers of certain behaviours and thus indicate ways to avoid particular scenarios from recurring (Omelan, 2006). Person-centred care planning has also been shown to reduce neuropsychiatric symptoms of dementia whilst leading to a reduction in psychotropic medication use in nursing homes (Li & Porock, 2014).

The electronic patient record

The advent of the electronic patient record (EPR) can be traced back to the 1960s. However, it was not until 1991 that the Institute of Medicine in the United States called for a shift from paper to computerised patient records (Hanson & Lubotsky Levin, 2013). This coincided with computers becoming more powerful and compact, as well as more affordable (Evans, 2016). EPRs were predicted to improve the safety, quality and efficiency of healthcare through the incorporation of a number of functionalities (Institute of Medicine, 2001). Key functionalities of a useful record system required for healthcare today include easy access and display of data at the point of care;

the possibility to share and integrate data amongst healthcare staff and disease surveillance and clinical decision support (Shortliffe & Blois, 2001). However, incorporating these components into the EPR successfully has been challenging.

The EPR has been described as 'underused and failed' across multiple health systems and countries (Obstfelder & Moen, 2006). This has been linked with a lack of standards in clinical and nursing terminology meaning that clinical decision support systems (CDSS) cannot be incorporated into the EPR, as well as concerns about data security and privacy, shortcomings in integrating records systems across healthcare settings and difficulties in data entry (Shortliffe & Blois, 2001). Furthermore, a lack of consideration has been given to the socio-technical issues associated with Health Information Technology (HIT) implementation, including technical, social and also environmental components (Obstfelder & Moen, 2006; Rogers et al., 2013; Sockolow et al., 2012).

Human factors engineering

Human Factors Engineering (HFE) has emerged from the various evaluation methods used in the field of Human Computer Interaction (Kushniruk & Patel, 2004). However, HFE is largely un-established in healthcare environments. HFE is distinct from traditional 'outcome-based evaluations', which have historically taken an objectivist approach, frequently using the randomised controlled trial to explore aspects such as the safety, accuracy and reliability of technology (Kushniruk & Patel., 2004). Issues with quantitative methods such as the RCT arise when results show a negative outcome, which does not usually reveal the reasons behind this outcome (Kushniruk & Patel., 2004). HFE may provide a more appropriate theoretical and methodical underpinning to address socio-technical issues (Rogers et al., 2013). Firstly, this approach emphasises the importance of iteration: the cyclical nature of designing, modifying and testing products and incorporating feedback from end users at each step (Rubin, 1994). Therefore, a human factors approach is also participatory, highlighting the importance of joint development (Rubin, 1994). Joint development has been frequently found to be valued by EPR users (Cherry et al., 2011; Wiederhold & Shortliffe, 2001). An HFE approach also takes into account three 'domains of system design': physical, cognitive and organisational (WHO, 2016). Therefore, HFE allows for an understanding of not only the device and software, but also the user, the task and the environment (Hanson & Lubotsky Levin, 2013). The importance of an HFE approach has been translated into policy guidance, whereby the WHO (2016) recommend that member states prioritise end user research when designing HIT, so that technology addresses information needs and matches with the preferences of healthcare providers and patients, as well as the context of use.

Aim

The aim of this study (Shiells et al., 2020) was to explore usability issues associated with the EPR for assessment and care planning for people with dementia in nursing homes, and to develop best practice guidelines accordingly.

Methods

Study design

Underpinned by HFE, this research used a multiple case study design, which enables the researcher to examine a phenomenon within its natural setting and explore differences and similarities across case studies (Baxter & Jack, 2008).

Data collection method

The Contextual Inquiry method was used, which allows the participant to perform relevant tasks whilst also providing an opportunity for the researcher to ask questions about processes and understand contextual issues (Martin & Crowe, 2010). Previous research found Contextual Inquiry to be an appropriate method for evaluating the usability of the EPR (Vitanen, 2011).

Interview guide

The interview guide was designed according to the components of the 'structural quality concept' of the Health Information Technology Framework (HITREF) (Sockolow et al., 2012). The HITREF is underpinned by the socio-technical paradigm (Lee, 2016), and was developed in response to a lack of consistent approaches to evaluating HIT, with previous frameworks commonly omitting contextual evaluation (Sockolow et al., 2015). The components explored included device, software functionality and organisational support. Two further components, 'structure and content', were added by the authors in order to elicit opinions on the language and structure of the EPR forms. Under each component, specific questions were developed from evidence collated from the authors' prior research (Shiells et al., 2019) and designed to elicit responses about the usability of the EPR for the task.

Setting

Data collection took place in three nursing homes in Belgium, Czech Republic and Spain between March 2018 and January 2019. In order to be eligible for this study, the nursing home had to have been using an EPR system for at least six months and provide care to people with dementia. Brief descriptions of the type of EPR system used in the nursing homes are provided in Box 14.1

Box 14.1   Descriptions of EPR systems used in the nursing homes

Belgium

The nursing home in Belgium introduced their EPR system in 2010. It was the role of the occupational therapist to complete the initial assessment on the EPR system. This involved completing an assessment template on a desktop computer, as well as filling out a separate paper assessment document that was created by the nursing home, as the assessment form on the EPR did not fully meet their documentation needs. This document was scanned and uploaded to the EPR as an attachment. Nursing staff had access to both a desktop computer and laptops which they used to complete the care plan template in the EPR. Auxiliary nurses had access to tablet devices which they could use to access a simpler version of the care plan.

Czech Republic

In the Czech nursing home, staff had recently transitioned to a new EPR application in March 2018, as the previous software was unsuitable for the nursing home environment. This meant that staff were then able to use the EPR to complete the assessments and care plans. In the Czech Republic, nursing home care is divided into two fields: 'health' and 'social care', and a dual approach to the assessment and care planning process took place. Staff members could only access documents in their respective fields. An art therapist working in the home was also involved in assessing residents' social needs and planning activities related to their hobbies and interests accordingly. Most staff had access to desktop computers although the nursing home had just introduced tablets for auxiliary nurses six weeks prior to the interviews.

Spain

In the Spanish nursing home, the EPR system had been introduced in 2010. When a resident moved into the nursing home, trained staff were required to fill out their own version of a needs assessment and an individualised plan of action in their field within a month. These documents were first filled out on paper, and then staff had to input information from this document into the respective sections of the EPR. A desktop device was used by trained staff to complete this process. Auxiliary nurses did not have access to the EPR and filled out documentation in notebooks.

Participants

Eight participants were recruited in Czech Republic (female $n=8$), seven in Spain (female $n=5$; male $n=2$) and six in Belgium (female $n=6$). Maximum variation sampling as characterised by job role was used. Participants were required to be a permanent member of staff who managed or provided care to residents with dementia; be involved in assessment and/or care planning; have worked in the nursing home for at least six months and been trained in how to use the EPR system.

Procedure

Participants were first provided with medical and social information about a fictional nursing home resident and were asked to show the researcher how they would create a new electronic file on the EPR and input the relevant information into the assessment or care plan template. Whilst carrying out this task, individuals were asked to use the 'think aloud' method in order to provide the researcher with an insight into their thought processes (Rubin, 1994). The participant was then invited to take part in a semi-structured interview to elaborate on the issues raised during the task.

Ethics

All participants gave written informed consent prior to participation. The study was approved by the Ethics Committee at the Centre of Gerontology, Prague, Czech Republic, and by the Medical Ethics Committee of the Vrije Universiteit Brussel, Belgium [2017/410]. The local ethics committee of the INTRAS Foundation, Valladolid, ruled that no formal ethics approval was required in this particular case in Spain.

Data analysis

Theoretical thematic data analysis was carried out, which allows data to be coded for a specific research question and according to a theoretical pre-conception (Braun & Clarke, 2006). Data were coded into sub-themes according to each of the a priori, overarching components from the Structural Quality evaluation concept of the HITREF Framework (Sockolow et al., 2012). Finally, in order to develop best practice guidelines, themes were compared and synthesised with an earlier integrative literature review conducted by the authors (Shiells et al., 2018) investigating the ways in which the EPR is facilitating or hindering care provision in nursing homes, and a scoping review exploring the self-reported needs and experiences of people with dementia in nursing homes (Shiells et al., 2019).

Results

Device

Type of device

A tablet device was preferred as it could be transported in the nurses' trolley for easy access to care plans, and also be used to record the assessment. However, when writing care plans, nurses preferred to use a desktop computer as they found the keyboard easier to use for long documents. Staff had mixed opinions on whether devices should be used in residents' rooms. In one home where they were using devices in rooms, the noise of the device made one participant uncomfortable:

> It's horrible. There is a human being, and you come and beep, beep like a robot. What is this, science fiction?
>
> (Auxiliary nurse)

Number of devices

Several staff complained about having to share devices and wait until they became available. This led to concerns that staff were prevented from viewing updated care plans before delivering care.

Software functionality

Drop-down menus

Participants across all three homes noted that it took time to type free text into the EPR. As such, despite having a portable device for data entry at the point of care, staff often carried out administrative work after delivering personal care to all residents, in order to prioritise time spent with individuals. This is even more crucial when caring for people with dementia:

> The tablet is extra work, and for people with dementia, it's very important for me to give them extra time.
>
> (Auxiliary nurse)

It was suggested that users would benefit from writing less if the software incorporated drop-down menus.

Customisable terminology

There were complaints that the terminology used in some EPRs was complex for staff with less training in the field. However, in the Czech home, where they had recently introduced a new programme, there was a customisable functionality that addressed this issue:

> It has an advantage, that you can adjust the phrases as you please so that everyone can understand.
>
> (Care Quality Manager)

Alerts about changes in a resident's condition

Staff in all homes used an internal messaging application within the EPR or hold regular meetings to communicate changes in a resident's condition and how to adjust care. However, there was no functionality to alert staff based on data entered into the EPR and staff would have liked alerts to show whether a resident had for instance, had a fall.

Alerts to update care plans

In the Czech home, staff were warned that the care plan needed updating when a red circle appeared next to a resident's name. In the two other homes, the EPR did not provide alerts and staff kept a record on paper.

Interoperability

In all three homes, the EPR was not interoperable. When residents moved to the home, they brought a paper report with details of medical history, which had to be manually entered into the EPR. Nurses found this frustrating and often needed to call the hospital to clarify unclear information.

Structure and content

Assessments for dementia

Core assessment scales were missing from the EPR and needed to be completed on paper. Scales that staff said they require for assessing people with dementia were the Quality of Life in Late-Stage Dementia Scale (QUALID), the Mini Mental State Examination (MMSE) and the Barthel Index. Furthermore, it was highlighted how staff also required access to assessment templates based on observations, which may be more appropriate for assessing people with advanced dementia with communication issues or those who become anxious during a typical assessment.

In the newly introduced system in the Czech home, many of the areas in the electronic assessment forms were said to be inappropriate for people with dementia:

> There are no options that we might like to have clicked, that the clients are, for example, chronically or acutely confused.
>
> (Nurse)

Care planning for dementia

Care planning plays an important role in the work of nurses, and the EPR should facilitate this process. In the Czech nursing home, the old EPR had been replaced, partly because it was inappropriate for nursing staff to develop their care plans:

> It's a programme for doctors . . . it's not suitable for nurses. . . . There was no space for a care plan, just to add medical history and a few assessment tests.
>
> (Care quality manager)

When asked about the most important information in a care plan that staff needed to know about a resident with dementia, a common answer was the need to be alerted to any deterioration in physical health. For example, changes in eating, drinking or bowel habits, and changes in temperature, all of which could indicate possible infection and explain recent behavioural changes. It was emphasised that such information is particularly valuable for those residents with difficulties communicating verbally. Information about the type of dementia is also needed.

In addition to information about physical health, a number of staff highlighted the importance of recording a life history in order to obtain a holistic picture of an individual:

> I want to put the stories in [the EPR] to remind people that this person who is lying on the bed was really a hero in his life.
>
> (Art therapist)

In order to create the most natural environment for the resident, knowledge about hobbies, past routines and professions is also important.

Improvements in structure

Specific improvements in structure included a table where all observations can be entered and viewed together. Trained staff also need to be able to access information recorded by each staff member.

Organisational support

Access

Access to the EPR differed across the homes. In Spain, auxiliary nurses could not access the EPR and were required to write notes by hand. In Belgium where auxiliary nurses had basic access to care plans via the tablet, they were frustrated with the limited amount of information they could access:

> [The tablet] shows what you have to do, but not how the person is. So, it doesn't show if the person has behavioural issues.
>
> (Auxiliary nurse)

Some trained staff felt that due to the complexity of the system, access should be restricted so that documentation is not accidentally deleted. One participant believed auxiliary nurses should not have access to dementia diagnosis, as they may treat the individual differently.

Others believed auxiliary nurses should have access to the full EPR, including dementia diagnosis, in order to provide the most person-centred care.

Training

When asked about training, the majority of participants said that learning 'on the job' was more useful than attending a course, as they found the EPR intuitive. However, one nurse felt overwhelmed when starting her role, and would have liked more time to learn to use the EPR.

System support

The importance of contact with developers on an ongoing basis was highlighted. In the Czech home, staff could write notes and feedback any problems directly to the developer, who also had remote access and could address any issues quickly. In all homes, there were allocated staff who were in charge of reporting issues to the developer; a system which worked well.

Discussion

Best practice guidelines for electronic patient records in nursing homes in Belgium, Czech Republic and Spain

The following section describes best practice guidelines for the development and implementation of EPR for use in the assessment and planning of dementia care in nursing homes.

Guideline 1: Nursing homes providing care for people with dementia should consider introducing portable devices in addition to desktop devices for EPRs. Devices should not disrupt or invade residents' privacy.

Portable devices may increase efficiency in some instances as they allow staff to record data into the EPR at the point of care. This enables staff to spend more time providing direct care to residents. Portable devices can support person-centred care by allowing immediate access to care plans with vital information about residents. However, staff may prefer desktop devices based on ease of use when completing substantial documents. The disruption that devices could have on residents should be taken into account.

Guideline 2: Applications promoting the effective use of electronic records are required.

A spell-check should be incorporated into the EPR in order to increase comprehension of documentation. A copy and paste function saves staff time by allowing easy transfer of information across documents, and a keyword search function allows for more efficient retrieval of information. Log-in processes should be rapid and secure to reduce barriers to using the EPR.

Guideline 3: Functionalities of electronic records should be tailored to the nursing home environment.

Developers should consider including a function allowing for the automated generation of graphs to show trends in data, increasing visibility of changes in a resident's condition and allowing staff to more rapidly identify and respond to changing care needs, for example graphs showing changes in weight. In addition, functions allowing for the automated generation of care plans from assessment data could save staff time on administration, and alerts to prompt staff to create or update a new document in the EPR may mean optimal care can be planned and provided to individuals with dementia. EPR systems should be interoperable so that staff can access and communicate relevant information efficiently with external healthcare providers, instead of using paper records.

Guideline 4: Electronic care documentation should meet the needs of nursing home staff caring for people with dementia.

EPR systems should include the necessary assessment templates for use in the care of people with dementia, such as the MMSE assessment, the QUALID scale and the Barthel Index of Activities of Daily Living. There should also be space to upload a photo of each resident. Electronic assessment forms and care plans for dementia care should use formalised nursing language to prompt the entry of correct information, and structured templates that guide staff through body systems, leading to comprehensive care plans. Staff require space to enter life stories, and space for free data entry for additional notes and observations.

Guideline 5: Electronic care documentation should meet the needs of people with dementia in nursing homes.

Electronic assessment forms and care plans used for planning dementia care should prompt staff to consider the following needs of residents: activities, maintaining previous roles, reminiscence, freedom and choice, appropriate environment, meaningful relationships, support with grief and loss, and end-of-life care.

Guideline 6: Nursing home managers should ensure the appropriate conditions for implementation of EPR systems.

Access to various parts of the EPR system should be considered, for instance, whether auxiliary staff should be allowed to access medical information, such as dementia diagnosis. Appropriate training in the EPR system according to individual staff needs is required. Developers should work alongside nursing homes during the design of EPR systems in order to ensure software is appropriate for their needs and continue to be involved in improving the EPR following implementation, as part of an iterative cycle.

Conclusion

This qualitative exploration of staff perspectives of EPR in three nursing homes revealed that the three EPR systems were both helping and hindering staff to plan and deliver care. All homes highlighted the importance of customisable systems, and the lack of specific characteristics needed to effectively plan and deliver care for people with dementia. People with dementia in nursing homes may have more complex needs in comparison to other residents. Therefore, EPR systems introduced into the nursing home environment should reflect best practice guidelines for dementia care, which may lead to improved outcomes and quality of life for people with dementia. Furthermore, all levels of nursing home staff should be consulted during the development, implementation and evaluation of EPR systems as part of an iterative, user-centred design process.

References

Alzheimer's Disease International. (2013). *World Alzheimer Report 2013. Journey of caring – An analysis of long-term care for dementia*. London: ADI. Retrieved from www.alz.co.uk/research/WorldAlzheimerReport2013.pdf

Ballantyne, H. (2016). Developing nursing care plans. *Nursing Standard, 30*(26), 51–57.

Baxter, P., & Jack, S. (2008). Qualitative case study methodology: Study design and implementation for novice researchers. *The Qualitative Report, 13*(4), 544–559.

Braun, V, Clarke V. (2006). Using thematic analysis in psychology. *Qualitative Research in Psychology, 3*(2), 77–101.

Brooker, D. (2003). What is person-centered care in dementia? *Reviews in Clinical Gerontology, 13*(3), 215–222.

Cherry, B, Carpenter, K. (2011). Evaluating the effectiveness of electronic medical records in a long-term care facility using process analysis. *Journal of Healthcare Engineering, 2*(1), 75–86.

Dellefield, M.E. (2006). Interdisciplinary care planning and the written care plan in nursing homes: A critical review. *The Gerontologist, 46*(1), 128–133.

Edelstein, J. (1990). A study of nursing documentation. *Nursing Management, 21*(1), 40–46.

Evans, R.S. (2016). Electronic health records: Then, now, and in the future. *Yearbook of Medical Informatics, 25*(S01), S48–S61.

Fazio, S., Pace D., Flinner, J., & Kallmyer, B. (2018). The fundamentals of person-centred care for individuals with dementia. *The Gerontologist, 58*(1), S10–S19.

Forster, S. (2003a). Nursing older people. In S. Carmody & S. Forster (Eds.), *Nursing older people: A guide to practice in care homes* (pp. 1–10). Melbourne: Ausmed Publications.

Forster, S. (2003b). Nursing assessments. In S. Carmody & S. Forster (Eds.), *Nursing older people: A guide to practice in care homes* (pp. 11–20). Melbourne: Ausmed Publications.

Forster, S. (2003c). Care plans. In S. Carmody & S. Forster (Eds.), *Nursing older people: A guide to practice in care homes* (pp. 189–198). Melbourne: Ausmed Publications.

Fossey, J. (2008). Care homes. In M. Downs & B. Bowers (Eds.), *Excellence in dementia care. Research into practice* (pp. 336–358). Maidenhead: Open University Press.

Fournier, D., Gosselin, D., & Rioux, N. (2006). The challenges of implementing an electronic medical record system in a long-term care facility. *Geriatric Nursing, 27*(1), 28–30.

Gibson, D.E., & Barsade, S.G. (2003). Managing organizational culture change: The case of long-term care. In A. S. Weiner & J.L. Ronch (Eds.), *Culture change in long-term care* (pp. 11–34). Philadelphia, PA: Haworth Press.

Hanesbo, G., Kihlgren, M., & Ljunggren, G. (1999). Review of nursing documentation in nursing home wards-changes after intervention for individualized care. *Journal of Advanced Nursing, 29*(6), 1462–1473.

Hanson, A., & Lubotsky Levin, B. (2013). *Mental health informatics.* New York, NY: Oxford University Press.

Hutchinson, A.M., Milke, D.L., Maisey, S., Johnson, C., Squires, J.E., Teare, G., & Estabrooks, C.A. (2010). The resident assessment instrument-minimum data set 2.0 quality indicators: A systematic review. *BMC Health Services Research, 10*(166).

Institute of Medicine. (2001). *Crossing the quality chasm: A new health system for the 21st century.* Washington, DC: National Academies Press.

Jeon, Y-H., Govett, J., Low, L-F., Chenoweth, L., McNeill, G., Hoolahan, A., Brodaty, H., & O'Connor, D. (2013). Care planning practices for behavioural and psychological symptoms of dementia in residential aged care: A pilot of an education toolkit informed by the Aged Care Funding Instrument. *Contemporary Nurse, 44*(2), 156–169.

Kushniruk, A.W., & Patel, V.L. (2004). Cognitive and usability engineering methods for the evaluation of clinical information systems. *Journal of Biomedical Informatics, 37*(1), 56–76.

Lee, T.T. (2016). Evaluation of health information technology-key elements in the framework. *Journal of Nursing Research, 24*(4), 283–285.

Li, J., & Porock, D. (2014). Resident outcomes of person-centred care in long-term care: A narrative review of interventional research. *International Journal of Nursing Studies, 51*(10), 1395–1415.

Martin J.L., & Crowe JA. (2010) Contextual inquiry for medical device development: A case study. In V. Duffy (Ed.), *Advances in human factors and ergonomics in healthcare.* Florida: CRC Press.

Minkman, M.M.N., Ligthart, S.A., & Huijsman, R. (2009). Integrated dementia care in The Netherlands: A multiple case study of case management programmes. *Health & Social Care in the Community, 17*(5), 485–494.

Nasso, J., & Celia, L. (2007). *Dementia care: In-service training modules for long-term care.* New York: Thomson Delmar Learning.

Obstfelder, A., & Moen, A. (2006). The electronic patient record in community health services-paradoxes and adjustments in clinical work. *Studies in Health Technology and Informatics, 122*, 626–631.

Omelan, C. (2006). Approach to managing behavioural disturbances in dementia. *Canadian Family Physician, 52*(2), 191–199.

Rogers, M.L., Sockolow, P.S., Bowles, K.H., Hand, K.E., & George, J. (2013). Use of human factors approach to uncover informatics needs of nurses in documentation of care. *International Journal of Medical Informatics, 82*, 1068–1074.

Rubin, J. (1994). *Handbook of usability testing.* Toronto: John Wiley & Sons.

Shiells, K., Diaz Baquero, A.A., Štěpánková, O., & Holmerová, I. (2020). Staff perspectives on the usability of electronic patient records for planning and delivering dementia care in nursing homes: a multiple case study. *BMC Medical Informatics and Decision Making, 20*(1).

Shiells, K., Holmerova, I., Steffl, M., & Stepankova, O. (2018). Electronic patient records as a tool to facilitate care provision in nursing homes: An integrative review. *Informatics for Health and Social Care, 44*(3), 262–277.

Shiells, K., Pivodic, L., Holmerová, I., & van den Block, L. (2019). Self-reported needs and experiences of people with dementia living in nursing homes: A scoping review. *Aging & Mental Health, 24*(10), 1553–1568.

Shortliffe, E.H., & Blois, M.S. (2001). The computer meets medicine and biology: Emergence of a discipline. In E.H. Shortliffe & L.E. Perreault (Eds.), *Medical informatics. Computer applications in health care and biomedicine* (pp. 41–75). New York, NY: Springer.

Sockolow, P.S., Bowles, K.H., Rogers, M. (2015). Health information technology evaluation framework (HITREF) comprehensiveness as assessed in electronic point-of-care documentation systems evaluations. *Studies in Health Technology and Informatics, 216*, 406–9.

Sockolow, P.S, Crawford P.R., Lehmann, H.P. (2012). Health services research evaluation principles. Broadening a general framework for evaluating health information technology. *Methods of Information in Medicine, 51*(2), 122–130.

Vitanen, J. (2011). Contextual inquiry method for user-Centred clinical IT system design. *Studies in Health Technology and Informatics, 169*, 965–9.

Wiederhold, G., & Shortliffe, E.H. (2001). System design and engineering. In E.H. Shortliffe & L.E. Perreault (Eds.), *Medical informatics. Computer applications in health care and biomedicine* (pp. 180–211). New York, NY: Springer.

World Health Organization. (2016). *Human factors: Technical series on safer primary care.* Geneva: World Health Organization. Retrieved from www.who.int/patientsafety/topics/primary-care/technical_series/en/

Chapter 15

PACE steps to success program — palliative healthcare technology for nursing home residents with and without dementia

Rose Miranda, Elisabeth Honinx, Tinne Smets, Lieve Van den Block, on behalf of the EU PACE consortium and trial collaborators

Introduction

Palliative care has been widely advocated for people living with dementia and their families, as this approach aims '*to improve the quality of life of patients and their families facing the problems associated with life-threatening illness, through the prevention and relief of suffering by means of early identification and impeccable assessment and treatment of pain and other problems, whether physical, psychosocial or spiritual*' (van der Steen et al., 2014; World Health Organization, 2002, p. 84).

Palliative care encompasses generalist palliative care and specialist palliative care. Generalist palliative care services are provided by healthcare providers with basic knowledge, competencies and skills in palliative care, while specialist palliative care is provided by a palliative care-trained multidisciplinary team, services or clinician. Specialist palliative care is highly applicable in times when the care needs of a person become so complex that generalist palliative care providers could no longer address them alone (Ryan & Johnston, 2019).

Earlier studies show the benefits of palliative care in improving the symptom burden and quality of life of adults with incurable conditions. Similarly, there is some evidence showing the benefits of palliative care for people living with dementia. However, existing literature on palliative care for nursing home residents with dementia remains scarce (Murphy et al., 2016; Walsh et al., 2021), and many nursing home residents with dementia remain at risk of dying with discomfort (Miranda et al., 2018; Miranda et al., 2021; Mitchell, 2015; Pivodic et al., 2018; Sampson et al., 2018). Throughout this chapter, 'nursing homes' are defined as collective institutional settings where on-site resident care is provided 24/7 (Froggatt et al., 2017).

DOI: 10.4324/9781003289005-19

Challenges of improving palliative care in nursing homes

Improving palliative care in nursing homes is challenging due to the complexity of the demographic and clinical characteristics of the population living in it and its context. In 2015, we conducted the PACE retrospective cross-sectional study in 322 nursing homes in Belgium, Finland, Italy, the Netherlands, Poland and the United Kingdom (Van den Block et al., 2016; Pivodic et al., 2018). On the basis of this study, we found that nursing home residents in Europe die on average at the age of 85 years, often with multiple comorbidities, poor functional and cognitive status, advanced dementia or other clinical complications (Honinx et al., 2019). We also found a general lack of understanding about the basic concept of palliative care among nurses and care assistants, which can have negative implications on the quality of care (Honinx et al., 2019). Examples of other factors that could complicate efforts to further improve palliative care in nursing homes include insufficient financial resources, staff and time, and high staff turnover (Froggatt et al., 2017a).

The palliative care needs of nursing home residents with dementia

People living with dementia often have complex physical, psychosocial and spiritual care needs that persist for months or years until the end of life. Because dementia has been associated with old age, comorbidity and frailty, pain, shortness of breath and other physical symptoms are prevalent in people living with dementia (Hendriks et al., 2013; Mitchell, 2015; Sampson et al., 2018). In all human beings, psychological and social needs are present, but these are likely to be heightened for people living with dementia. The functional and cognitive impairment inherent in dementia makes it difficult for these people to take actions to satisfy these needs. If these needs remain unmet, this could result in social isolation, loneliness and depression (Hansen et al., 2017). The life-limiting nature of dementia could also evoke people to question their illness, spirituality and existence (Bernard et al., 2020).

In addition, the disease trajectory and symptoms of dementia pose another layer of complexity in providing palliative care services to people living with dementia. For instance, as dementia has an unpredictable disease trajectory, disability and death might occur at any stage of dementia (Pivodic et al., 2018). Such unpredictability poses added challenges for clinicians in determining prognosis and in deciding on whether or not the benefits of certain medical treatments and interventions that are considered aggressive outweigh the potential harm. This puts people living with dementia at risk of receiving burdensome and futile interventions and potentially avoidable hospitalisations (Hendriks et al., 2013; Houttekier et al., 2014; Mitchell, 2015; Sampson et al., 2018). The cognitive impairment that often results in communication difficulties may also leave affected people unable to verbalise their care needs (Mitchell, 2015; Sampson et al., 2018). Overall, due to the different layers of these palliative care needs, providing care to nursing home residents with dementia is a highly complex work that requires dementia-specific knowledge and skill sets from health and social care professionals and family caregivers.

The European PACE Steps to Success palliative care programme — A complex health technology for nursing home residents with and without dementia

To improve palliative care for nursing home residents with and without dementia, we developed 'PACE Steps to Success'. PACE Steps to Success is a multicomponent complex health technology aiming to integrate generalist and non-disease-specific palliative care into nursing homes (Payne et al., 2019). The WHO defines health technology as an '*application of organized knowledge and skills in the form of medicines, medical devices, vaccines, procedures and systems developed to solve a health problem and improve quality of life*' (World Health Organization, 2021).

Ultimately, PACE Steps to Success aims to optimise the delivery of palliative care in nursing homes in Europe by developing tools to assist practitioners and policy- and decision-makers to make evidence-based decisions regarding best palliative care practices in this setting (Payne et al., 2019; Smets et al., 2018). PACE Steps to Success comprises six steps:

- **Step 1**: Discussions about current and future care through advance care planning discussions with residents and/or families to elicit wishes and preferences around end-of-life care using the Looking and Thinking Ahead document. This communication process usually takes place in the context of an anticipated deterioration in the individual's condition in the future, with attendant loss of capacity to make decisions and/or ability to communicate wishes to others.
- **Step 2:** Assessment and review: Completion of a prognostic register to prompt appropriate advance care planning discussions, and 'do not attempt cardio-pulmonary resuscitation' – orders alongside regular symptoms assessments for pain and depression.
- **Step 3**: Coordination of care through monthly multidisciplinary review meetings where residents identified as having less than six months to live are discussed in detail, with specific invitations sent to GPs.
- **Step 4:** Delivery of high-quality palliative care through symptom management focusing on pain and depression. General staff education concerning principles of palliative care for frail nursing home residents (including those with dementia), symptom control and complex communication skills.
- **Step 5:** Care in the last days of life using an integrated care plan for the last days of life to empower staff to provide high-quality care to the dying resident and their family.
- **Step 6:** Care after death, in which monthly reflective debriefings were conducted to support staff following a death and encourage experiential learning.

Using a train–the–trainer approach, PACE Steps to Success was implemented over the course of one year, including two months for pre-implementation phase, six months training for nursing home staff in the six steps and four months consolidation. All countries had one or more country trainers. Each nursing home assigned one to six staff members as PACE coordinators. After being trained by two experienced trainers, the country trainers trained and supported the PACE coordinators who were in turn responsible for training and supporting fellow nursing home staff. During the pre-implementation phase, PACE coordinators got a 'pre-intervention training' given by the Country trainer. During the six-month implementation of the programme, each step of the programme was delivered every month. The implementation phase consists of six 90-minute workshops for nursing home staff provided by the Country trainer. Each workshop covers one of the six steps. In the consolidation phase, the tools and actions introduced in the workshops are further implemented and monthly meetings are led by the PACE coordinator and supported by the Country trainer (Payne et al., 2019; Smets et al., 2018).

PACE Steps to Success also includes three dementia-specific elements, including:

- Communication training in advanced dementia for the PACE coordinators during the pre-implementation phase
- Training for all nursing home staff with an emphasis on dementia as a life-limiting illness as a part of Step 2
- Training for all nursing home staff regarding symptom control strategies for residents with and without dementia in Step 4

Method

The PACE cluster-randomised controlled trial

The effects of PACE Steps to Success were evaluated in a cluster-randomised controlled trial (RCT) in 78 nursing homes in Belgium, the Netherlands, the United Kingdom, Finland, Italy, Poland and Switzerland (2015–2017) (Smets et al., 2018). As the programme involved the training of nursing home staff, stratified randomisation was performed at the nursing home level. One contact person per nursing home identified all residents who had died in the previous four months. After-death structured questionnaires for each resident were sent to the nursing home staff most involved in care (preferably a nurse), the nursing home administrator and the general practitioner (GP) at baseline (month 0) and twice post-intervention (at months 13 and 17). Outcome measures included comfort in the last week of life measured using the validated Comfort Assessment in Dying-End of Life Care in Dementia (CAD-EOLD) (primary outcome) and quality of care and dying in the last month of life measured using the Quality of Dying-Long Term Care (QOD-LTC) (secondary outcome).

We also performed cost–effectiveness analyses. Direct medical costs, quality-adjusted life years (QALYs) based on the 5-level EQ-5D version (EQ-5D-5L) and costs per quality increase measured with the QOD-LTC were outcome measures. Process evaluation was also conducted to explore the level of implementation of PACE Steps to Success (according to the RE-AIM framework – that is Reach, Adoption, Implementation and intention to Maintenance) and the factors that may have affected this implementation. It involved various participants and used mixed methods, including structured diaries, registries on training attendance, document adoption, individual and group interviews and evaluation questionnaires.

Because PACE Steps to Success was originally designed for all residents and included only three dementia-specific elements, we hypothesised a priori that its effects might differ between those with and without dementia in favour of those with mild/moderate or no dementia compared with advanced dementia. It has been widely argued that for palliative care programmes to be effective for people living with dementia, they should address the specific needs of this population (Goodman et al., 2010; Mitchell, 2015). However, no study has yet investigated this assumption. Hence, we planned a subgroup analysis at the outset of the PACE cluster-RCT to investigate whether the effects of PACE Steps to Success differ between residents with advanced, non-advanced and no dementia (Van den Block et al., 2020). Whether or not residents died with dementia was based on the judgement of the GP and/or the nursing home staff, while the severity of their dementia was estimated based on the combination of two validated instruments that measure cognitive and functional status, Cognitive Performance Scale and Global Deterioration Scale (Smets et al., 2018).

Results

Effects of PACE steps to success for the overall nursing home population

The primary analyses of the PACE cluster-RCT showed that PACE Steps to Success did not improve the comfort in the last week of life (primary outcome) in the overall nursing home population, but it appeared to improve quality of care and dying in the last month of life for this population, although the latter was the secondary outcome. We did not find any negative effects (Van den Block et al., 2020).

Differential effects for nursing home residents with and without dementia

The subgroup analyses showed that contrary to the hypothesis, the effects of PACE Steps to Success did not differ between residents with advanced, non-advanced and no dementia. For the primary outcome – comfort in the last week of life – PACE Steps to Success did not achieve better outcomes for residents without dementia or with non-advanced dementia than for those with advanced dementia. This finding confirmed the lack of improvement of the primary trial analyses on comfort at the end of life. Nevertheless, for the secondary outcome, analyses showed that PACE Steps to Success improved quality of care and dying in the last month of life equally for those with dementia (regardless of the stage) and those without dementia (Miranda et al., 2021a).

Cost-effectiveness of PACE steps to success

The cost-effectiveness analysis showed that costs decreased and QoL was retained due to PACE Steps to Success. The implementation of PACE Steps to Success realised substantial medical cost savings, mainly due to lower hospitalisation-related costs. In particular, there was a total of 80.6% decrease in hospitalisations on the geriatric, general and intensive care unit (ICU) ward. A clinically relevant difference of almost 3 nights shorter (from nine to six nights; a decrease of 30%) hospitalisations in favour of the intervention group was found, indicating residents are returning to nursing homes earlier. Although the length of hospitalisation and the cost decrease on the mentioned wards did not decrease significantly, the combination of both components of the composite outcome pointing in the same direction resulted in a significant cost decrease (Wichmann et al., 2020).

Factors influencing the implementation of PACE steps to success

The performance of PACE Steps to Success on the different Re-AIM components was highly variable within and across countries, with generally a better performance on the components Implementation and Maintenance than on the components Reach and Adoption. We also identified factors that may have influenced the implementation of PACE Steps to Success. These factors could be classified into three major categories, namely (1) the PACE Steps to Success programme and its way of delivery, (2) people working in the programme and (3) contextual factors. The first category includes factors such as the time between and duration of training sessions, high amount of paperwork, the vocabulary used in the PACE documents and the practical experience of the trainer and his/her way of teaching. The second category relates to the manager, PACE coordinators and nursing home staff involved in delivering the programme. In-depth analysis showed that organisational problems may have played a part here. Difficulty in planning the meetings and absent or unreachable PACE coordinators complicated implementation in some nursing homes. In addition, the experience and approach of the PACE trainers highly affected staff motivation. Elements such as nursing home management, communication, current methods and staff skills and readiness, influenced how the facilities adopted the programme. Factors related to the nursing homes that may have also affected implementation include staff turnover, changes within organisation or upcoming inspection visit. Finally, the third category entails important contextual factors affecting implementation, such as the fit of the programme with the nursing home staff needs, expectations and work setting; or whether or not the nursing home staff prioritise their involvement in the programme, which include the release of resources, in terms of budget or dedicated time for PACE coordinators. The international scope of the PACE cluster-RCT added another layer of complexity, as country-specific facilitators and barriers have also been identified. For instance, prevailing taboos on discussing death or limited knowledge on palliative care have been identified in some of the countries, which may have impacted the staff's ability to implement the programme (Oosterveld-Vlug et al., 2019).

Discussion

Towards better palliative care for nursing home residents with and without dementia

The primary analyses of the PACE cluster-RCT combined with the process evaluation showed a number of potential factors that can explain why PACE Steps to Success did not affect the primary outcome. These factors include (1) the content of the intervention itself, (2) a possible mismatch between the intervention and the primary outcome, (3) the quality of its implementation in several nursing homes, or a combination of these factors. First, it is possible that PACE Steps to Success included too many components to implement during a period of one year. Earlier research stated that interventions that focus on one component at a time are more likely to produce positive outcomes than those requiring broader practice changes (Low et al., 2015). Second, there might have been a mismatch between the primary outcome and the components of the programme. For instance, the only programme step that was aimed at improving care in the last days of life was implemented at the very end of the programme (Step 5), which was not implemented optimally in some of the nursing homes. Third, when a trial fails, one should also question the implementation and the setting and not only the (effectiveness of) the programme. How it was conducted, introduced, delivered and received and by whom are important questions to consider, especially in a care setting as complex as nursing homes. The process evaluation highlighted a number of factors that should be addressed in future developments of palliative care programmes in nursing homes (Oosterveld-Vlug et al., 2019; Van den Block et al., 2020).

While PACE Steps to Success clearly needs further improvement, its apparent positive effects on quality of care and dying at the end of life for nursing home residents both with and without dementia and its medical cost-saving potential showed that this generalist non-disease-specific palliative care programme can be a useful starting point for the further development of palliative care in nursing homes (Van den Block et al., 2020; Wichmann et al., 2020).

Such a generalist palliative care approach is a promising way forward to increase the timely access and improve the quality of palliative care for nursing home residents, including those living and dying with dementia. This would mean that for all nursing home residents, regardless of whether they are dying or in their final months of life, a palliative care approach that focuses on the quality of life, needs and preferences of residents and their families can be a suitable approach. Such an approach would be innately complementary to a high-quality dementia care approach that includes person-centred care, optimal symptom management, psychosocial and spiritual support, advance care planning, continuity of care, multidisciplinary collaborations, education and support of healthcare professionals, and support and bereavement counselling for family carers (van der Steen et al., 2014).

Health and social care professionals play a pivotal role in identifying and managing the palliative care needs of nursing home residents with dementia. If they are to carry out these roles effectively, they need continuous education and training to provide them with a wide range of up-to-date skills and knowledge related to palliative care in dementia (Artioli et al., 2019; Smets, Pivodic, et al., 2018; Teixeira et al., 2019). While this recommendation in itself is not unique, it is essential to repeat and further emphasise it in order to better integrate a comprehensive palliative care approach in the knowledge and skills of care professionals delivering care on a daily basis to residents with and without dementia.

Dementia-specific trainings for specialist palliative care services working in nursing homes can also contribute to improving the quality of and access to optimal palliative care of nursing home residents with dementia, especially in times when their care needs become too complex to be managed by other healthcare professionals. Such collaborative practice might result in reciprocal sharing of knowledge and skills, and in the long run, this might further improve the capabilities of generalist palliative care providers in delivering complex palliative care services in dementia. Of course, the operationalisation of such a generic model might differ between countries, depending on the care services available and accessible for this setting. Enhancing collaboration between palliative care, nursing home care and dementia care, and between nursing home, hospitals and/or home care settings seems crucial for the future (van der Steen et al., 2014).

Comprehensive management of residents with dementia also requires the building of partnership between health and social care professionals and family carers. Family carers of nursing home residents with dementia are critical to provide care to maintain or improve the quality of life of people living with dementia. Finally, to ultimately improve the quality of life of nursing home residents with dementia, it is imperative to instil a mind shift among patients and their families, healthcare professionals, policymakers and the general public from 'recognizing palliative care as an alternative to life-prolonging treatments' to 'promoting palliative care as a complementary approach that can be offered alongside *life-prolonging treatments*'. We also need to spread the word that palliative care is not only about dying but also about living well until death, as well as to highlight the benefits of palliative care for nursing home residents with dementia (van der Steen et al., 2014).

Conclusion

While PACE Steps to Success needs further improvement, its apparent positive effects on quality of care and dying for nursing home residents both with and without dementia and its medical cost-saving potential showed that such a generalist palliative care approach is a promising way forward to further improve palliative care for nursing home residents, including those living and dying with dementia. We also highlighted a number of factors that should be addressed in future developments of palliative care programmes in nursing homes. These factors are categorised into (1) the PACE Steps to Success programme and its way of delivery, (2) people working in the programme and (3) contextual factors.

Abbreviations

CAD-EOLD	Comfort Assessment in Dying-End of Life Care in Dementia
EQ-5D-5L	5-level EQ-5D version
GP	General Practitioner
QALYs	Quality-adjusted Life Years
QOD-LTC	Quality of Dying-Long Term Care
RE-AIM	Reach, Adoption, Implementation, and intention to Maintenance
RCT	Randomised controlled trial
WHO	World Health Organization

References

Artioli, G., Bedini, G., Bertocchi, E., Ghirotto, L., Cavuto, S., Costantini, M., & Tanzi, S. (2019). Palliative care training addressed to hospital healthcare professionals by palliative care specialists: A mixed-method evaluation. *BMC Palliative Care*, *18*(1), 1–10. https://doi.org/10.1186/s12904-019-0476-8

Bernard, M., Berchtold, A., Strasser, F., Gamondi, C., & Borasio, G.D. (2020). Meaning in life and quality of life: Palliative care patients versus the general population. *BMJ Supportive & Palliative Care*, bmjspcare-2020–002211. https://doi.org/10.1136/bmjspcare-2020-002211

Froggatt, K., Arrue, B., Edwards, M., Finne-Soveri, H., Morbey, H., Payne, S., . . . Van den Block, L. (2017). *Mapping palliative care systems and current practices in long term care facilities in Europe*. European Association of Palliative Care Taskforce. Retrieved from https://www.endoflifecare.be/sites/default/files/atoms/files/mapping_palliative_care_systems_in_european_ltcfs_eapc_report_2016.pdf

Froggatt, K., Payne, S., Morbey, H., Edwards, M., Finne-Soveri, H., Gambassi, G., . . . Van den Block, L. (2017a). Palliative care development in European care homes and nursing homes: Application of a typology of implementation. *Journal of the American Medical Directors Association*, *18*(6), 550.e7–550.e14. https://doi.org/10.1016/j.jamda.2017.02.016

Goodman, C., Evans, C., Wilcock, J., Froggatt, K., Drennan, V., Sampson, E., . . . Iliffe, S. (2010). End of life care for community dwelling older people with dementia: An integrated review. *International Journal of Geriatric Psychiatry*, *25*(4), 329–337. https://doi.org/10.1002/gps.2343

Hansen, A., Hauge, S., & Bergland, Å. (2017). Meeting psychosocial needs for persons with dementia in home care services – A qualitative study of different perceptions and practices among health care providers. *BMC Geriatrics*, *17*(1), 1–10. https://doi.org/10.1186/s12877-017-0612-3

Hendriks, S.A., Smalbrugge, M., Hertogh, C., & van der Steen, J. (2013). Dying with dementia: symptoms, treatment, and quality of life in the last week of life. *Journal of Pain and Symptom Management*. https://doi.org/10.1016/j.jpainsymman.2013.05.015

Honinx, E., Dop, N. Van, Smets, T., Deliens, L., Noortgate, N. Van Den, Froggatt, K., . . . Szczerbińska, K. (2019). Dying in long-term care facilities in Europe: the PACE epidemiological study of deceased residents in six countries. *BMC Public Health*, *19*, 1199.

Honinx, E., Smets, T., Piers, R., & Deliens, L. (2019). Agreement of nursing home staff with palliative care principles : A PACE cross-sectional study among nurses and care assistants in five European countries. https://doi.org/10.1016/j.jpainsymman.2019.06.015

Houttekier, D., Reyniers, T., Deliens, L., Van Den Noortgate, N., & Cohen, J. (2014). Dying in hospital with dementia and pneumonia: A nationwide study using death certificate data. *Gerontology*, *60*(1), 31–37. https://doi.org/10.1159/000354378

Low, L.F., Fletcher, J., Goodenough, B., Jeon, Y.H., Etherton-Beer, C., Macandrew, M., & Beattie, E.R.A. (2015). A systematic review of interventions to change staff care practices in order to improve resident outcomes in nursing homes. *PLoS ONE*, *10*(11), 1–60. https://doi.org/10.1371/journal.pone.0140711

Miranda, R., Penders, Y., Smets, T., Deliens, L., Miccinesi, G., Vega Alonso, T., . . . Van den Block, L. (2018). Quality of primary palliative care for older people with mild and severe dementia: an international mortality follow-back study using quality indicators. *Age and Ageing*, *47*(6), 824–833. https://doi.org/10.1093/ageing/afy087

Miranda, R., Smets, T., Van Den Noortgate, N., Deliens, L., & Van den Block, L. (2021). Higher prevalence of dementia but no change in total comfort while dying among nursing home residents with dementia between 2010 and 2015: Results from two retrospective epidemiological studies. *International Journal of Environmental Research and Public Health*, *18*(4), 1–14. https://doi.org/10.3390/ijerph18042160

Miranda, R., Smets, T., Van Den Noortgate, N., van der Steen, J.T., Deliens, L., Payne, S., . . . de Paula, E.M. (2021a). No difference in effects of 'PACE steps to success' palliative care program for nursing home residents with and without dementia: a pre-planned subgroup analysis of the seven-country PACE trial. *BMC Palliative Care*, *20*(1), 1–10. https://doi.org/10.1186/s12904-021-00734-1

Mitchell, S.L. (2015). Advanced dementia. *New England Journal of Medicine*, *372*(26), 2533–2540. https://doi.org/10.1056/NEJMcp1412652

Murphy, E., Froggatt, K., Connolly, S., O'Shea, E., Sampson, E.L., Casey, D., & Devane, D. (2016). Palliative care interventions in advanced dementia. *The Cochrane Database of Systematic Reviews*, *12*, CD011513. https://doi.org/10.1002/14651858.CD011513.pub2

Oosterveld-Vlug, M., Onwuteaka-Philipsen, B.D., Ten Koppel, M., Van Hout, H., Smets, T., Pivodic, L., & Tanghe, M. (2019). Evaluating the implementation of the PACE Steps to Success Programme in long-term care facilities in seven countries according to the REAIM framework. *Implementation Science, 14,* 107.

Payne, S., Froggatt, K., Hockley, J., Sowerby, E., Moore, D.C., Kylänen, M., . . . Van den Block, L. (2019). *PACE steps to success intervention FINAL for translation.* Retrieved from www.eapcnet.eu/Portals/0/PDFs/1. PACE Steps to Success Information Pack ÔÇô English 31012019.pdf

Pivodic, L., Smets, T., Van den Noortgate, N., Onwuteaka-Philipsen, B.D., Engels, Y., Szczerbińska, K., . . . Van Den Block, L. (2018). Quality of dying and quality of end-of-life care of nursing home residents in six countries: An epidemiological study. *Palliative Medicine, 32*(10), 1584–1595.

Ryan, K., & Johnston, B. (2019). Generalist and specialist palliative care. *Textbook of Palliative Care,* 503–516. https://doi.org/10.1007/978-3-319-77740-5_42

Sampson, E.L., Candy, B., Davis, S., Gola, A.B., Harrington, J., King, M., . . . Jones, L. (2018). Living and dying with advanced dementia: A prospective cohort study of symptoms, service use and care at the end of life. *Palliative Medicine, 32*(3), 668–681. https://doi.org/10.1177/0269216317726443

Smets, T., Onwuteaka-Philipsen, B.B.D., Miranda, R., Pivodic, L., Tanghe, M., Van Hout, H., . . . PACE trial group (2018). Integrating palliative care in long-term care facilities across Europe (PACE): Protocol of a cluster randomized controlled trial of the "PACE Steps to Success" intervention in seven countries. *BMC Palliative Care, 17*(1), 1–11. https://doi.org/10.1186/s12904-018-0297-1

Smets, T., Pivodic, L., Piers, R., Pasman, H.R.W., Engels, Y., Szczerbińska, K., . . . Van den Block, L. (2018). The palliative care knowledge of nursing home staff: The EU FP7 PACE cross-sectional survey in 322 nursing homes in six European countries. *Palliative Medicine, 32*(9), 1487–1497. https://doi.org/10.1177/0269216318785295

Teixeira, M.J.C., Alvarelhão, J., Neri de Souza, D., Teixeira, H.J.C., Abreu, W., Costa, N., & Machado, F.A.B. (2019). Healthcare professionals and volunteers education in palliative care to promote the best practice – an integrative review. *Scandinavian Journal of Caring Sciences, 33*(2), 311–328. https://doi.org/10.1111/scs.12651

Van den Block, L., Honinx, E., Pivodic, L., Miranda, R., Onwuteaka-Philipsen, B.D., van Hout, H., . . . Smets, T. (2020). Evaluation of a palliative care program for nursing homes in 7 countries the PACE cluster-randomized clinical trial. *JAMA Internal Medicine, 180*(2), 233–242.

Van den Block, L., Smets, T., van Dop, N., Adang, E., Andreasen, P., Collingridge, D. van der Steen, J.T. (2016). Comparing Palliative Care in Care Homes Across Europe (PACE): Protocol of a cross-sectional study of deceased residents in 6 EU Countries. *Journal of the American Medical Directors Association, 17,* 566.e1–566.e7. https://doi.org/10.1016/j.jamda.2016.03.008

van der Steen, J.T., Radbruch, L., Hertogh, C.M.P.M., de Boer, M.E., Hughes, J.C., Larkin, P., . . . Volicer, L. (2014). White paper defining optimal palliative care in older people with dementia: A Delphi study and recommendations from the European Association for Palliative Care. *Palliative Medicine, 28*(3), 197–209. https://doi.org/10.1177/0269216313493685

Walsh, S., Murphy, E., Devane, D., Sampson, E., Connolly, S., Carney, P., & O'Shea, E. (2021). Palliative care interventions in advanced dementia. *Cochrane Database of Systematic Reviews, 9,* CD011513. https://doi.org/10.1002/14651858.CD011513.pub2

Wichmann, A.B., Adang, E.M.M., Vissers, K.C.P., Szczerbińska, K., Kylänen, M., Payne, S., . . . Tanghe, M. (2020). Decreased costs and retained QoL due to the "PACE Steps to Success" intervention in LTCFs: Cost-effectiveness analysis of a randomized controlled trial. *BMC Medicine*, *18*(1), 1–9. https://doi.org/10.1186/s12916-020-01720-9

World Health Organization. (2002). *National cancer control programmes: Policies and managerial guidelines* (2nd ed., p. 84). Geneva, Switzerland: World Health Organization.

World Health Organization. (2021). *Health technology assessment*. Retrieved from https://www.who.int/teams/health-product-policy-and-standards/assistive-and-medical-technology/medical-devices/assessment#:~:text=Health%20technology%20assessment%20(HTA)%20refers,health%20intervention%20or%20health%20technology (last accessed 10.11.21).

Chapter 16

A complex healthcare technology to improve advance care planning (ACP) in nursing homes

Annelien van Dael-Wendrich, Lara Pivodic,
Lieve Van den Block, Joni Gilissen

Introduction

Large need but limited uptake of advance care planning (ACP) in dementia and nursing homes

Advance care planning (ACP) is defined as a continuous, early initiated process of communication between healthcare providers, patients and families about the goals and desired direction of future healthcare (Rietjens et al., 2017). It can empower people living with dementia as it aims to enable them to exercise their autonomy regarding options for future care, consistent with their values and preferences (Prince et al., 2016). Timely initiation of ACP is recognised as an important part of routine nursing home care, especially since many people living with dementia reside there and given it's a care setting where still a large proportion receives inappropriate (and often unwanted) aggressive treatment at the end of life (Honinx et al., 2019, 2021). Studies have shown that older adults are willing to be involved in this shared decision-making process, including those living with dementia (Mignani et al., 2017; Wendrich-van Dael et al., 2019). Research shows that the process of ACP is associated with decreased hospitalisations, increased concordance between care received and prior wishes, and increased completion of care directive documents (Wendrich-van Dael et al., 2020). Nevertheless, its uptake among people living with dementia, and its implementation in nursing homes, remains low and difficult. For example, it has been estimated that worldwide less than 40% of people living with dementia have the opportunity to participate in an ACP conversation and recorded their preferences (Sellars et al., 2019; Tjia et al., 2018). In addition, research has shown that in nursing homes across Europe, reaching a significant proportion of residents to engage in the ACP process is still difficult (Andreasen et al., 2019).

Barriers that are often reported to hinder implementation of ACP in nursing homes exist at several levels (the resident and their families, the professional, the nursing home and the broader community/healthcare system).

DOI: 10.4324/9781003289005-20

Most barriers are related to the level of the healthcare professional (Frechman et al., 2020; Gilissen et al., 2017), and include, among others: not feeling confident to start a conversation about ACP and end-of-life-related issues (Evenblij et al., 2019), being unsure about their role in ACP or who is responsible (Beck et al., 2017; Lo et al., 2017; McGlade et al., 2017; Tilburgs et al., 2018), lack of knowledge (Kermel-Schiffman & Werner, 2017), fear of not being able to comply with future wishes (Flo et al., 2016; McGlade et al., 2017), or feeling that it would emotionally burden residents with dementia (Albers et al., 2014). Hence, future initiatives to improve practice could therefore focus on investing in the capacities and confidence of the professionals involved to engage in ACP.

The complexity of ACP (implementation) warrants detailed description of interventions

To improve current practice, a diverse spectrum of ACP intervention models have been developed and tested in various care settings (McMahan et al., 2021). ACP is an umbrella term including a wide variety of definitions and operationalisations. The concept has evolved considerably over time from a focus on documentation intended to honour the wishes of incompetent patients at the very end of life, to a much broader concept of communication and consultation of various aspects related to the future treatment and care planning (Van den Block, 2019).

As the definition of ACP changed over time (e.g. from focusing on treatment decisions to focusing more on ACP as a *process* that tries to elicit *values, life goals* and *preferences* for future care), it became more complex to implement in clinical practice and to evaluate (Gilissen et al., 2020; Rietjens et al., 2017). As a result, interventions that are aimed at improving ACP uptake and other desired outcomes that come from ACP have progressed from single-component interventions, such as a new advance directive document, to complex interventions consisting of multiple components that may lead to various changes in skills, behaviours, organisation, healthcare use etc (McMahan et al., 2021).

There is a lack of information about current ACP interventions. The limited level of detail on provided interventions is a generally acknowledged phenomenon in ACP research and non-pharmacological intervention research in general (Gilissen et al., 2021; Hoffmann et al., 2013). Intervention components are usually vaguely described or defined, and although intervention manuals are usually produced, they are often only available in a certain language or are not properly referenced, leaving the readers with little understanding of what the intervention entailed. More transparency about the content of interventions is the first important step towards more insight into ACP implementation and what is needed for it to be successful (McMahan et al., 2021).

The complexity of nursing home setting warrants for an in-depth investigation of how outcomes can be achieved in real-world practice

In addition to the limited detail in descriptions of ACP interventions, the limited understanding of what led to certain outcomes is named as an important cause of the lack of translation of research evidence regarding ACP into practice. When ACP trials (failed to) show effectiveness, researchers found it challenging to understand the reasons why (Overbeek et al., 2018).

There is an inevitable interplay between fundamental standardised science and the complexity of an intervention such as ACP, as outlined earlier, as well as the complexity presented by the nursing home setting (i.e. high rates of staff turnover, clinicians having limited bandwidth, an increasingly complex patient population, lack of cognitive capacity in residents, access to medical files, documentation (Kane et al., 2017; Lam et al., 2018; Shepherd et al., 2015)). This urges current researchers to not only focus on what is impacted but also provide more insights into 'how' and 'why' an intervention is effective in its context (Gilissen et al., 2021a; Skivington et al., 2021).

For research conducted in the 'real-life' setting of a nursing home, it cannot be assumed that the delivery of a complex intervention or its evaluation will be exactly as planned or intended in the design stage of a trial. Literature on process evaluation points to the importance of a systematic approach to documenting and accounting for this deviation, reporting on the actual implementation, delivery and setting of an intervention to interpret its effects (May et al., 2016; Skivington et al., 2021).

Aim

The ACP+ project aimed to improve the implementation of ACP in nursing homes in Flanders, Belgium. In this chapter, we describe the different components and tools of the ACP+ intervention and summarise results of the outcome and process evaluation.

Methods

Study design

The ACP+ project is constructed according to the conceptual framework outlined by the 2012 UK Medical Research Council (MRC) Framework to guide the development and evaluation of complex health interventions, following the first three phases of the 2008 update by Craig et al., the extension on process evaluations and on the Theory of Change (ToC) approach (Craig et al., 2008; De Silva et al., 2014; Moore & Evans, 2017).

The trial is registered at clinicaltrials.gov (NCT03521206) (Gilissen et al., 2020b). The methods and research procedures in the development, modelling and feasibility stage were approved by the Medical Ethics Committee, University Hospital Brussels (Vrije Universiteit Brussels (VUB), 2017/31 B.U.N. 143201732133). The trial was approved by the Medical Ethics Committee of University Hospital Brussels (VUB, 22/02/2018, ref: 18–003 – B.U.N. 143201834759). The protocol of the study and results have been published elsewhere (Pivodic et al., 2022).

PHASE 1: Development of the ACP+ intervention

In a first phase, we developed and tested the ACP+ intervention for its acceptability and feasibility, applying multiple study methods (Gilissen et al., 2019).

Step 1. Identification of essential preconditions for optimal implementation

In our systematic review (Gilissen et al., 2017), we identified preconditions related to successful ACP in the nursing home setting. By specifying those, we were able to make well-founded choices for the future design and planning of our ACP intervention programme.

Step 2. Programme theory and prototype intervention

It has been stressed within the MRC framework as well as other recent guidelines that researchers should start making explicit the underlying theory behind the intervention early on. This would enable them to start with a particular focus on the most important uncertainties that need to be addressed and will advance understanding of the implementation and functioning of the intervention later. Within this study, we embedded the Theory of Change (ToC) approach (De Silva et al., 2014) into the MRC phases to improve the design and evaluation of our intervention, and as such increase the likelihood that the intervention would be effective, sustainable and scalable. A ToC is 'a (programme) theory of how and why an initiative works which can be empirically tested by measuring indicators for every expected step on the hypothesised causal pathway to impact' (De Silva et al., 2014). We developed this theoretical model, together with stakeholders through workshops, while integrating the evidence of a systematic review (Gilissen et al., 2017) and a contextual analysis of the nursing home setting in Flanders, Belgium. The ToC displays all intermediate steps necessary to achieve desired long-term outcomes for nursing home residents and their families while highlighting organisational factors that potentially facilitate the implementation of ACP (i.e. support from management). The key intervention components, identified as part of a previously developed theoretical model on how ACP is expected to lead to its desired outcomes in nursing homes, were converted into a prototype intervention including specific activities and accompanying materials.

Step 3. Refining intervention to enhance acceptability and feasibility

A prototype ACP+ intervention was then evaluated for feasibility and acceptability in five nursing homes by the nursing home management and staff and expert discussions with a multidisciplinary expert group and a palliative care nurse-trainer. This resulted in the final ACP+ intervention (Gilissen et al., 2019).

PHASE 2: Evaluation of the ACP+ intervention

We performed a cluster-randomised controlled trial with embedded process evaluation (Gilissen et al., 2020b). An overview of the study design can be found in Figure 16.1.

Outcome evaluation: cluster randomised controlled trial

A multi-facility cluster randomised controlled trial was conducted in Flanders, Belgium, to compare the effects of the ACP+ intervention (intervention group) with usual care (control group) between February 2018 and January 2019 (prior to the COVID-19 pandemic) (Pivodic et al., 2022). Healthcare staff (including nurses, care assistants and other allied care staff such as social workers or physiotherapists) of the 14 included nursing homes (seven in the intervention arm, seven in the control arm) filled out questionnaires on ACP knowledge and self-efficacy (primary outcomes) and ACP practices (secondary outcome). All outcomes were assessed at baseline (month zero) and after the intervention (month eight).

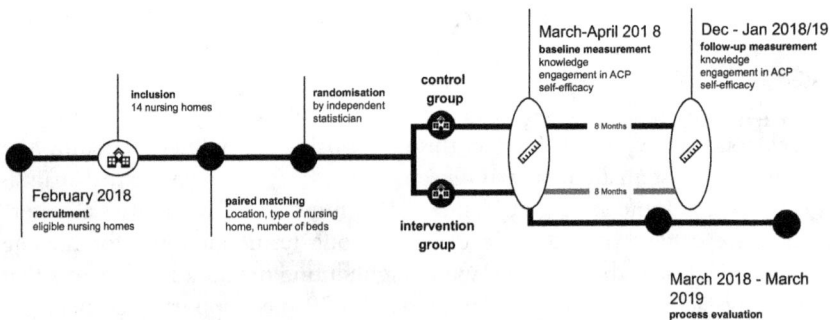

Figure 16.1 Overview of the ACP+ study design

Box 16.1   Outcomes and measures in outcome evaluation

Outcomes

1   Primary outcome 1: Improved care staff's knowledge of ACP
2   Primary outcome 2: Improved care staff's self-efficacy (confidence in own skills) concerning ACP
3   Secondary outcome: Improved care staff's self-reported engagement in ACP communication and documentation practices (this measure should be interpreted as the number of clinicians that do ACP conversations, rather than the number of ACP conversations at patient level)

Measurement instruments

Because no validated measures were available to assess staff's ACP knowledge, self-efficacy and engagement in communication/documentation, we developed new measures. Measures were tested for internal consistency and face validity through cognitive testing with several care professionals (Gilissen et al., 2020).

1   Knowledge: eleven statements (e.g. concerning applicability of advance directives) with response options 'true', 'false' and 'I don't know'. The responses were scored as 0 ('incorrect'; 'I don't know') and 1 ('correct').
2   Self-efficacy: twelve items, rated on a ten-point Likert-type scale ranging from 'not at all confident' (scored as 0) to 'very confident' (scored as 10) or 'not applicable' (coded as missing).
3   Engagement in ACP: list of six practices asking staff whether they performed this practice yes or no, over the past six months (e.g. initiating an ACP conversation). Responses were scored as 0 ('not performed') or 1 ('performed').

Rationale for using knowledge and self-efficacy in different types of care staff as primary outcomes

In our systematic review, we identified that prominent factors inhibiting care staff to engage in ACP are low knowledge and self-efficacy (Gilissen et al., 2017). In a preliminary cross-sectional study among nurses in nursing homes, we additionally found that self-efficacy is positively associated with the number of ACP practices that nurses carry out (Gilissen et al., 2020). Considering current literature about successful ACP in nursing homes, sufficient self-efficacy is an important precondition for staff to be able to carry out ACP in practice (Gilissen et al., 2018; Sudore et al., 2018). This finding also complies with the social cognitive theory that assumes an individual's knowledge translates through self-efficacy into action (Bandura, 1993). Therefore, there is an argument for raising knowledge and self-efficacy because it can be essential to increase staff's uptake of ACP. However, since we cannot conclude a causal relationship from this cross-sectional study, the results may also suggest that carrying out a variety of ACP practices leads to greater confidence, and thus it may have been the act of carrying out ACP practices that increased confidence in performing ACP (e.g. self-efficacy is in that case influenced by prior experiences of the action that is required, as is also stipulated in cognitive theory).

We focused on different care staff working in the nursing home instead of only nurses, who are previously been put forward to take the lead in ACP. Increasingly, a team-based approach has been advocated for (Dixon & Knapp, 2018), especially in nursing homes where important time constraints and inadequate staffing levels of nurses are reported. In addition, care in nursing homes is most often conducted by a multidisciplinary healthcare team. Although there are significant differences between care assistants, nurses and other allied staff in their knowledge regarding ACP, a preliminary study reported no significant differences in self-efficacy, albeit that the overall level of self-efficacy was low (Gilissen et al., 2021). To explore and honour resident preferences, competency in providing ACP and feeling confident to do so might therefore be considered key requirements for all frontline nursing home staff, regardless of their profession.

Process evaluation: mixed-methods study

Concurrently with the cluster RCT, a process evaluation was conducted in the intervention nursing homes. Quantitative and qualitative data were collected throughout and after the intervention implementation period. Participants were nursing home staff, managers and external ACP trainers hired by the research team to implement ACP. Methods included were weekly structured diaries filled out by the ACP trainers, attendance lists of all training activities, observation forms of the training sessions, post-training surveys, facility-level data (e.g. number of staff employed) and individual and group interviews with trained care staff, at least one member of the management and the trainers.

Box 16.2   Outcomes in process evaluation

1   *Implementation:* the process through which interventions are delivered, and what is delivered in practice. Outcomes involve how delivery is achieved and what is delivered (dose, reach, fidelity, adaptations).

2 *Mechanisms of impact:* the intermediate mechanisms through which intervention activities produce intended (or unintended) effects.

3 *Context:* factors external to the intervention that may influence its implementation or whether mechanisms of impact act as intended, including outcomes such as contextual moderators (barriers and facilitators) and participant's intention or commitment to continuing and maintaining the implemented intervention programme.

Analysis

In trial analysis, ACP knowledge was treated as a rate of correct statements relative to the total number of statements responded to (Pivodic et al., 2022). For ACP self-efficacy, the mean score of all items was used. ACP engagement was considered as a dichotomous variable (at least one activity performed versus none). Outcomes were set as missing if a respondent had not answered more than 25% of statements or items. We conducted intention-to-treat analyses using linear mixed models. Process evaluation of mixed-methods data is currently being analysed, applying descriptive statistics and thematic inductive and deductive qualitative analysis.

Results

We first describe the ACP+ intervention. Next, the results of the outcome and process evaluation are summarised.

The ACP+ program theory and intervention

The final ACP+ program includes ten intervention components and several materials to support delivery into routine nursing home care. The key components are ongoing training and coaching; management engagement; different roles and responsibilities for organising ACP; conversation; documentation and information transfer; integration of ACP into multidisciplinary meetings; auditing and tailoring it to the specific setting. Components are implemented step-wise, over a period of eight months (Figure 16.2, reprint from Gilissen et al., 2020b), with the help of two external ACP trainers: a GP specialised in nursing home care and a nursing home nurse specialised in palliative care and dementia (assigned to four and three nursing homes in the intervention group, respectively).

We list as follows the key features of the ACP+ intervention.

A tiered-roles system

At the core of the intervention is a tiered-roles system (Table 16.1). These roles include, apart from the ACP trainers, a wide range of staff and identify distinct responsibilities in ACP. Each staff member is assigned to a role within

INTERVENTION ACTIVITY	Selection and preparation ACP Trainers	Meeting(s) with ACP Trainer with management, BoD, head nurses and CAP	Training of ACP Ref Persons (session 2)	Information for residents and family / Information for FPs	In-house training of ACP Conversation Facilitators (session 2)		Specialization session 1: Dementia	Specialization session 2: Communication with other healthcare professionals	ACP audit meeting
		Training of ACP Ref Persons (session 1)		In-house training of ACP Conversation Facilitators (session 1)	In-house training of ACP Antennas		Comeback seminar for ACP Ref Persons / Follow-up meeting(s) with management		
		Tailoring-meetings with ACP Ref Person, management, and decision-makers†					Multidisciplinary meeting		
		ACP Trainer 'shadows' ACP Ref Persons					One-to-one coaching		
							Planned ACP conversations		
TIMING	3 months before the start of the program	Month 1	Month 2	Month 3	Month 4	Month 5	Month 6	Month 7	Month 8
PHASE	Before the start of the program	Preparation and training phase				Follow-up phase			
PERSON WITH MAIN RESPONSIBILITY	Research team	ACP Trainer takes the lead. As soon as ACP Reference Persons are trained, they are involved in the organization of each activity				ACP Ref Persons take the lead and are supported by the ACP Trainer			

ACP advance care planning; CAP coordinating advisory physician within the nursing home; BoD board of directors

Figure 16.2 Overview of the ACP+ intervention components and timeframe

ACP, advance care planning; CAP, coordinating advisory physician within the nursing home; BoD board of directors

their competencies and roles and considering their willingness to act according to this role: ACP Reference Persons, ACP Conversation Facilitators and ACP Antennas.

Tailoring

At the start and during implementation, tailoring of several components to the existing nursing home context was permitted. Tailoring means that the timing and order of implementing components of the complex health technologies may not be applicable in all situations, so interventions should be flexible for nursing staff to decide when to implement certain intervention components. Tailoring in our study aimed to increase staff engagement, make the intervention easier to implement and ensure the sustainability of ACP. During the recruitment of nursing homes, we started with assessing existing ACP policies and procedures. We considered existing routines, practices and guidelines that were already in place, at baseline or at inclusion. An ACP+ tailoring checklist was developed by the researchers in the development phase of the project (Gilissen et al., 2019) in which it was listed what could be changed and what had to be minimally standardised (e.g. a monthly team meeting that is part of the intervention could become a bi-weekly meeting because it could be integrated in a meeting framework that already existed). Management and ACP Reference Persons met regularly to discuss the ACP intervention steps outlined in the protocol that had to be implemented in the upcoming weeks/month and what was to be adapted to local procedures, using this list as guidance. Examples of tailoring included: the multidisciplinary meeting component was integrated in existing in-house professional meetings, information sessions about ACP were integrated within in-house existing resident or family meetings, ACP+ documents were integrated into existing (electronic) documentation systems.

Table 16.1 Tiered roles and responsibilities within the ACP+ intervention

ACP+ Trainers	Trainers have clinical practice experience in nursing homes and in performing ACP conversations. They support staff and management in implementing ACP. Their support is intensive at the beginning but decreases throughout. They are external and not employed by the facilities. In the future, regional palliative care networks and trainers working within these networks might take up this role.
ACP+ Reference Persons Training: four full days at the start of implementation and one come-back seminar at four months	Reference Persons are responsible for implementing ongoing ACP within the nursing home, by marketing its high priority and organising and conducting ACP conversations. These are professionals employed by the nursing home who have roles in daily resident care (e.g. head nurses, team coordinators, nurses, palliative care reference persons, reference persons for dementia, psychologists, members of the palliative care team), who are experienced and have a genuine interest in ACP. These people are required to be enthusiastic and motivated to stimulate their colleagues and have sufficient organisational skills. After a while, following train-the-trainer principles, these Reference Persons should be able to train their colleagues in subsequent roles. The number of ACP Reference Persons per nursing home was estimated in this project to be at least two 0.10 FTE's per 30 beds, which was the study's average number of beds at one ward.
ACP+ Conversation Facilitators Training: two days (two hours)	The Conversation Facilitators support the Reference Persons in planning and performing regular ACP conversations with designated residents and family. In the ACP+ study, these were often linked to one ward and a specific team lead, cf. ACP Reference Person. There were on average three or four people per ward.
ACP+ Antennas Training: one day (two hours)	The Antennas are all other staff, including support staff (administrative, technical, cleaning staff) and volunteers, who were offered a short training session to enable them to recognise and signal triggers that might indicate a persons' readiness, need or willingness to engage in ACP.

ACP advance care planning; FTE full-time equivalent

Tools to support ACP conversations and documentation of care wishes and preferences

The nursing home-specific ACP+ tools that were developed as part of the intervention aimed to avoid a purely document-driven or 'tick-box' approach to the ACP process and to involve residents, including those living with dementia according to their capacity, their families and healthcare professionals. These tools aim to aid care staff in discussing and documenting wishes and preferences for future treatment and care and include (1) an extensive ACP conversation guide, (2) a one-page conversation tool and (3) an ACP document to record outcomes of conversations. The tools are built around the same sections that are deemed important as part of one or more ACP conversations (Box 16.3). The content of these tools is described in full elsewhere (Wendrich-van Dael et al., 2021).

Box 16.3   Preparation, engagement and follow-up of ACP discussion(s)

Preparation

1   Inform the resident and family about ACP.
2   Assess decision-making capacity.
3   Identify a loved one/family.
4   Contact the GP.
5   Collect background information.

Engaging in discussion(s)

How often/when?

Planned (after nursing home admission (>6 weeks), yearly, when change (in health or living situation) occurs, when resident/family asks) or at informal occasions

With whom?

The nursing home resident (as much as possible), the nursing home staff who is most involved in the care of the resident, the GP, family most involved in the care of the resident (cf. assigned loved one or legal representative)

What?

Section A: Ideas about a good life/broadly asking about values (e.g. 'What is important to you?')
    Section B: Preferences for current care and treatment (e.g. 'How do you consider your current quality of life'?
    Section C: Preferences for future care and care goals/Ideas and worries about the future and the end of life (e.g. 'When considering the future, what do you hope for/are you worried about'?)

Section D: Appointing a legal representative 'In case you would become so ill, you could no longer decide you care for yourself, is there someone you trust enough to make these decisions for you'?

Section E: Documenting end-of-life wishes – which may include Advance Directives (e.g. 'There are several ways to document your wishes. Some people think it is useful to compose an Advance Directive. You don't have to do this if you don't want to, and you should certainly not rush into this. Shall we discuss all the options together'?)

Section F: Place of care/death (e.g. 'Where would you like to be cared for at the end of life'?

Section G: Other preferences (e.g. 'Are there other preferences you would like to take us into account'?

Section H: Preferences regarding dying (e.g. 'Are there specific (religious) wishes that we should consider'? 'Would you like to make funeral arrangements'?)

Section I: Revising preferences and wishes (e.g. 'Which circumstances would be a reason for you to revise your wishes and preferences about the care'?

Summarise the conversation (e.g. 'So today you told me about . . . Is that correct?' 'Do I correctly understand that today we decide on the following . . . '?)

Documenting wishes and preferences

1   Document the conversation (cf. ACP+ Document).
2   Translate wishes and preferences into care goals that are summarised in ACP Summary, which may include also care codes (e.g. ABC, DNR).
3   Document Advance directives if wanted.
4   Double-check consistency all documents, provide a date and signature if applicable.

Plan a follow-up conversation

For example, 'A while ago we spoke about . . . Is this still applicable'?

For example, 'A year ago, we spoke about . . . I was just wondering how you feel about this now. Would it be alright for you to discuss this'?

> **Communication to other involved healthcare professionals**
>
> 1   Note/copy in the (digital) nursing home file of the resident.
> 2   Mention during the (monthly) multidisciplinary meetings to inform all healthcare staff.
> 3   Inform the general practitioner.

Effects on staff-level outcomes

Fourteen nursing homes were included and randomised to intervention or control after baseline data collection. All clusters received the intended intervention, none were lost to follow up, and all were included in the analyses of data from the outcome evaluation (Pivodic et al., 2022). Both study arms taken together, we received questionnaires from 694 of 1,017 care staff (68% response rate) at baseline and 491 of 989 care staff (50% response rate) post-intervention. Care staff and management from the seven intervention nursing homes, and the external ACP+ Trainers participated in the process evaluation. Final analysis of the process evaluation is currently underway.

The results of the outcome evaluation showed that ACP+ was able to improve staff's self-efficacy in performing ACP but not their ACP knowledge. Care staff's mean knowledge about ACP after the intervention did not differ significantly between groups (ratio 1.04; 95% CI, 0.95 to 1.15; $p = 0.339$). Their mean self-efficacy in ACP was significantly higher in the intervention group than in the control group (baseline-adjusted mean difference, 0.57; 95% CI, 0.20 to 0.94; $p = 0.003$; effect size (Cohen's d) = 0.3) (Figure 16.3). We found no difference between the intervention and control groups for staff's engagement in ACP (ratio 1.47; 95% CI 0.88 to 2.46; $p = 0.145$).

Preliminary process evaluation results

Preliminary results point to low reach of staff in the ACP+ training sessions *(implementation)*. Although they seemed highly motivated to attend the training *(mechanism of impact)*, they were hampered by contextual difficulties such as lack of time and human resources *(context)*. We noticed that ACP conversations were mainly initiated by ACP Reference Persons and only to the limited extent by other roles identified *(implementation)*. Staff pointed to the fact that a four-day training was too limited in time, and they did not have the opportunity for 'real-life' experiences, or on-the-job learning *(mechanism of impact)*. As is highlighted earlier, the ACP+ Trainer's support was supposed to gradually decrease once the nursing home became more independent in organising ACP. However, trainers highlighted their support was highly needed *(mechanism of*

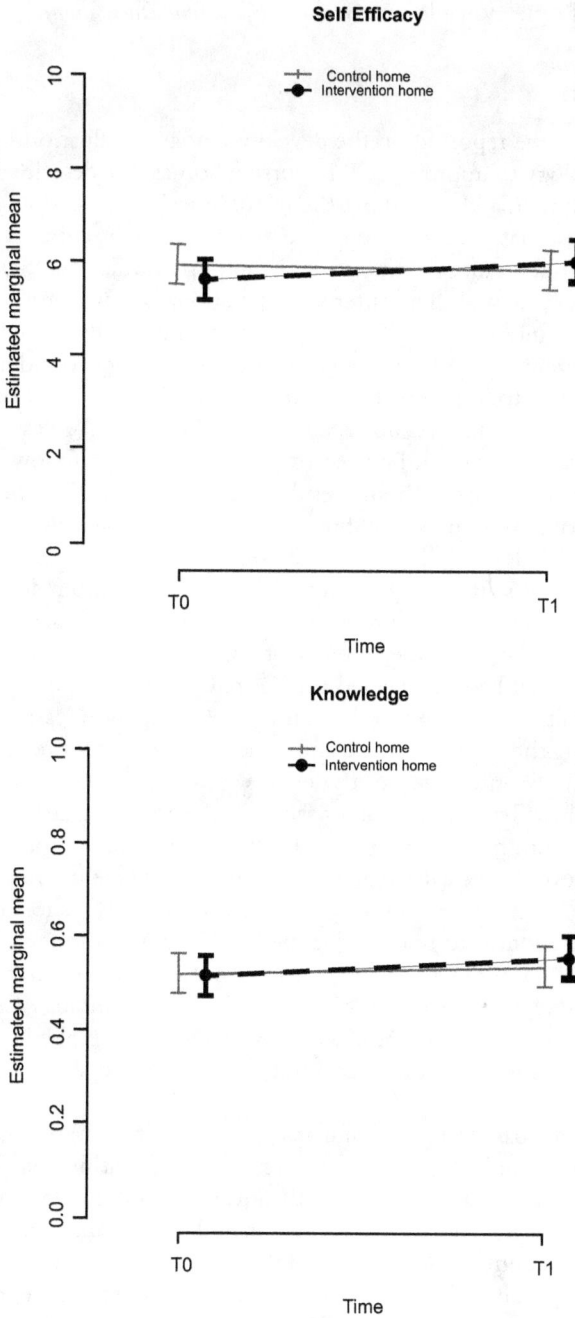

Figure 16.3 Estimated marginal means for ACP self-efficacy and ACP knowledge at T0 and T1 in intervention and control groups

impact) as most nursing homes struggled with implementing the steps outlined in the limited time available within the project *(implementation)*.

Discussion

In this chapter, we reported on the development and evaluation of a complex health technology to improve ACP in nursing homes. We described the underlying program theory that outlines the hypothetical causal pathway of ACP in nursing homes, that is what changes are expected, using which processes, and under what circumstances – stipulating the important role of sufficiently skilled and knowledgeable staff. The latter was operationalised within the multicomponent ACP+ intervention. This intervention specifically aimed to support and train different types of care staff so that they felt more confident to engage in ACP, as well as to implement a systematic procedure to do so. Emphasis was on external trainer support, management buy-in, a tiered-roles system and a proposed structure that can be used to plan, execute and follow up on ACP conversations with nursing home residents and/or family. Preliminary results of the evaluative study however showed limited effect on self-efficacy and no effect on knowledge. We found no difference between the intervention and control groups for staff's engagement in ACP communication/documentation. This measure should be interpreted as the number of clinicians who do ACP conversations, rather than the number of ACP conversations at patient level. Although this trial has not yielded the desired positive outcomes, it still adds important additional context to the considerable body of research in ACP.

Considering the comprehensive and multi-component training component within the ACP+ intervention, the effects were smaller than expected. This can be explained by a multitude of factors. Methodological factors include: First, the medium baseline scores for both primary and secondary outcomes might be part of the explanation, as improving a low baseline might be easier. Second, the chosen follow-up period might have been too short because staff only had four months to practice planned ACP conversations and documentation. Third, a poor match between the contents of the intervention and the survey items may also have played a role. For example, ACP+ training sessions focused on communication and organisational embedment of ACP, while constructs measured mainly evaluated knowledge about legal requirements of ADs.

Furthermore, based on preliminary process evaluation results, additional reasons might be linked to the limited reach of staff within the ACP+ trainings, most probably due to high staff turnover and competing work and time demands. At T1 we therefore may have included new and untrained staff in follow-up measurement. In addition, although much applied in ACP educational models (Chan et al., 2019; Dixon et al., 2018), the train the trainer model might have been too ambitious in the short timeframe of eight months, considering that we expected healthcare staff to both engage in ACP conversations and become trainers in a short time frame. A longer implementation period with sufficient and continuous training might have improved outcomes.

Within the ACP+ project, we have put strong emphasis on ACP implementation and facilitation by in-house staff themselves (with the support from trainers) rather than by external facilitators, as was often done in other similar ACP interventions (Korfage et al., 2015; Rietjens et al., 2017). This requires a prolonged and substantial input of human and other (i.e. training/education, physical space and time) resources within the nursing home to both ensure implementation of the intervention and sustain ongoing operations. It also requires continued professional motivation. Policy support and buy-in from the nursing home management to ensure staff has the time and space to engage in ACP are therefore essential prerequisites. Implementing a new service model is always interchanged with changing existing practices or adding new ones. Basic principles from change management are therefore at play here. Develop urgency with key stakeholders, build a guiding team and create a common vision and explicit buy-in (cf. agreement/support to do something).

Although the challenge of staff turnover is a well-known given for the nursing home setting, which was accounted for in our ACP+ intervention by introducing a tiered roles system, additional support measures are warranted for future interventions and implementation attempts. Trained facilitators may not continuously be employed and a training session at the start of the intervention implementation period, of which the effect is evaluated four to eight months later among all staff employed at that point in time, might significantly affect trial outcomes.

The above-described complexity makes it difficult to evaluate ACP in nursing homes using traditional experimental designs (Skivington et al., 2021). Embedded process evaluations are a good way forward, but researchers are additionally encouraged to explore other research designs and methods that might be more suitable to capture real-world endeavours (e.g. pragmatic trials (Palmer et al., 2018) and embedding ethnographic case studies (Steele Gray et al., 2021; Côté-Boileau et al., 2020)).

Strengths and limitations

The main strength of this study is that it is the first to present a theory-based choice of outcomes and components of an ACP intervention in nursing homes, based on an extensive program theory and in-depth development process. It thereby answers a frequent call made by important research bodies to include the rationale, theory or goals that underpin the intervention and study design (Gilissen et al., 2021; Moore & Evans, 2017; Skivington et al., 2021; Higginson et al., 2013). The preliminary in-depth process evaluation provided insight into implementation process (the 'how' and 'what', to 'whom'), mechanisms of impact (intermediate processes which explain subsequent changes in outcomes) and contextual factors (factors external to the intervention that might have impacted the outcomes). Its absence would have complicated our interpretation of the trial results, whereas we now have several sources of information available. Full analyses of the process evaluation data may point to important factors that should be considered when trying to improve staff-level outcomes such as knowledge and self-efficacy. Hence, results of this study will inform both researchers and implementers.

The evaluative study had several limitations. First, the study duration of eight months may have been too short when considering we were expecting to complete whole-setting changes on staff level. We were confronted with a trade-off between attrition (i.e. staff turnover) and length of time of the intervention to show effect. Secondly, outcomes of the trial were limited to staff level outcomes, which are very well rationalised but might have only limited value for the residents and family themselves. In recent debate about the value of ACP, it was also raised that other outcomes might be more appropriate (e.g. feelings of involvement among the patient/family, empowerment) (Tishelman et al., 2021). In retrospect, the study might have profited if we had considered several constructs on the resident level as secondary outcomes. However, at the time, we particularly aimed to minimise the measurement burden for the nursing homes and staff and hence focused on the predominant outcomes identified in our theory of change. Finally, as appropriately validated measures to evaluate staff outcomes were lacking, we used measures which we developed ourselves and which were only tested for face validity.

Conclusion

We need to make explicit how interventions are expected to work and explore what happened while implementing them. This will contribute to greater accuracy and quality of our research activities, enhance comparing existing ACP interventions more adequately, promote more meaningful interpretations of the effects and better inform future reliable implementation in real world practice.

List of acronyms

ACP+   Name of intervention program to improve advance care planning
ACP   Advance care planning
AD   Advance directive
GP   General practitioner (Family physician)
MRC   Medical Research Council
ToC   Theory of Change
FTE   Fulltime equivalent
CI   Confidence interval

References

Albers, G., Van den Block, L., & Vander Stichele, R. (2014). The burden of caring for people with dementia at the end of life in nursing homes: A postdeath study among nursing staff. *International Journal of Older People Nursing, 9*(2), 106–117. https://doi.org/10.1111/opn.12050

Andreasen, P., Finne-Soveri, U.H., Deliens, L., Van den Block, L., Payne, S., Gambassi, G., . . . Szczerbińska, K. (2019). Advance directives in European long-term care facilities: A cross-sectional survey. *BMJ Supportive & Palliative Care,* bmjspcare-2018-001743. https://doi.org/10.1136/bmjspcare-2018-001743

Bandura, A.C. (1993). Perceived Self-Efficacy in Cognitive Development and Functioning. *Educational Psychologist, 28*(2), 117–148.

Beck, E.R., McIlfatrick, S., Hasson, F., & Leavey, G. (2017). Health care professionals' perspectives of advance care planning for people with dementia living in long-term care settings: A narrative review of the literature. *Dementia, 16*(4), 486–512. https://doi.org/10.1177/1471301215604997

Chan, C.W.H., Ng, N.H.Y., Chan, H.Y.L., Wong, M.M.H., & Chow, K.M. (2019). A systematic review of the effects of advance care planning facilitators training programs. *BMC Health Services Research, 19*(1), 362. https://doi.org/10.1186/s12913-019-4192-0

Côté-Boileau, É., Gaboury, I., Breton, M., & Denis, J.L. (2020). Organizational ethnographic case studies: Toward a new generative in-depth qualitative methodology for health care research? *International Journal of Qualitative Methods, 19,* 1–17.

Craig, P., Deippe, P., Macintyre, S., Michie, S., & Nazareth, I. (2008). *Medical research framework's guidance on developing and evaluating complex interventions: New guidance.* Medical Research Council (MRC). Retrieved from http://internationalmidwives.org/assets/uploads/documents/News%20Archive%202011/News%20Archive%202010/Research%20Methods%20and%20Reporting.pdf

De Silva, M.J., Breuer, E., Lee, L., Asher, L., Chowdhary, N., Lund, C., & Patel, V. (2014). Theory of change: A theory-driven approach to enhance the Medical Research Council's framework for complex interventions. *Trials, 15*(1), 267.

Dixon, J., Karagiannidou, M., & Knapp, M. (2018). The effectiveness of advance care planning in improving end-of-life outcomes for people with dementia and their carers: A systematic review and critical discussion. *Journal of Pain and Symptom Management, 55*(1), 132–150.e1.

Dixon, J., & Knapp, M. (2018). Whose job? The staffing of advance care planning support in twelve international healthcare organizations: A qualitative interview study. *BMC Palliative Care, 17*(1), 78. https://doi.org/10.1186/s12904-018-0333-1

Evenblij, K., Ten Koppel, M., Smets, T., Widdershoven, G.A.M., Onwuteaka-Philipsen, B.D., & Pasman, H.R.W. (2019). Are care staff equipped for end-of-life communication? A cross-sectional study in long-term care facilities to identify determinants of self-efficacy. *BMC Palliative Care, 18*(1), 1–11. https://doi.org/10.1186/s12904-018-0388-z

Flo, E., Husebo, B.S., Bruusgaard, P., Gjerberg, E., Thoresen, L., Lillemoen, L., & Pedersen, R. (2016). A review of the implementation and research strategies of advance care planning in nursing homes. *BMC Geriatrics, 16*(1). https://doi.org/10.1186/s12877-016-0179-4

Frechman, E., Dietrich, M.S., Walden, R.L., & Maxwell, C.A. (2020). Exploring the uptake of advance care planning in older adults: An integrative review. *Journal of Pain and Symptom Management, 60*(6), 1208–1222.e59. https://doi.org/10.1016/j.jpainsymman.2020.06.043

Gilissen, J., Pivodic, L., Wendrich-van Dael, A., van, Gastmans, C., Stichele, R.V., Humbeeck, L.V., Deliens, L., & Block, L.V. den. (2019). Implementing advance care planning in routine nursing home care: The development of the theory-based ACP+ program. *PLOS ONE*, *14*(10), e0223586. https://doi.org/10.1371/journal.pone.0223586

Gilissen, J., Pivodic, L., Gastmans, C., Vander Stichele, R., Deliens, L., Breuer, E., & Van den Block, L. (2018). How to achieve the desired outcomes of advance care planning in nursing homes: A theory of change. *BMC Geriatrics*, *18*(1), 47. https://doi.org/10.1186/s12877-018-0723-5

Gilissen, J., Pivodic, L., Smets, T., Gastmans, C., Vander Stichele, R., Deliens, L., & Van den Block, L. (2017). Preconditions for successful advance care planning in nursing homes: A systematic review. *International Journal of Nursing Studies*, *66*, 47–59. https://doi.org/10.1016/j.ijnurstu.2016.12.003

Gilissen, J., Pivodic, L., Wendrich-van Dael, A., Cools, W., Vander Stichele, R., Van den Block, L., Deliens, L., & Gastmans, C. (2020a). Nurses' self-efficacy, rather than their knowledge, is associated with their engagement in advance care planning in nursing homes: A survey study. *Palliative Medicine*, 0269216320916158. https://doi.org/10.1177/0269216320916158

Gilissen, J., Pivodic, L., Wendrich-van Dael, A., Gastmans, C., Vander Stichele, R., Engels, Y., . . . Van Den Block, L. (2020b). Implementing the theory-based advance care planning ACP+ programme for nursing homes: Study protocol for a cluster randomised controlled trial and process evaluation. *BMC Palliative Care*, *19*(1), 1–18. https://doi.org/10.1186/s12904-019-0505-7

Gilissen, J., Van den Block, L., & Pivodic, L. (2021a). Complexities and outcomes of advance care planning. *JAMA Internal Medicine*, *181*(1), 142–143. https://doi.org/10.1001/jamainternmed.2020.5539

Gilissen, J., Wendrich-van Dael, A., Gastmans, C., Vander Stichele, R., Deliens, L., Detering, K., Van den Block, L., & Pivodic, L. (2021b). Differences in advance care planning among nursing home care staff. *Nursing Ethics*, 1–18.

Higginson, I.J., Evans, C.J., Grande, G., Preston, N., Morgan, M., McCrone, P., . . . Todd, C. (2013). Evaluating complex interventions in End-of-Life Care: The MORECare statement on good practice generated by a synthesis of transparent expert consultations and systematic reviews. *BMC Medicine*, *11*(111), 1–11. https://doi.org/10.1186/1741-7015-11-111

Hoffmann, T.C., Erueti, C., & Glasziou, P.P. (2013). Poor description of non-pharmacological interventions: Analysis of consecutive sample of randomised trials. *BMJ*, *347*, f3755–f3755. https://doi.org/10.1136/bmj.f3755

Hoffmann, T.C., Glasziou, P.P., Boutron, I., Milne, R., Perera, R., Moher, D., . . . Michie, S. (2014). Better reporting of interventions: Template for intervention description and replication (TIDieR) checklist and guide. *BMJ (Online)*, *348*, 1–12. https://doi.org/10.1136/bmj.g1687

Honinx, E., Van den Block, L., Piers, R., Van Kuijk, S.M.J., Onwuteaka-Philipsen, B.D., Payne, S.A., . . . PACE. (2021). Potentially inappropriate treatments at the end of life in nursing home residents: Findings from the PACE cross-sectional study in six European Countries. *Journal of Pain and Symptom Management*, *61*(4), 732–742.e1. https://doi.org/10.1016/j.jpainsymman.2020.09.001

Honinx, E., van Dop, N., Smets, T., Deliens, L., Van Den Noortgate, N., Froggatt, K., Gambassi, G., Kylänen, M., Onwuteaka-Philipsen, B., Szczerbińska, K., Van den Block, L., Gatsolaeva, Y., Miranda, R., Pivodic, L., Tanghe, M., van Hout, H., Pasman, R.H.R.W., Oosterveld-Vlug, M., Piers, R., . . . on behalf of PACE. (2019). Dying in long-term care facilities in Europe: The PACE epidemiological study of deceased residents in six countries. *BMC Public Health*, *19*(1), 1199. https://doi.org/10.1186/s12889-019-7532-4

Kane, R.L., Huckfeldt, P., Tappen, R., Engstrom, G., Rojido, C., Newman, D., Yang, Z., & Ouslander, J.G. (2017). Effects of an intervention to reduce hospitalizations from nursing homes: A randomized implementation trial of the INTERACT program. *JAMA Internal Medicine*, *177*(9), 1257–1264. https://doi.org/10.1001/jamainternmed.2017.2657

Kermel-Schiffman, I., & Werner, P. (2017). Knowledge regarding advance care planning: A systematic review. *Archives of Gerontology and Geriatrics*, *73*, 133–142. https://doi.org/10.1016/j.archger.2017.07.012

Korfage, I.J., Rietjens, J.A.C., Overbeek, A., Jabbarian, L.J., Billekens, P., Hammes, B.J., . . . Van Der Heide, A. (2015). A cluster randomized controlled trial on the effects and costs of advance care planning in elderly care: Study protocol. *BMC Geriatrics*, *15*(87), 1–6. https://doi.org/10.1186/s12877-015-0087-z

Lam, H.R., Chow, S., Taylor, K., Chow, R., Lam, H., Bonin, K., Rowbottom, L., & Herrmann, N. (2018). Challenges of conducting research in long-term care facilities: A systematic review. *BMC Geriatrics*, *18*(1), 242. https://doi.org/10.1186/s12877-018-0934-9

Lo, T.J., Ha, N.H.L., Ng, C.J., Tan, G., Koh, H.M., & Yap, P.L.K. (2017). Unmarried patients with early cognitive impairment are more likely than their married counterparts to complete advance care plans. *International Psychogeriatrics*, *29*(3), 509–516. https://doi.org/10.1017/S1041610216001903

May, C.R., Johnson, M., & Finch, T. (2016). Implementation, context, and complexity. *Implementation Science*, *11*(1), 141. https://doi.org/10.1186/s13012-016-0506-3

McGlade, C., Daly, E., McCarthy, J., Cornally, N., Weathers, E., O'Caoimh, R., & Molloy, D.W. (2017). Challenges in implementing an advance care planning programme in long-term care. *Nursing Ethics*, *24*(1), 87–99. https://doi.org/10.1177/0969733016664969

McMahan, R.D., Tellez, I., & Sudore, R.L. (2021). Deconstructing the complexities of advance care planning outcomes: What do we know and where do we go? A scoping review. *Journal of the American Geriatrics Society*, *69*(1), 234–244. https://doi.org/10.1111/jgs.16801

Mignani, V., Ingravallo, F., Mariani, E., & Chattat, R. (2017). Perspectives of older people living in long-term care facilities and of their family members toward advance care planning discussions: A systematic review and thematic synthesis. *Clinical Interventions in Aging*, *12*, 475–484. https://doi.org/10.2147/CIA.S128937

Moore, G., Audrey, S., Barker, M., Bond, L., Bonell, C., Cooper, C., . . . Baird, J. (2014). Process evaluation in complex public health intervention studies: The need for guidance. *Journal of Epidemiology & Community Health*, *68*(2), 101–102. https://doi.org/10.1136/jech-2013-202869

Moore, G., Audrey, S., Barker, M., Bond, L., Bonell, C., Hardeman, W., Moore, L., O'Cathain, A., Tinati, T., Wight, D., & Baird, J. (2012). *Process evaluation of complex interventions. UK Medical Research Council (MRC) guidance.* London: UK Medical Research Council (MRC).

Moore, G.F., & Evans, R.E. (2017). What theory, for whom and in which context? Reflections on the application of theory in the development and evaluation of complex population health interventions. *SSM – Population Health*, *3*, 132–135. https://doi.org/10.1016/j.ssmph.2016.12.005

Overbeek, A., Korfage, I.J., Jabbarian, L.J., Billekens, P., Hammes, B.J., Polinder, S., . . . Rietjens, J.A.C. (2018). Advance care planning in frail older adults: A cluster randomized controlled trial. *Journal of the American Geriatrics Society*, *66*(6), 1089–1095. https://doi.org/10.1111/jgs.15333

Palmer, J.A., Mor, V., Volandes, A.E., McCreedy, E., Loomer, L., Carter, P., Dvorchak, F., & Mitchell, S.L. (2018). A dynamic application of PRECIS-2 to evaluate implementation in a pragmatic, cluster randomized clinical trial in two nursing home systems. *Trials*, *19*(1), 453. https://doi.org/10.1186/s13063-018-2817-y

Pivodic, L., Wendrich-van Dael, A., Gilissen, J., De Buyser, S., Deliens, L., Gastmans, C., Vander Stichele, R., & Van den Block, L. (2022). Effects of a theory-based ACP intervention for nursing homes: A cluster randomized controlled trial. *Palliative Medicine*, *36*(7), 1059–1071.

Prince, M., Comas-Herrera, A., Knapp, M., Guerchet, M., & Karagiannidou, M. (2016). World Alzheimer Report 2016 Improving healthcare for people living with dementia. Coverage, Quality and costs now and in the future. *Alzheimer's Disease International (ADI)*, 1–140.

Rietjens, J.A.C., Korfage, I.J., Dunleavy, L., Preston, N.J., Jabbarian, L.J., Christensen, C.A., de Brito, M., Bulli, F., Caswell, G., Červ, B., van Delden, J., Deliens, L., Gorini, G., Groenvold, M., Houttekier, D., Ingravallo, F., Kars, M.C., Lunder, U., Miccinesi, G., . . . van der Heide, A. (2016). Advance care planning – A multi-centre cluster randomised clinical trial: The research protocol of the ACTION study. *BMC Cancer*, *16*(1). https://doi.org/10.1186/s12885-016-2298-x

Rietjens, J.A.C., Sudore, R.L., Connolly, M., Delden, J.J. van, Drickamer, M.A., Droger, M., . . . Korfage, I.J. (2017). Definition and recommendations for advance care planning: An international consensus supported by the European Association for Palliative Care. *The Lancet Oncology*, *18*(9), e543–e551. https://doi.org/10.1016/S1470-2045(17)30582-X

Sellars, M., Chung, O., Nolte, L., Tong, A., Pond, D., Fetherstonhaugh, D., McInerney, F., Sinclair, C., & Detering, K.M. (2019). Perspectives of people with dementia and carers on advance care planning and end-of-life care: A systematic review and thematic synthesis of qualitative studies. *Palliative Medicine*, *33*(3), 274–290. https://doi.org/10.1177/0269216318809571

Shepherd, V., Nuttall, J., Hood, K., & Butler, C.C. (2015). Setting up a clinical trial in care homes: Challenges encountered and recommendations for future research practice. *BMC Research Notes*, *8*(1), 306. https://doi.org/10.1186/s13104-015-1276-8

Skivington, K., Matthews, L., Simpson, S.A., Craig, P., Baird, J., Blazeby, J.M., . . . Moore, L. (2021). A new framework for developing and evaluating complex interventions: Update of Medical Research Council guidance. *BMJ (Clinical Research Ed.)*, *374*, n2061. https://doi.org/10.1136/bmj.n2061

Steele Gray, C., Chau, E., Tahsin, F., Harvey, S., Loganathan, M., McKinstry, B., . . . Wodchis, W.P. (2021). Assessing the implementation and effectiveness of the electronic patient-reported outcome tool for older adults with complex care needs: Mixed methods study. *Journal of Medical Internet Research*, *23*(12), e29071. https://doi.org/10.2196/29071

Sudore, R.L., Heyland, D.K., Lum, H.D., Rietjens, J.A.C., Korfage, I.J., Ritchie, C.S., . . . You, J.J. (2018). Outcomes that define successful advance care planning: A Delphi panel consensus. *Journal of Pain and Symptom Management*, *55*(2), 245–255.e8. https://doi.org/10.1016/j.jpainsymman.2017.08.025

Tilburgs, B., Vernooij-Dassen, M., Koopmans, R., van Gennip, H., Engels, Y., & Perry, M. (2018). Barriers and facilitators for GPs in dementia advance care planning: A systematic integrative review. *PLoS ONE*, *13*(6), 1–21. https://doi.org/10.1371/journal.pone.0198535

Tishelman, C., Eneslätt, M., Menkin, E.S., & Van Den Block, L. (2021). Tishelman et al.'s response to Morrison: Advance directives/care planning: Clear, simple, and wrong

(DOI: 10.1089/jpm.2020.0272). *Journal of Palliative Medicine, 24*(1), 16–17. https://doi.org/10.1089/jpm.2020.0540

Tjia, J., Dharmawardene, M., & Givens, J.L. (2018). Advance directives among nursing home residents with mild, moderate, and advanced dementia. *Journal of Palliative Medicine, 21*(1), 16–21. https://doi.org/10.1089/jpm.2016.0473

Van den Block, L. (2019). Advancing research on advance care planning in dementia. *Palliative Medicine, 33*(3), 259–261. http://dx.doi.org/10.1177/0269216319826411

Vernooij-Dassen, M., & Moniz-Cook, E. (2014). Raising the standard of applied dementia care research: Addressing the implementation error. *Aging & Mental Health, 18*(7), 809–814. https://doi.org/10.1080/13607863.2014.899977

Wendrich-van Dael, A., Bunn, F., Lynch, J., Pivodic, L., Van den Block, L., & Goodman, C. (2020). Advance care planning for people living with dementia: An umbrella review of effectiveness and experiences. *International Journal of Nursing Studies, 107*, 103576. https://doi.org/10.1016/j.ijnurstu.2020.103576

Wendrich-van Dael, A., Gilissen, J., Van Humbeeck, L., Deliens, L., Vander Stichele, R., Gastmans, C., Pivodic, L., & Van den Block, L. (2021). Advance care planning in nursing homes: New conversation and documentation tools. *BMJ Supportive & Palliative Care, 11*(3), 312–317. https://doi.org/10.1136/bmjspcare-2021-003008

Wendrich-van Dael, A., Pivodic, L., Cohen, J., Deliens, L., Van den Block, L., & Chambaere, K. (2019). End-of-life decision making for people who died of dementia: A mortality follow-back study comparing 1998, 2007, and 2013 in Flanders, Belgium. *Journal of the American Medical Directors Association, 20*(10), 1347–1349.

Chapter 17

Conclusion

Best Practice Guidance human interaction with technology in dementia[1]

Rose-Marie Dröes, Martin Orrell, Frans R.J. Verhey

Technology and dementia

Technologies are increasingly vital in today's activities in homes and communities. Yet, little attention is paid to the consequences of the increasing complexity and reliance on them, for example at home, in shops, traffic situations, meaningful activities and healthcare services. The users' ability to manage products and services has been largely neglected or taken for granted. People with dementia often do not use the available technology because it does not match their needs and capacities (Rosenberg et al., 2009; Wallcook et al., 2019).

Although the evidence is still limited, policymakers, care professionals and researchers often see technology applications as promising solutions to promote independence and autonomy in people with dementia.

The rapid growth of the technological landscape and related new services have the potential to improve the overall effectiveness and cost-effectiveness of health and social services and facilitate social participation and engagement in activities. But which technology is effective and how is this evaluated best?

Successful implementation of technology in dementia care depends not merely on its effectiveness but also on other facilitating or impeding factors on a micro, meso and macro level, related to, for example the personal living environment (privacy, autonomy and obtrusiveness); the outside world (stigma and human contact); design (personalisability, affordability and safety), (co)financing (laws and regulations) and ethics on these subjects.

Best practice guidance on human interaction with technology in dementia

To guide and stimulate the further development, evaluation and implementation of usable technology for people with dementia, a web-based Best Practice Guidance on Human Interaction with technology (www.dementiainduct.eu/guidance/) was composed based on literature studies and field research conducted within the 15 projects of the Marie Sklodowska Curie funded Innovative Training Network INDUCT (2016–2020).

DOI: 10.4324/9781003289005-21

The recommendations in the Best Practice Guidance are divided into three sections, in accordance with the three main objectives of INDUCT:

- Practical, cognitive and social factors that improve the usability of technology for people with dementia;
- Evaluating the effectiveness of specific contemporary technology; and
- Implementation of technology in dementia care: facilitators and barriers.

Each section is divided into three sub-sections, concerning technology in daily life, technology for meaningful activities and technology for healthcare. A search engine helps to find relevant recommendations based on keywords. Where available and allowed, materials that support the recommendation, such as scientific publications and factsheets, can be downloaded, and videos explaining the recommendation can be watched.

As the recommendations are meant to be helpful for different target groups, such as people with dementia, their formal and informal carers, managers of care organisations, policymakers, designers and researchers, representatives of these target groups were consulted and involved in all individual INDUCT projects, whenever relevant, for example by patient and public involvement (PPI) groups, individual expert consultations and/or surveys. Within the Best Practice Guidance it is possible to search for recommendations relevant to specific target groups by means of a target group search engine.

Recommendations in the best practice guidance

Practical, cognitive & social factors that improve usability of technology for people with dementia

In this section of the Best Practice Guidance, recommendations are provided to improve the *usability* of technology in daily life, for meaningful activities and healthcare services for people with dementia. Below some examples are given.

Technology for everyday life should be needs-based and prevent stigmatisation

In order to improve the usability of everyday technology, users, carers, clinicians and researchers are strongly recommended that the individual needs of people with cognitive impairments and their carers are taken into account when developing or using it, as is also recommended for the development of surveillance technology and, for example digital cognitive training (Vermeer et al., 2019) and digital self-monitoring interventions (Bartels et al., 2019). These needs will differ between people with dementia and carers, and also depend on the type and severity of the cognitive impairments, and the assistance needed by users, that is both the person with dementia and the carer.

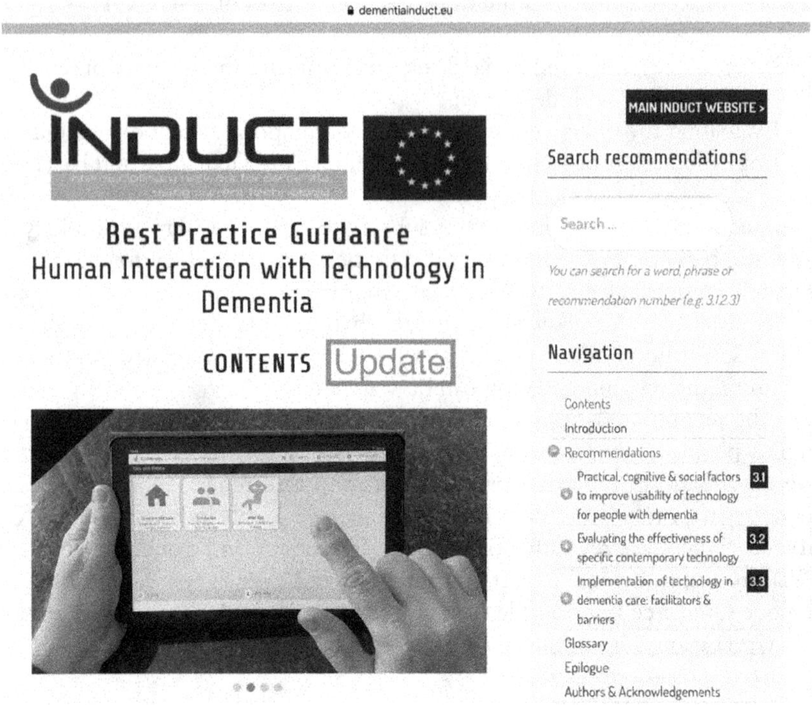

Figure 17.1 Navigation page of the web-based Best Practice Guidance for Human Interaction with Technology in Dementia

To the providers and marketers of surveillance technology, it is advised to consider selling empowering products for people with dementia and carers and to avoid stigmatising stereotypes in their communication, such as a 'wanderer with dementia' (Vermeer et al., 2020). Researchers and policymakers should pay more attention to the undesired side effects of dementia prevention technologies, such as brain training, and to discourses that may reinforce the fear of dementia and imply a moral responsibility for people who cannot maintain their cognition in later life due to the progression of the disease (Libert et al., 2020).

To transportation planners, operators and policymakers, it is advised to become more aware of barriers to access public transport by means of everyday technologies, and to consider adaptations to enable better accessibility for people with cognitive disabilities or living with dementia. A similar recommendation is made to service providers of, for example eHealth or online banking. Without face-to-face or written options people with dementia are at risk of stigma associated with digital exclusion and of social isolation (Gaber et al., 2019). In general, developers of everyday Information and Communication Technologies should be aware that the challenges to use these technologies can be high for older adults and people with dementia. They therefore should use inclusive design that addresses cognitive usability (Wallcook et al., 2019).

In order to understand the ability of older people with cognitive impairments to use everyday technology developers, clinicians and researchers are recommended to both observe their interaction with the technology and ask for their opinion (Bartels et al., 2020a). Through self-perception, the individual can reflect on a wider range of technologies and identify the effect of technology use to perform well in everyday life. For example, if someone has problems using the ticket machine for public transport, this might impact visiting family and friends and, more generally, participating in society.

The usability of technology for meaningful activities should be tested with working prototypes

Developers of digital applications for meaningful activities are recommended to test their usability with working prototypes with people with dementia as they find it hard to imagine paper prototypes (Rai et al., 2021a). Also, it is recommended to ensure an optimal user experience and to focus on sophisticated, mature design including clear signposting, an easy and intuitive navigation, and clearly orientated to adults not children (Rai et al., 2020, 2021a).

Healthcare technology should meet the needs of nursing home staff

Regarding healthcare services, nursing homes for people with dementia and developers of Electronic Patient Records (EPR) are recommended to consider introducing portable devices in addition to desktop devices for EPR (Shiells et al., 2018). Portable devices can support person-centred care by allowing immediate access to care plans with vital information about residents. This is especially important for staff retrieving information about individuals who are at the nursing home temporarily on respite; for those residents who may be unable to recall personal information; and for staff who work infrequently in the nursing home and are unfamiliar with residents. Developers of EPR systems for dementia care should consider that the system meets the needs of nursing home staff (e.g. assessment templates and space to entry free text) and the needs of people with dementia (i.e. activities, maintaining previous roles, reminiscence, freedom and choice, appropriate environment, meaningful relationships, support with grief and loss, and end-of-life care) (Shiells et al., 2020a). Furthermore, it is recommended to include additional functions, such as automated generation of graphs to show trends in data and to prompt staff about changes in a resident's condition, as well as functions allowing for the automated generation of care plans from assessment data, and alerts to prompt staff to create or update a new document in the EPR, which may be of value to nursing homes (Shiells et al., 2020b).

Evaluating the effectiveness of specific contemporary technology

In this section of the Best Practice Guidance recommendations are provided to evaluate the *effectiveness* of technology for everyday life, meaningful activities and healthcare services for people with dementia and examples of proven effective technologies in some of these areas are provided.

Ecological validity and cultural context of technology for everyday life should be taken into account

When evaluating technology for daily life, researchers, developers and policy makers are recommended to take into account the ecological validity and cultural context in which the technology will be implemented, to ensure its applicability to the 'real-life situation' of the person with dementia (Diaz-Baquero, 2020).

Studies evaluating technology for meaningful activities should also investigate contextual, implementation and psychological factors and cost-effectiveness

Researchers and industry evaluating meaningful activities interventions, for example aimed at improving the self-management of people with mild dementia living at home, are recommended to also evaluate how people succeed in coping psychologically and emotionally with the consequences of dementia in their daily life (Mangiaracina et al., 2019), as adaptation problems and mood can influence the evaluation outcomes. It is suggested to use additional instruments for this. Furthermore it is recommended to conduct pilot studies to help inform and reduce technical problems and improve accuracy prior to evaluating the effectiveness of, for example new tablet interventions (Beentjes et al., 2020a,b).

Besides conducting pilots before a definitive effectiveness trial, it is recommended to conduct a process evaluation alongside the effectiveness evaluation to understand the possible influence of contextual, implementation and mechanisms of impact factors that may have influenced the intervention outcomes (Beentjes et al., 2020a). This will also provide useful information on the conditions for successful implementation of the intervention.

In addition to evaluating the effectiveness of eHealth interventions, it is recommended to also conduct cost-effectiveness research. This will help policy makers to make the right decisions when deploying eHealth interventions (van Santen et al., 2021).

Regarding apps for self-management, meaningful activities and social participation, a tool is recommended that helps people with dementia and carers find such apps in the Google Play store and Apple store, that match their needs, interests and abilities. Within INDUCT, a previous developed tool, called FindMyApps, was piloted. The study showed that people with dementia who were offered this tool more frequently downloaded and used apps for self-management and meaningful activities than people who did not have access to this tool. This confirmed the usefulness of the tool (Beentjes et al., 2020b).

An example of an intervention that is recommended to day-care centres, care organisations and people with dementia and carers, based on an effectiveness study carried out within INDUCT, is Exergaming. This is an innovative way of exercising in a gaming environment, for example interactive cycling. This movement activity may be experienced as meaningful by persons with dementia, is generally considered fun to do and has shown to have benefits for people with dementia, that is improved cognitive and social functioning, as well as for their relatives, who showed less distress and improved sense of competence (van Santen et al., 2020).

High-quality evaluation of healthcare technology, such as online carer support, personalised services and palliative care interventions needed

Regarding healthcare services, policy makers and healthcare providers are recommended to implement Internet training programmes for family carers as they have potential to increase carers' well-being, to reduce distress, depression and anxiety symptoms and to increase knowledge skills (Egan et al., 2018). Good examples of informative websites and Internet training programmes for family carers are 'Mastery over Dementia', iSupport, 'iCARE: Stress management eTraining programme' and the STAR e-Learning course. Researchers are encouraged to further investigate the moderation effect of demographic characteristics of the carers and other characteristics of the person with dementia on the Internet training programmes outcomes as well as the mechanisms of change in carers.

When researchers or clinicians are using smartphone-based digital self-monitoring/experience sampling in carers of people with dementia, they are advised to consider providing personalised feedback to promote carers' emotional well-being and encourage them to engage in more activities they enjoy (e.g. relaxation activities) (Bartels et al., 2020b).

On the basis of a systematic review that showed that the existing evidence base of palliative care interventions for people with dementia living at home is insufficient and generally too weak to robustly assess the effects, high-quality studies are recommended to develop, implement and evaluate complex palliative care interventions (Miranda et al., 2019).

Implementation of technology in dementia care: facilitators & barriers

In this section recommendations are provided on the *implementation* of technology in everyday life, meaningful activities and healthcare technology. Below are some examples.

Involve diverse professional and user groups when developing and implementing technologies for everyday life

In all stages of design, development and implementation of everyday life technologies, technology companies and developers are advised to involve more diverse groups of people living with dementia or caring for people with dementia. They should also consider existing contexts before introducing the technologies (Gaber et al., 2020).

Health and social care planners and policy makers are recommended to consider involving occupational therapists in providing interventions that enable people with dementia to effectively use the everyday information and communication technologies they have (Wallcook et al., 2019).

Service providers and service developers are recommended to provide alternative non-ICT options when they deliver services and interventions that rely on smartphones, tablets and computers, to avoid excluding some people with dementia (Wallcook et al., 2019).

Ensure that technologies for meaningful activities match the interests of users and that the implementation in care settings is feasible for staff and supported by the management of the organisation

Regarding the implementation of technologies for meaningful activities in care organisations, it is recommended to professional carers to ensure the support of the management, and for example in the case of implementing Exergaming (see section 'Evaluating the effectiveness of specific contemporary technology'), to ensure that multiple employees are responsible for the intervention to make the implementation successful (van Santen et al., 2019).

In general it is advised, when introducing new application (app) technology, to focus on aspects that are of interest to people with dementia, such as family photographs, video calls with friends and family, music, games or art applications (Cavalcanti Barroso et al., 2020) and to ensure that the technology is compatible with a range of relevant platforms to promote implementation (Rai et al., 2021). At the same time it is important to investigate the needs of the people who will be implementing e-Health interventions after a trial phase (such as case managers, hospital workers, volunteers or professionals associated with advocacy groups) and to start making financing and business plans already at the start of the development phase (Christie et al., 2018).

The implementation of healthcare technologies should be adaptive to context and professional working processes on multiple levels and easily accessible, also in rural areas

With regard to the implementation of healthcare technology researchers and policy makers should ensure that the technology, such as cognitive rehabilitation technology, is physically accessible at the home of persons with dementia, especially for people living in rural areas and with mobility problems, and available at low cost (Fumero Vargas et al., 2009; Diaz-Baquero, 2020).

Healthcare providers, patient organisations, policy makers and researchers are recommended to inform family carers about the potential benefits of online interventions for them and to actively promote their use (Egan et al., 2018)

Regarding the implementation of complex health technologies, like Advance care planning, in nursing homes, it is advised to make them flexible to existing situations and processes, such as the specific context of the nursing home, the needs and roles of nursing staff and the timing and order of implementation of different intervention components (e.g. training on specific subjects). In addition, it is important to ensure that multiple levels are targeted (management, nurses, care staff, volunteers, physicians, families, cleaning and other staff), a dedicated trainer is involved, and that the nursing home management, is actively engaged. This will help to ensure staff have sufficient time and other resources (Oosterveld-Vlug et al., 2019; Gilissen et al., 2019; Wendrich-van Dael et al., submitted).

Developers of electronic patient records (EPR) and nursing home managers are recommended to ensure that issues such as access to various parts of the EPR system, appropriate training 'on the job' according to individual staff needs, and system development and support are considered by nursing homes before and during the implementation of EPR system (Shiells et al., 2020b).

Conclusion

The recommendations that were included in this Best Practice Guidance for Human Interaction with Technology in Dementia were based on the findings of research done by 15 Early Stage Researchers in the INDUCT Innovative Training Network (2016–2020) funded by the European Marie Sklodowska Curie Programme.

Each of the early stage researchers systematically investigated part of the literature to get a comprehensive insight in the state of the art of science regarding the usability of technology for people with dementia in daily life and in meaningful activities as well as in the application of technology in the organisation of dementia care. All researchers did also scientific field work, systematically collecting new data in these areas, with a special focus on the usability of technology, the evaluation of its impact on people with dementia and their carers and/or tracing facilitators and barriers for the implementation of technologies in daily practice. Moreover, during their field work they involved different types of stakeholders, such as people with dementia and carers, professional healthcare workers, managers of care organisations, developers of technology, policy makers and researchers to get feedback on their work and findings and to get informed on the different stakeholders' perspectives. All together this resulted in a comprehensive knowledge base and in total 56 recommendations to improve the development, usage and implementation of technology for people with dementia and their application in dementia care. More specifically 21 recommendations on Practical, cognitive and social factors to improve the usability of technology for people with dementia, 15 recommendations on Evaluating the effectiveness of specific contemporary technology, and 20 recommendations on facilitators and barriers in the implementation of technology in dementia care. Although this set of recommendations is not exhaustive, it provides different stakeholders with useful state-of-the-art information to promote the use of technology in dementia.

Following the recommendations in this Best Practice Guidance will help technical developers to develop technology for daily life and meaningful activities that is usable and useful for people with dementia, matches their needs, abilities and wishes, and therefore can contribute to their daily functioning, quality of life and digital inclusion. Better evaluation and understanding of the effectiveness and cost-effectiveness of technologies will help users make informed choices and policy and decision makers decide which applications and healthcare technologies to promote and financially support. Finally, following the recommendations for successful implementation will contribute to more effective use, dissemination and assurance of technology, thus improving the quality of dementia care and the quality of life of the rapidly growing number of people with dementia and their families in Europe and worldwide in the coming decades.

This Best Practice Guidance should be seen as a dynamic document that can, and will have to, be updated when new insights are available in the continuously developing technological landscape. The recommendations should therefore always be interpreted with caution. This Best Practice Guidance paves the way for a new Marie Sklodowska Curie funded ITN project DISTINCT (2019–2023) in which 15 new Early Stage Researchers will investigate the usability, impacts and implementation of technology in three domains of Social health in dementia, that is supporting/promoting their ability to fulfil their potential in the society, supporting/promoting self-management in daily life and supporting/promoting social participation and meaningful activities.

Research into the usability, impact and implementation of technology is still in its infancy. With this Best Practice Guidance we hope to inspire and stimulate many researchers, policy makers and investors in the development of technology for people with dementia and innovation of dementia care to effectively contribute to the further development and implementation of user-friendly, useful and easy implementable technology for people with dementia and carers and dementia care in general.

Acknowledgements

We thank all Early Stage Researchers and their supervisors involved in INDUCT for their contributions to this Best Practice Guidance: Rose-Marie Dröes, Yvette Vermeer (ESR 1), Sébastien Libert (ESR2), Sophie N. Gaber (ESR3), Sarah Wallcook (ESR4), Harleen Kaur Rai (ESR5), Aline Cavalcanti Barroso (ESR6), Joeke van Santen (ESR7), Floriana Mangiaracina (ESR8), Kim Beentjes (ESR 8), Sara Laureen Bartels (ESR9), Hannah Christie (ESR10), Rose Miranda (ESR11), Annelien Wendrich-van Dael (ESR12), Kate Shiells (ESR 13), Ángel C. Pinto Bruno (ESR 14), Angie A. Diaz-Baquero (ESR15), and the ESRs supervisors Lieve Van den Block, Lara Pivodic, Louise Nygard, Manuel Franco Martin, Maria Victoria Perea Bartolomé, Paul Higgs, Iva Holmerová, Camilla Walles Malinowsky, Franka Meiland, Henriëtte G. van der Roest, Justine Schneider, Annemieke van Straten, Frans Verhey, Marjolein de Vugt, Martin Orrell. We also thank the 2nd level partners involved in INDUCT: Alzheimer Europe, Alzheimer Disease International, World Federation of Occupational Therapists, University of Hertfordshire, University of Witten, Silverfit BV and EuMediaNet. We thank the web designing company Pixelshrink for designing an easily accessible web-based version of the Best Practice Guidance.

Note

1 Parts of this chapter were previously published in the INDUCT deliverable D6.2 Best Practice Guidance Human interaction with technology in dementia (update Dröes et al., 2020) and its webbased version www.dementiainduct.eu/guidance/

References

Bartels, S.L., Assander, S., Patomella, A.H., Jamnadas-Khoda, J. & Malinowsky, C. (2020a). Do you observe what I perceive? The relationship between two perspectives on the ability of people with cognitive impairments to use everyday technology, Aging & Mental Health, 24(8), 1295–1305, DOI: 10.1080/13607863.2019.1609902

Bartels, S.L., Van Knippenberg, R.J., Dassen, F.C., Asaba, E., Patomella, A.-H., Malinowsky, C., Verhey, F.R., & de Vugt, M.E. (2019). A narrative synthesis systematic review of digital self-monitoring interventions for middle-aged and older adults. Internet Interventions, 18, 100283.

Bartels, S.L., Van Knippenberg, R.J.M., Viechtbauer, W., Simons, C.J.P., Ponds, R.W., Myin-Germeys, I., Verhey, F.R.J., & de Vugt, M.E. (2020b). Intervention mechanisms of an experience sampling intervention for spousal carers of people with dementia: A secondary analysis. Aging & Mental Health, 24(9), 1–9. doi: 10.1080/13607863.2020.1857692.

Beentjes, K.M.,. Kerkhof Y.J.F., Neal D.P., Ettema, T.P., Koppelle, M.A., Meiland, F.J.M., Graff, M., Dröes, R.M. (2020a). Process evaluation of the FindMyApps program trial among people with dementia or MCI and their caregivers based on the MRC guidance. *Gerontechnology*, *20*(1), 1–15. https://doi.org/10.4017/gt.2020.20.1.406.11

Beentjes, K.M., Neal, D.P., Kerkhof, Y.J.F., Broeder, C., Moeridjan, Z.D.J., Ettema, T.P., Pelkmans, W., Muller, M.M., Graff, M.J.L., Dröes, R.M. (2020b). Impact of the Find-MyApps program on people with mild cognitive impairment or dementia and their caregivers; an exploratory pilot randomised controlled trial. *Disabil Rehabil Assist Technol.*, *27*, 1–13. https://doi.org/10.1080/17483107.2020.1842918

Cavalcanti Barroso, A., Rai, H.K., Sousa, L., Orrell, M., Schneider, J. (2020). Participatory visual arts activities for people with dementia: A review. *Perspectives in Public Health*, *20*(10), 1–10.

Christie, H.L., Bartels, S.L., Boots, L.M., Tange, H.J., Verhey, F.R., & de Vugt, M.E. (2018). A systematic review on the implementation of eHealth interventions for informal caregivers of people with dementia. *Internet interventions*, *13*, 51–59.

Diaz-Baquero, A.A. (2020). Ecological validity contributes to the effectiveness of a technology. In Dröes et al. (Eds.), *Best practice guidance for human interaction with technology in dementia* (p. 22). INDUCT Deliverable 6.5 [recommendation 3.2.1.1].

Egan, K.J., Pinto-Bruno, A.C., Bighelli, I., Berg-Weger, M., van Straten, A., Albanese, E., & Pot, A.M. (2018). Online training and support programs designed to improve mental health and reduce burden among caregivers of people with dementia: A systematic review. *Journal of the American Medical Directors Association*, *19*(3), 200–206.e201. doi: 10.1016/j.jamda.2017.10.023

Fumero Vargas, G., Franco Martin, M.A., & Perea Bartolomé, M.V. (2009). *Start-up and study of usability of a computer cognitive rehabilitation program "Gradior" in the treatment of neurocognitive deficits* [Doctoral thesis, Department of Basic psychology, psychobiology and methodology of behavioural sciences - Faculty of Psychology, University of Salamanca], Spain.

Gaber, S.N., Nygård, L., Brorsson, A., Kottorp, A., Charlesworth, G., Wallcook, S., Malinowsky, C. (2020). Social participation in relation to technology use and social deprivation: A mixed methods study among older people with and without dementia. *International Journal of Environmental Research and Public Health*, *17*, 4022. www.mdpi.com/1660-4601/17/11/4022#

Gaber, S.N., Nygård, L., Brorsson, A., Kottorp, A., & Malinowsky, C. (2019). Everyday technologies and public space participation among people with and without dementia. *Canadian Journal of Occupational Therapy*, *86*(5), 400–411. https://doi.org/10.1177/0008417419837764

Gilissen, J., Pivodic, L., Wendrich-van Dael, A., Gastmans, C., Vander Stichele, R., Van Humbeeck, L., Deliens, L., & Van den Block, L. (2019). Implementing advance care planning in routine nursing home care: The development of the theory-based ACP+ program. *PloS One*, *14*(10), e0223586. https://doi.org/10.1371/journal.pone.0223586

Libert, S., Charlesworth, G., & Higgs, P. (2020). Cognitive decline and distinction: A new line of fracture in later life? *Ageing and Society*, *40*(12), 2574–2592. doi:10.1017/S0144686X19000734

Mangiaracina, F., Meiland, F., Kerkhof, Y., Orrell, M, Graff, M, Dröes, R.M. (2019). Self-management and social participation in community-dwelling people with mild dementia: a review of measuring instruments. *International Psychogeriatrics*, *31*(9), 1267–1285. doi: 10.1017/S1041610218001709.

Miranda, R., Bunn, F., Lynch, J., Van den Block, L., Goodman, C. (2019). Palliative care for people with dementia living at home: A systematic review of interventions. *Palliative Medicine, 33*(7), 726–742.

Oosterveld-Vlug, M., Onwuteaka-Philipsen, B.D., Ten Koppel, M., Van Hout, H., Smets, T., Pivodic, L., et al. (2019). Evaluating the implementation of the PACE Steps to Success Programme in long-term care facilities in seven countries according to the REAIM framework. *Implementation Science, 14*, 107.

Rai, H.K., Griffiths, R., Yates, L., Schneider, J., & Orrell, M. (2021a). Field-testing an iCST touch-screen application with people with dementia and carers: A mixed method study. *Aging & Mental Health, 25*(6), 1008–1018, doi.org/10.1080/13607863.2020.1783 515.

Rai, H.K., Prasetya, V.G.H., Sani, T.P., Theresia, I., Tumbelaka, P., Turana, Y., Schneider, J., & Orrell, M. (2021). Exploring the feasibility of an individual cognitive stimulation therapy application and related technology for use by people with dementia and carers in Indonesia: A mixed-method study. *Dementia, 20*(8), 2820–2837. https://doi.org/10.1177/14713012211018003

Rai, H.K., Schneider, J., Orrell, M. (2020). An Individual Cognitive Stimulation Therapy App for People with Dementia: Development and Usability Study of Thinkability. *JMIR Aging, 3*(2), e17105. doi: 10.2196/17105

Rosenberg, L., Kottorp, A., Winblad, B., & Nygård, L. (2009). Perceived difficulty in everyday technology use among older adults with or without cognitive deficits. *Scandinavian Journal of Occupational Therapy, 16*(4), 216–226. https://doi.org/10.3109/11038120802684299

Santen, J. van, Dröes, R.M., Schoone, M., Blanson Henkemans, O.A., Bosmans, J.E., van Bommel, S., Hakvoort, E., Valk, R., Scholten, C., Wiersinga, J., Smit, M., Meiland, F. (2019). *FACTSHEET Exergaming for people living with dementia: Can you move along? Recommendations to promote successful implementation* [in Dutch: FACTSHEET Exergaming voor mensen met dementie: beweeg je mee? Adviezen ter bevordering van succesvolle implementatie]. Amsterdam: UMC, Locatie VUmc, afdeling Psychiatrie, Amsterdam

Shiells, K., Diaz Baquero, A.A., Stepankova, O., & Holmerova, I. (2020b). Staff perspectives on the usability of electronic patient records for planning and delivering dementia care in nursing homes: a multiple case study. *BMC Medical Informatics and Decision Making, 20*, 159 https://doi.org/10.1186/s12911-020-01160-8

Shiells, K., Holmerova, I., Steffl, M., Stepankova, O. (2018). Electronic patient records as a tool to facilitate care provision in nursing homes: an integrative review. *Informatics for Health and Social Care, 44*(3), 262–277. DOI: 10.1080/17538157.2018.1496091

Shiells, K., Pivodic, L., Holmerova, I., Van den Block, L. (2020a). Self-reported needs and experiences of people with dementia in nursing homes: A scoping review. *Aging & Mental Health, 24*(10), 1553–1568, DOI: 10.1080/13607863.2019.1625303

Van Santen, J., Dröes, R.M., Twisk, J.W., Henkemans, O.A.B., van Straten, A., & Meiland, F.J. (2020). Effects of exergaming on cognitive and social functioning of people with dementia: A randomized controlled trial. *Journal of the American Medical Directors Association, 21*, 1958–1967. doi.org/10.1016/j.jamda.2020.04.018.

Van Santen, J., Meiland, F.J.M., Dröes, R.M., Straten, A, Bosmans, J.E. (2021). Cost-effectiveness of exergaming compared to regular Day care activities in dementia: Results of a randomised controlled trial in the Netherlands. *Health and Social Care in the Community*, 1–11. doi.org/10.1111/hsc.13608

Vermeer, Y., Higgs, P., Charlesworth, G. (2019). What do we require from surveillance technology? A review of the needs of people with dementia and informal caregivers.

Journal of Rehabilitation and Assistive Technologies Engineering, 2(6), 2055668319869517. doi: 10.1177/2055668319869517.

Vermeer, Y., Higgs, P., & Charlesworth, G. (2020). Selling surveillance technology: Semiotic themes in advertisements for ageing in place with dementia, *Social Semiotics*. DOI: 10.1080/10350330.2020.1767399

Wallcook, S., Nygård, L., Kottorp, A. & Malinowsky, C. (2019). The use of Everyday Information Communication Technologies in the lives of older adults living with and without dementia in Sweden. *Assistive Technology*. DOI: 10.1080/10400435.2019.1644685

Wendrich-van Dael, A., Gilissen, J., Deliens, L., Vander Stichele, R., Gastmans, C., Pivodic, L. & Van den Block, L. (Submitted). Implementation of advance care planning in nursing homes in Flanders, Belgium: A mixed-methods process evaluation of the ACP+ trial.

Index

For Product Safety Concerns and Information please contact our EU
representative GPSR@taylorandfrancis.com
Taylor & Francis Verlag GmbH, Kaufingerstraße 24, 80331 München, Germany

www.ingramcontent.com/pod-product-compliance
Lightning Source LLC
Chambersburg PA
CBHW052122230326
41598CB00080B/4012